Evidence-Based Medical Exercise Therapy

Sandro Wolfram · Robin Bauer

Evidence-Based Medical Exercise Therapy

Springer

Sandro Wolfram
BWS Education GmbH
Thalheim, Germany

Robin Bauer
BWS-Education GmbH
Thalheim, Germany

Translation from the German language edition: "Evidenzbasierte medizinische Trainingstherapie" by Sandro Wolfram and Robin Bauer, © Der/die Herausgeber bzw. der/die Autor(en), exklusiv lizenziert an Springer-Verlag GmbH, DE, ein Teil von Springer Nature 2024. Published by Springer Berlin Heidelberg. All Rights Reserved.

This book is a translation of the original German edition "Evidenzbasierte medizinische Trainingstherapie" by Sandro Wolfram and Robin Bauer, published by Springer-Verlag GmbH, DE in 2024. The translation was done with the help of an artificial intelligence machine translation tool. A subsequent human revision was done primarily in terms of content, so that the book will read stylistically differently from a conventional translation. Springer Nature works continuously to further the development of tools for the production of books and on the related technologies to support the authors.

ISBN 978-3-662-70773-9 ISBN 978-3-662-70774-6 (eBook)
https://doi.org/10.1007/978-3-662-70774-6

This Springer imprint is published by the registered company Springer-Verlag GmbH, DE, part of Springer Nature.
The registered company address is: Heidelberger Platz 3, 14197 Berlin, Germany

Preface

Dear readers,
In the course of an ever-aging society and the constant endeavor to improve quality of life through preventive and therapeutic measures, we, Sandro Wolfram and Robin Bauer, have decided to compile our knowledge and many years of experience in the book "Evidence-based Medical Training Therapy". Our motivation is to give you a profound insight into the world of medical training therapy, based on solid scientific facts, and to illuminate its physiological effects as well as its influences on the aging process of organ systems.

This book aims to increase attention to the importance and benefits of medical training therapy. It is intended to provide you with specific guidance on how to determine and improve the current status of strength, endurance, and coordination. To ensure the reliability of our content, our arguments are based on meta-analyses and randomized controlled trials, thereby best excluding effects that are merely due to chance or placebo.

A central concern of this book is to guide medical/therapeutic practice towards active forms of therapy. We see passive measures as an important basis for preparing for regular and targeted training therapy. The contents of the book not only cover the proven therapeutic effects for orthopedic, surgical, and internal diseases, but can also be used preventively to promote health and well-being.

In addition, this book contains supplementary information on the influence of mental training, nutrition, and sleep on health and performance. We thoroughly discuss all types of strength as well as endurance training, proprioceptive training, and flexibility training, to create a comprehensive understanding of the complexity and effectiveness of medical training therapy. The theory is made clear through several hundred illustrations, which refines and deepens the understanding of the conveyed content.

Our goal is not only to impart knowledge, but also to inspire and motivate you to integrate the principles and methods into your daily life or professional practice. We hope that this book will be a valuable companion for you, whether you are a professional or an interested layperson.

In conclusion, we wish you much enjoyment and success in reading and implementing the contents of this book. May it positively influence your life and that of your fellow human beings.

Strong and enduring greetings,
Sandro Wolfram
Robin Bauer

Contents

Glossary of Abbreviations

1RM	one repetition maximum
BDNF	Brain-derived neurotrophic factor
BMI	Body Mass Index
bzw.	respectively
et al.	et alii in English, “and others”
IGF-1	insulin-like growth factor 1
kg	Kilogram
M	Torque from the Latin “momentum”
m	Meter
MPa	Megapascal
N	Newton
Nm	Newton meter
P	Pressure from the Latin “pressura”
TNF-α	Tumor Necrosis Factor Alpha
VEGF	Vascular Endothelial Growth Factor
vgl.	Comparison
VO_2max	Maximum Oxygen Uptake

Basics of Medical Exercise Therapy

1

Contents

▶ **Trailer**
Dive into the fascinating world of medical training therapy, where science and movement meet to reveal the secrets of our muscular system. Starting with a gripping introduction to evidence-based training therapy, this chapter navigates through the complex anatomy and vital functions of skeletal muscle. Learn how muscle and fat mass influence body weight and discover the diversity and uniqueness of muscle types.

S. Wolfram and R. Bauer, *Evidence-Based Medical Exercise Therapy*,
https://doi.org/10.1007/978-3-662-70774-6_1

With a deep dive into muscle physiology, a window opens to the world of the sensorimotor system, the processes of muscle contraction, and the vital energy supply processes that drive our movements. Be fascinated by the functioning of muscle spindles, Golgi tendon organs, and other key receptors that make our myofascial system a marvel of nature.

Explore the differences between muscle fiber types and their specific roles in our body. Deepen your understanding of the various forms of muscle work and how they shape our physical performance. Dive into the world of training-related biomechanics, explore the nature of torque in strength training, and learn how biomechanical principles can help you avoid injuries and achieve your training goals more efficiently.

In conclusion, the difference between the open and closed system in training is discussed, an essential aspect for optimizing your training routine. This chapter promises not only a profound understanding of the basics of medical training therapy but also exciting insights that will revolutionize your view of movement and health. Get ready to expand your knowledge and take your training practice to the next level.

1.1 Introduction to Evidence-Based Training Therapy

The core of successful medical training therapy is as individual as possible and stimulus setting adapted to the target position. Only through a supra-threshold stimulus are the structures of the human organism able to adapt in the sense of performance enhancement. The resulting central question deals with the most optimal type of stimulus and its intensity.

If the required stimulus intensity, which is necessary for maintaining or improving the performance of the skeletal muscles, is not achieved, muscular atrophy is the logical consequence. This adaptation reaction, based on lack of use, offers the human body the avoidable advantage of energy saving through reduced consumption of adenosine triphosphate (cf. Lacour 2011). Atrophy of the skeletal muscles is defined as an imbalance of protein synthesis or protein degradation. From a functional point of view, it is characterized by a weakening of the muscle. If the structural level is considered, a shrinkage and a reduction of the muscle mass are evident. Additionally, from a histological perspective, a decrease in the fiber cross-sectional area must be noted (cf. Yin et al. 2021). The described change mechanisms can not only be evoked by a sub-threshold stimulus but also by a too strong stimulus. During excessive stimulus, injuries such as muscle strains, muscle fiber tears, muscle bundle tears, or even tendon tears can occur (cf. Walters et al. 2018).

In addition to the stimulus intensity, the intervening recovery time plays a key role. If the recovery time from one supra-threshold stimulus to the next is too short, this can lead to the state of muscular overtraining. The intramuscular chemical reaction of overtraining, which is comparable to the atrophy mechanism, manifests itself through both oxidative and inflammatory stress and also leads to gradual performance loss (cf. Cheng et al. 2020; cf. Yin et al. 2021).

The person responsible for the training distinguishes their quality through the most current training-specific knowledge. In acquiring this knowledge, one should not rely solely on "expert opinions" or on tried and tested training methods. The highest value of available information is provided by the research results of medical training science. These should be used as a fundamental basis for arguments. If the person responsible for training manages to absorb this information, critically question it, and implement it in practice, the training takes place based on the best available information. Within medical training science, there is literature that includes measurement methods of different validity, objectivity, and reliability. Practitioners are thus faced with the challenge of qualitatively classifying different publications or

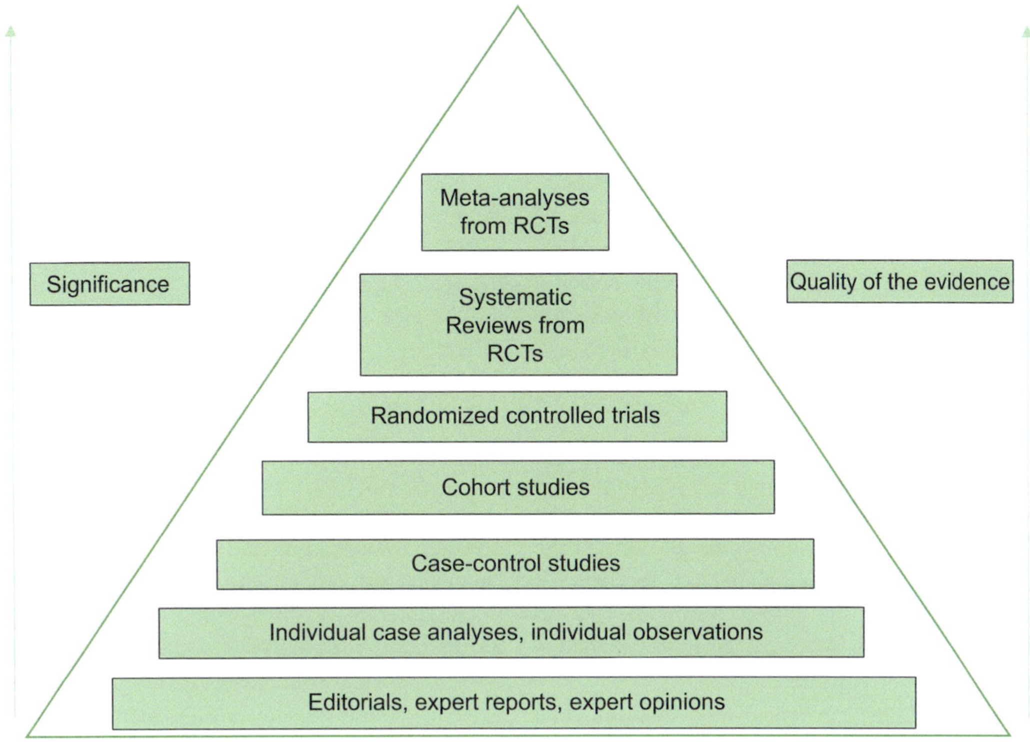

Fig. 1.1 Simplified representation of an evidence pyramid. (Own illustration 2022)

types of literature. With the aim of hierarchically arranging different research designs, so-called evidence pyramids were created (Fig. 1.1). The validity of the statement from randomized controlled studies can only be surpassed by systematic reviews or meta-analyses (cf. Murad et al. 2016).

The study design of the randomized controlled study offers the possibility to classify the sample chosen by means of defined inclusion or exclusion criteria into groups through the implementation of randomization. This structure allows the academic professional staff to check various individual or combination interventions or placebo applications against each other for effectiveness. During the defined study period, quantitative values are collected by applying predetermined measurement methods. These values are subsequently objectively evaluated and interpreted using statistical methods. The advantage of this approach lies in the central effectiveness check of the intervention, while at the same time excluding other influencing factors as much as possible. Randomized controlled studies represent the gold standard of primary literature (cf. Mad et al. 2008).

The rapid growth of publications in the field of medical training therapy leads to a lack of clarity. For people who are active in practice and only have limited time windows for acquiring new evidence-based knowledge, summaries of literature dealing with similar research questions are of great value. Both systematic reviews and meta-analyses fulfill this task. Systematic reviews are thus to be understood as qualitative summaries of primary literature. The synopsis of randomized controlled studies with the highest possible homogeneity of data represents the optimal case of systematic information synthesis (cf. Gartlehner et al. 2008). If there is sufficient homogeneity of the data originating from the primary literature, the level of meta-analysis can be reached through statistical evaluation. In contrast to the systematic review, the meta-analysis is to be understood as a quantitative summary of primary literature (cf. Rosenthal and DiMatteo 2001).

If training-specific information originates from the mentioned research designs, these are to be interpreted as the most valuable information available. Within the mentioned research designs, a finer quality determination can be realized through the use of so-called appraisal tools (cf. Zeng et al. 2015). Due to the strongly diverging methodological quality of research work, the use of these instruments is indispensable with regard to determining the validity of the literature.

Training research is subject to a desired constant dynamic. New research findings modulate earlier hypotheses and at the same time new views or research questions emerge. Due to the plasticity of the training-specific theorem, it is essential from the author's point of view to be able to access the most current knowledge through lifelong learning.

Based on the presented explanations, this book is intended to provide a contemporary and valuable evidence-based contribution to the theoretical understanding and practical implementation of medical training therapy. At the same time, readers should be motivated to critically question information. Through continuous self-reflection within practice, the best available training therapeutic intervention can be realized.

1.2 Anatomy of the Skeletal Muscle

1.2.1 Muscle and Fat Mass in Relation to Body Weight

The musculature of the human body can be divided into smooth and striated muscle. By evaluating 500,000 data sets, the values of fat and muscle tissue in relation to body weight were determined in a gradation of every four years (see AG Science 2019). While the muscle mass in women between the ages of 16 and 20 fluctuates by the value of 36 percentage points, this decreases to 22% in the age group between 76 and 80 years. During the same period, the proportion of fat mass increased from 26% to 37%. The trend of decreasing muscle mass in relation to body weight over the course of life is also evident in males. Between the ages of 16 and 20, men had an average muscle mass of 43%. This value dropped to 32 percentage points in the age group between 76–80 years. At the same time, the fat mass increased from 16% to 28% (see AG Science 2019).

1.2.2 Classification and Differences of Muscle Types

When considering the types of muscles, a subdivision into smooth and striated muscles can be made. Smooth muscle is found in the area of the internal organ systems. It is innervated by the autonomic nervous system and is therefore largely not voluntarily recruitable. For this reason, smooth muscle is only mentioned here for the sake of completeness, but is not further discussed in the course of the book. The focus is therefore on the anatomy of striated muscle. This can in turn be divided into skeletal muscle and cardiac muscle. Essential distinguishing features between cardiac and skeletal muscle are characterized by differences in the number of cell nuclei, the presence of motor end plates and a syncytium, and the fiber arrangement (Fig. 1.2). While cardiac muscle has only one cell nucleus but no motor end plates, skeletal muscle has many cell nuclei and motor end plates. The cylindrical arrangement of the muscle fibers of the skeletal muscle and the existence of a syncytium also differs from the branched fiber arrangement and the non-anatomical, but merely functional syncytium of the cardiac muscle, which is realized through gap junctions. Skeletal muscles have an anatomical connection to the skeletal system, whereas the cardiac muscle represents a layer of the heart wall. The cardiac muscle is controlled by the heart's own excitation formation system and the autonomic nervous system. The control of the skeletal muscle is carried out by the somatic nervous system (see Prabhat 2011).

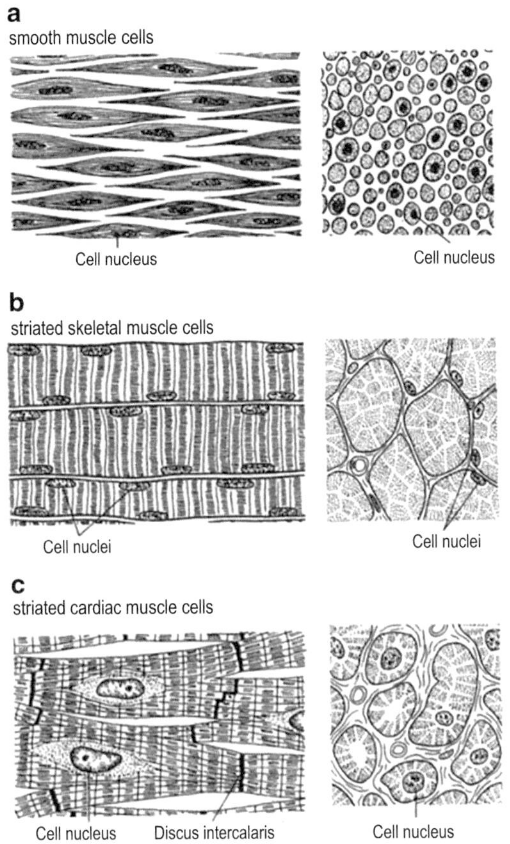

Fig. 1.2 Structural differences of skeletal muscle, cardiac muscle and smooth muscle from "Zilles, K., & Tillmann, B. (2010). Anatomy. Berlin, Heidelberg: Springer-Verlag. doi: 10.1007/978-3-540-69483-0."—Fig. 2.21a–c

1.2.3 Detailed Anatomy of the Skeletal Muscle

The skeletal muscle is characterized by tendinous material in the origin and insertion area as well as by an intervening muscle belly or muscle bellies. The muscle origin is determined by the proximal location or by the fixed point. Accordingly, the insertion tendon is characterized by the distal location or by the mobile point. In the transition zone between the tendons and the bony skeleton, a distinction can be made between a chondral-apophyseal and a diaphyseal-periosteal transition zone. More information on the anatomy of the tendon can be found in Sect. 1.2.3.2.

1.2.3.1 Anatomy of the Muscle Belly

When the skeletal muscle is viewed in cross-section, a visual distinction can be made between red muscular components and whitish appearing envelope tissue. The whitish appearing parts represent connective tissue, which is often also referred to as fascial tissue.

The following explanations describe the muscular anatomy from the outside in, or from the macroscopic to the microscopic anatomy. The muscle fascia surrounds the entire skeletal muscle in a circular manner and transitions into the origin or insertion tendon at the ends. The body fascia consists of firm, net-like collagen tissue and elastin. In a fluid transition, the epimysium follows the body fascia inward. This is a layer of loose connective tissue that also surrounds the muscle in a circular manner. Further into the depth of the skeletal muscle, there is another layer of connective tissue deep to the epimysium, the so-called perimysium. The main characteristic of the perimysium is the pull into the interior of the muscle. This fascial layer is capable of enveloping muscle bundles. The external perimysium is responsible for enveloping secondary bundles, while the internal perimysium surrounds primary bundles. Secondary bundles are composed of several primary bundles. Primary bundles, in turn, consist of several muscle fibers. These muscle fibers are encased by endomysium, a connective tissue layer that runs circularly around individual muscle fibers. The basal membrane, which also surrounds the muscle fiber in a circular manner, follows the endomysium inward. Satellite cells are encased between the endomysium and the basal membrane. The sarcolemma, which follows inward, is the cell membrane of the muscular tissue. The muscle fiber itself consists of many fused myoblasts and is therefore multinucleated. Within the muscle fiber, there are several myofibrils, which run parallel. The myofibril, in turn, consists of longitudinally arranged sarcomeres (see Müller-Wohlfahrt et al. 2010).

The sarcomere represents the smallest unit of a skeletal muscle, which is capable of performing a contraction. The sarcomere is composed of various structural proteins (see Rassier 2017).

The lateral boundaries of the sarcomere are provided on both sides by the Z-lines. The contractile actin filaments are attached to the Z-discs by the anchoring protein actinin and pull on both sides towards the center of the sarcomere. The binding sites of the actin filaments are covered by tropomyosin threads during muscular inactivity. After every seven actin filaments, there are three horizontally oriented troponin peptides on the tropomyosin threads. The structural protein nebulin surrounds the actin filaments helically and thus contributes to the stabilization of the actin (see Henderson et al. 2017).

The myosin filaments are found between the actin filaments. The contractile structural protein myosin can be subdivided into a head part, a neck part, and a tail part (see Ojima 2019). The myosin filaments are elastically fixed to the Z-lines by the structural protein titin (see Kellermayer 2019). The titin, in turn, is attached to the Z-lines by telethonin. Myomesin is attributed a stabilizing function between the titin and the myosin (see Lange et al. 2020).

Desmin extends between the individual Z-discs. It surrounds the myofibril in a net-like manner and extends over the sarcolemma. This establishes a connection between the myofibrils (see Dayal et al. 2020).

Within a sarcomere, different areas can be distinguished from each other. The I-band is the area of the actin filaments, which is free of myosin filaments. The Z-lines are located in the middle of the I-band. The A-band is the area within a sarcomere where the myosin filaments and the actin filaments protruding into the myosin filaments are located. The area of the sarcomere center, which is free of actin filaments, is titled the H-zone. The M-line marks the midpoint of the A-band (see Henderson et al. 2017).

Useful visualizations can be found in Figs. 1.3 and 1.4.

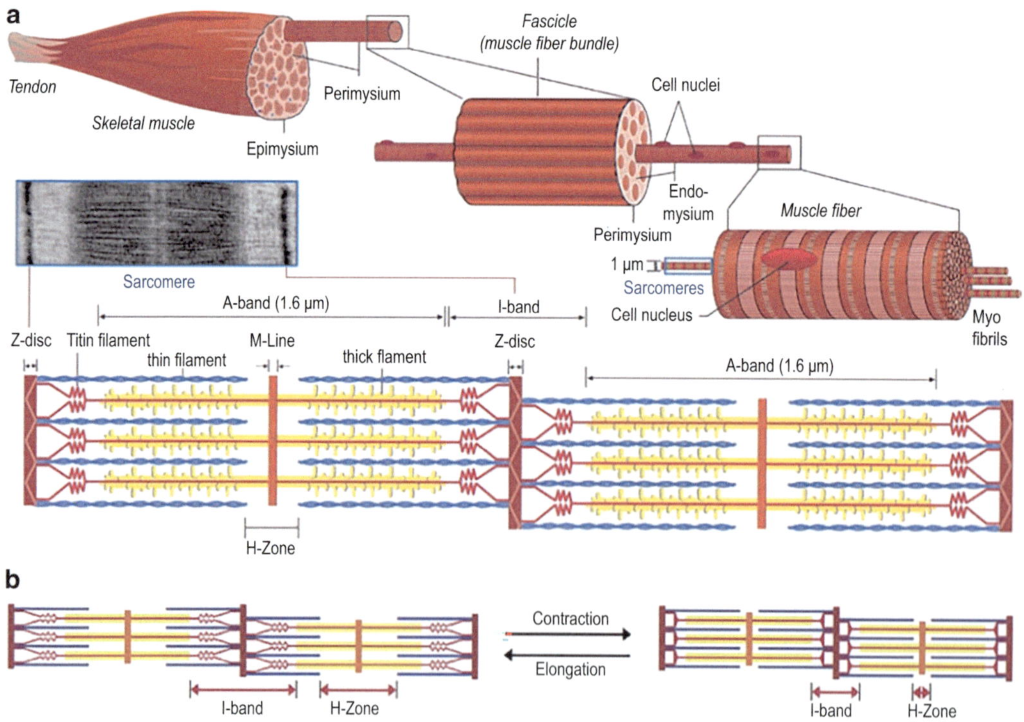

Fig. 1.3 Cross-section of the skeletal muscle and anatomical representation of the sarcomere from "Ferrauti, A. (2020). Training science for sports practice. Berlin, Heidelberg: Springer-Verlag. doi: 10.1007/978-3-662-58227-5"—Fig. 4.7a–b

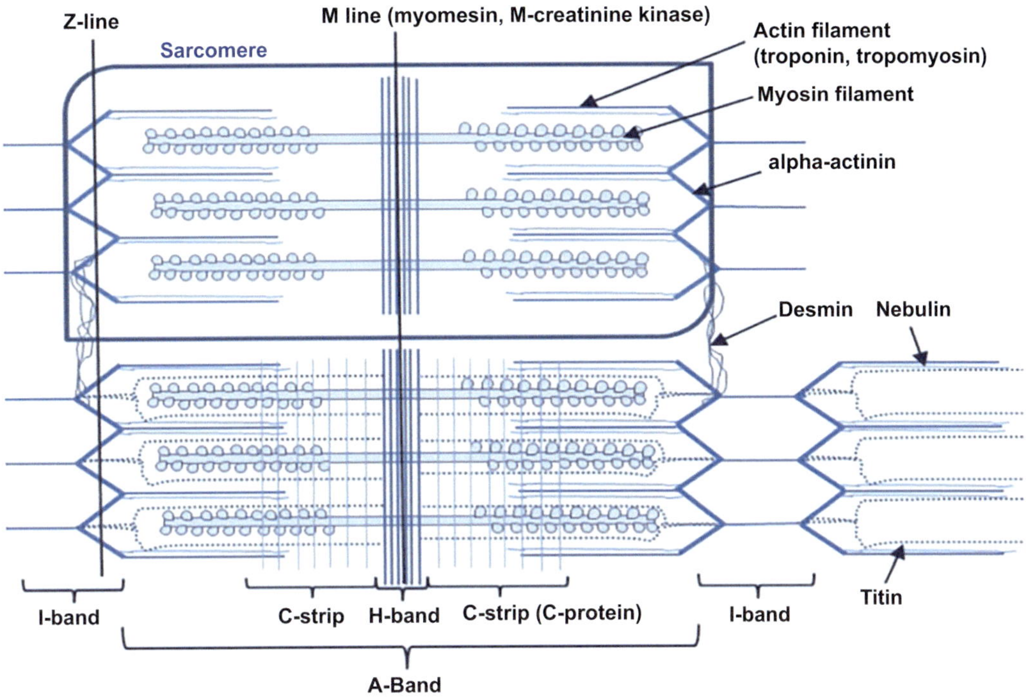

Fig. 1.4 Schematic representation of the sarcomere from "Bachl, N., Löllgen, H., Tschan, H., Wackerhage, H., & Wessner, B. (2018). Molecular sports and performance physiology. Vienna: Springer-Verlag. doi: 10.1007/978-3-7091-1591-6"—Fig. 5.3

1.2.3.2 Anatomy of the Tendon

Within the tendon, type 1 collagen molecules bundle together to form collagen microfibrils. These, in turn, combine to form collagen fibrils (see Silver et al. 2003). Due to a staggered arrangement of the collagen molecules, the so-called fibril periodicity can be observed longitudinally (see Canty and Katler 2002). The collagen fibrils join together to form collagen fibers. Between the collagen fibers, tenocytes are positioned in long rows. A cellular network is formed by the cellular extensions of the tenocytes (see Zschäbitz 2005). In the resting state, the collagen fibers appear slightly wavy due to the tension of the elastic fibers (Fig. 1.5). A tendon is surrounded from the outside by the so-called paratendineum. This is a layer of loose and well-vascularized connective tissue that encircles the tendon. For the purpose of reducing friction, the paratendineum can develop fluid-filled sliding layers in longer tendons (see O'Brien 1997). The paratendineum is followed inwardly by a layer of strong connective tissue, the so-called epitendineum. The peritendineum that follows inward can be understood as a denser sheath tissue. This layer can be subdivided into an external peritendineum and an internal peritendineum. The external peritendineum encircles the tendon. The internal peritendineum extends from the external peritendineum with several strands into the depths of the tendon. This surrounds variously sized bundles of collagen fibers. Bundles with a diameter of 1–3 mm are referred to as tertiary bundles, while bundles with a diameter between 150–1000 μm are understood to be secondary bundles. Both tertiary and secondary bundles are encircled by the components of the peritendineum. The primary bundles, which are characterized by a diameter of 15–400 μm, are surrounded by the endotendineum (Fig. 1.6). This is a layer of loose connective tissue (see Zschäbitz 2005). The water content of the tendon can be quantified as 60–70%. This high

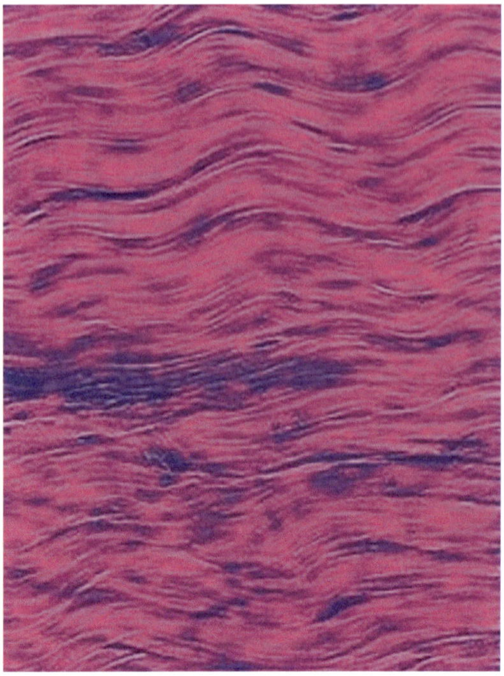

Fig. 1.5 Wavy arrangement of the collagen fibers within the tendon bundles from "Zschäbitz, A. (2005). Anatomy and behavior of tendons and ligaments. The Orthopedist, 34, pp. 516–525. doi: 10.1007/s00132-005-0799-4"—Fig. 1.8

water-binding capacity is due to the high number of proteoglycans within the tendon structure (see Benjamin and Ralphs 2000).

Tendon sheaths are found in the area of the forearm or hand as well as in the area of the lower leg or foot. When tendons are deflected near the bone in their course, tendon sheaths are found in those regions. Anatomically, a tendon sheath consists of the outer stratum fibrosum and the inner stratum synoviale. In the area of the wrist or the upper ankle joint, the stratum fibrosum is reinforced by the retinaculum extensorum or the retinaculum musculorum extensorum inferius. The ligamenta anularia of the fingers are also to be interpreted as reinforcing facilities. The inner leaf of the stratum synoviale is fused with the epitendineum. The outer leaf of the stratum synoviale is structurally connected to the stratum fibrosum. The cavitas synoviales of the stratum synoviale is filled with synovia. The mesotendineum serves at some points for the linear connection between the two leaves of the stratum synoviale (Fig. 1.7). In the area of the fingers, several narrow bands are anatomically connected to the mesotendineum. These are referred to as vincula breve or longum. Blood vessels and nerves manage to pull into the

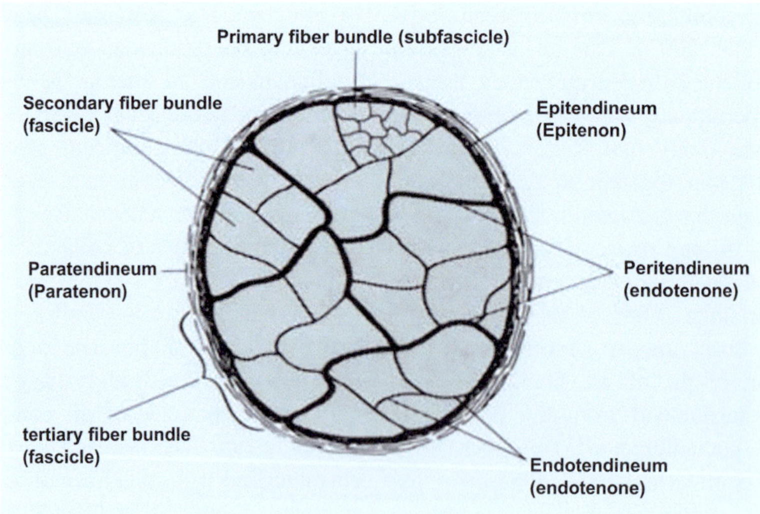

Fig. 1.6 Schematic representation of the anatomy of the tendon in cross-section from "Zschäbitz, A. (2005). Anatomy and behavior of tendons and ligaments. The Orthopedist, 34, pp. 516–525. doi: 10.1007/s00132-005-0799-4"—Fig. 1.9

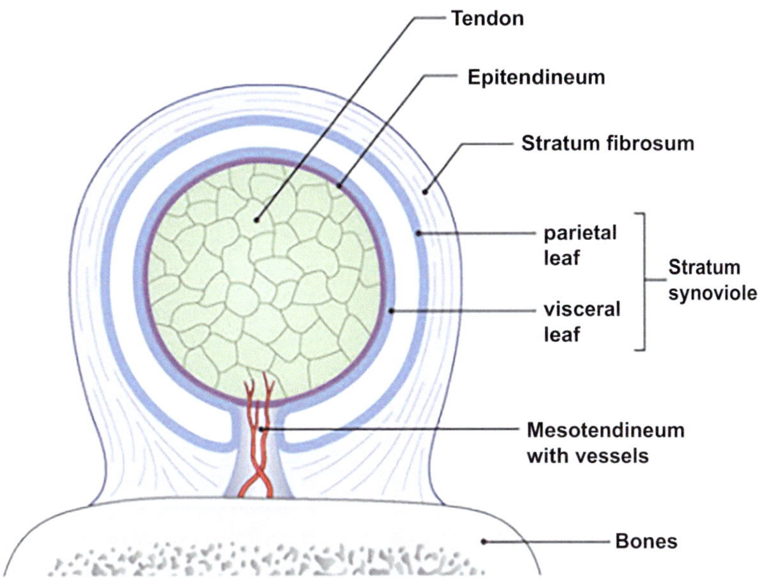

Fig. 1.7 Schematic representation of a cross-section of a tendon sheath from Zilles, K., & Tillmann, B. (2010). Anatomy. Berlin, Heidelberg: Springer-Verlag. doi: 10.1007/978-3-540-69483-0"—Fig. 4.18.

tendon via the connective tissue bridges of the mesotendineum or the vincula breve et longum (cf. Zschäbitz 2005).

In the area of the transition between the muscle belly and the origin or insertion tendon, the muscle cells fan out and thus serve to expand the contact surface. This is increased by the described circumstance by 10–20 times. There is an interweaving of the muscular and tendinous parts (cf. Ovalie 1987, Fig. 1.8).

In the area of the tendon origins or the tendon insertions, a distinction can be made between a periosteal-diaphyseal and a chondral-apophyseal transition into the bone. Fig. 1.9 presents the chondral-apophyseal tendon-bone transition of the triceps brachii muscle into the olecranon. In comparison, elastic connective tissue would be found in the periosteal-diaphyseal bone-tendon transition instead of cartilage tissue.

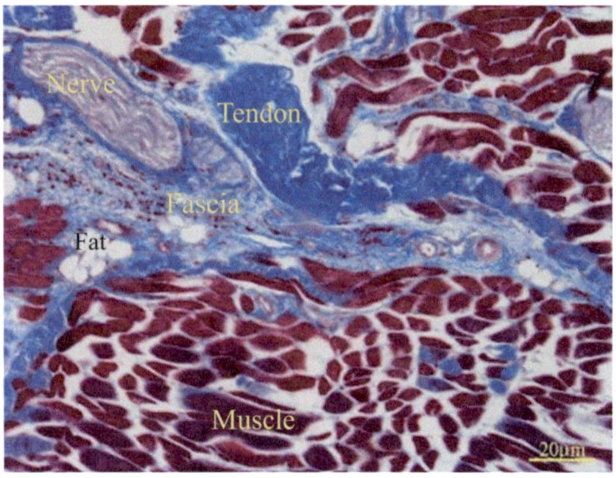

Fig. 1.8 Anatomy of the myotendinous transition from "Jirikowski, G. (13. January 2016). Fasciae and aponeuroses of the musculoskeletal system. Manual Medicine, 54, p. 10–13. doi: 10.1007/s00337-015-0086-3"—Fig. 1.1

1.2.3.3 Vascular Supply and Drainage of the Muscle

For the arterial supply of the skeletal muscle with blood, larger arteries initially branch off, which run in the epimysium. From there, interconnected arcade arterioles extend into the depths of the perimysium. From there, transversely running arterioles penetrate into the endomysium. These in turn branch off into asymmetrically arranged terminal arterioles. From these terminal arterioles, arterial capillaries, which run parallel to the muscle fibers, emerge. The arterial capillaries, which originate from a terminal alveolus, are referred to as

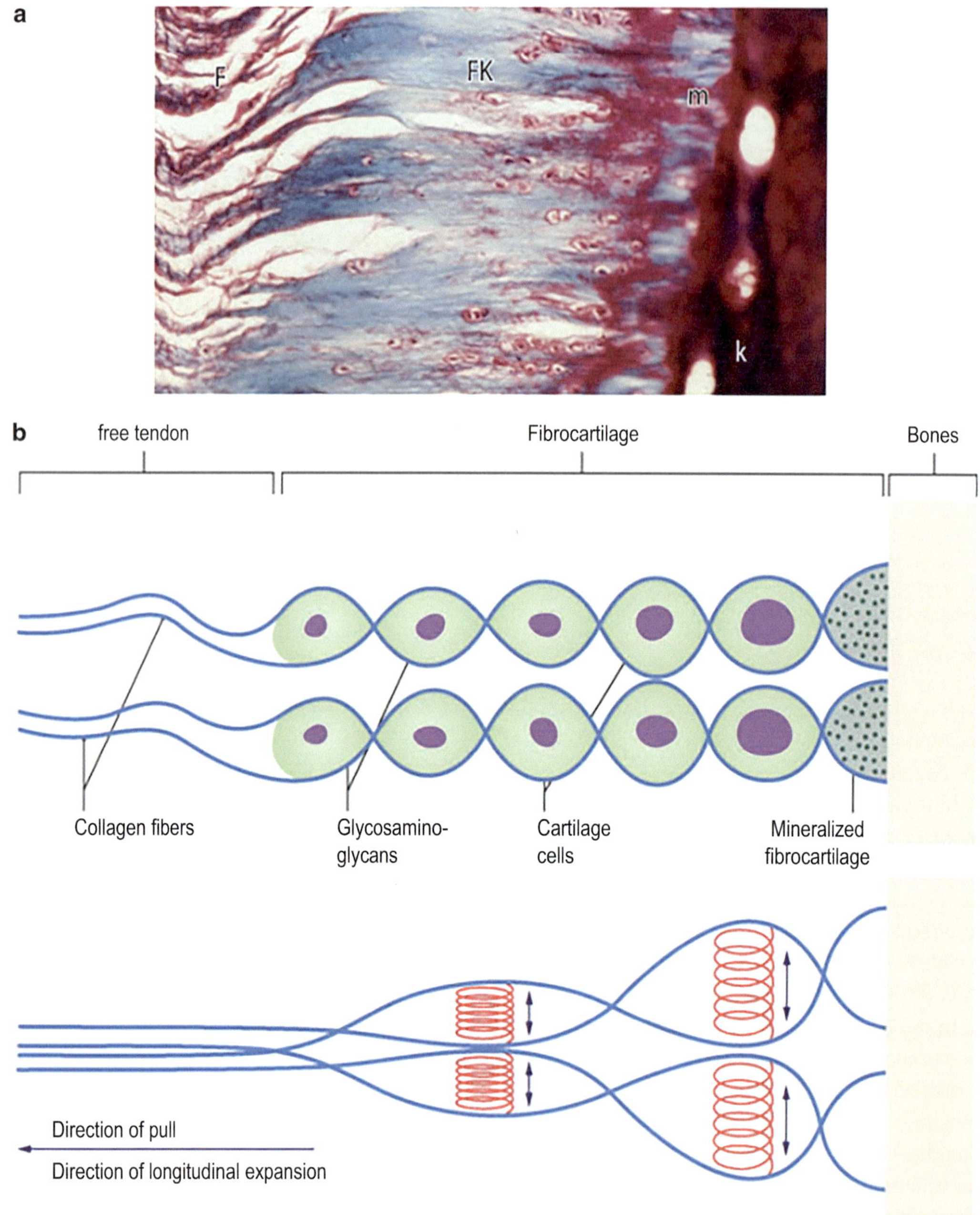

Fig. 1.9 Anatomy of the chondral-apophyseal tendon transition using the example of the insertion of the triceps brachii muscle into the olecranon from "Zilles, K., & Tillmann, B. (2010). Anatomy. Berlin, Heidelberg: Springer-Verlag. doi: 10.1007/978-3-540-69483-0"—Fig. 4.17a–b

a microvascular unit (Fig. 1.10). This represents the smallest functional unit, which is subject to blood flow control. Each microvascular unit consists of 15–20 arterial capillaries, which run in both directions at a distance of less than one millimeter.

The subsequent venous capillaries lead the blood into a receiving venule. The further

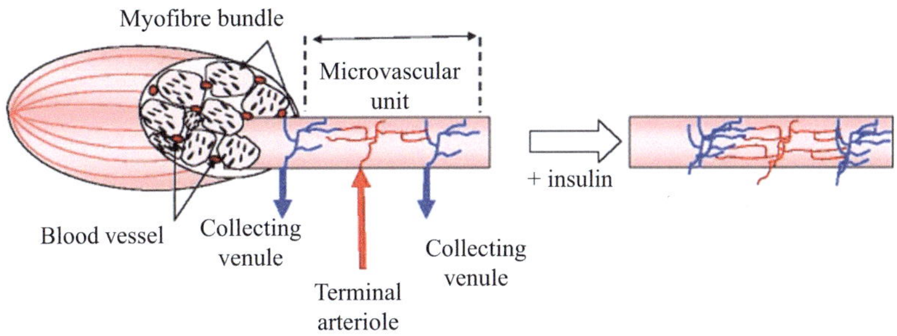

Fig. 1.10 Schematic representation of a microvascular unit from "Barrett, E., Eggleston, E., Inyard, A., Wang, H., Li, G., Chai, W., & Liu , Z. (13. March 2009). The vascular actions of insulin control its delivery to muscle and regulate the rate-limiting step in skeletal muscle insulin action. Diabetologia, 52, p. 752–764. doi: 10.1007/s00125-009-1313-z"—Fig. 4

venous outflow corresponds to the described arterial inflow (cf. Latroche et al. 2015). The lymphatic drainage, with the initial lymph vessels as the starting point, also runs within the described connective tissue layers (cf. Causey et al. 2012).

1.2.3.4 Vascular Supply and Drainage of the Tendon

The blood vessels responsible for feeding the tendon initially run in the paratendineum or, in the presence of tendon sheaths, in the mesotendineum or the vinculi. From the paratendineum, the blood vessels extend over the peritendineum to the endotendineum. The course of the blood vessels can be described as parallel to the collagen fibers (cf. Petersen et al. 2000). The intensity of vascularization within the tendon depends on the area of the tendon and its individual anatomy. In the area of the myotendinous transition, the blood supply is intense. If the tendon anchoring takes place in the bone via a periosteal-diaphyseal transition, the supply of blood vessels is considered high. In comparison, the blood supply via the perichondrium at chondral-apophyseal tendon-bone transition zones is significantly reduced (cf. Benjamin and Ralphs 2000).

1.2.3.5 Nervous Innervation of the Musculature or the Tendon

The innervation of the skeletal musculature is carried out via so-called motor units. Starting from motor alpha-motoneurons, which are located in the anterior horn of the spinal cord, a certain number of axons extending into the periphery are controlled per neuron (cf. Murrant et al. 2021). The combination of an alpha-motoneuron and the axons under its control is referred to as a motor unit (Fig. 1.11). The number of motor units can range between 10 and 1000. The number of muscle fibers recruited by a motor unit can vary between 5 and 1500 depending on the muscle (cf. Heckman and Enoka 2012).

Comparable to the vascular supply, the nerve structures innervating the muscle also extend within the connective tissue structures. They end via the synapses at the motor end plate in the area of the sarcolemma (cf. Nishimune and Shigemoto 2018).

Nerves supplying the tendon enter the interior of the tendon via the paratenon or the epitendon. In the existence of tendon sheaths, nerve structures enter the tendon tissue via the mesotenon. Subsequently, the nerve branches extend via the peritenon to the endotenon (cf. O'Brien 2005).

1.2.3.6 Receptor Supply of the Musculature

Muscle spindles can be found within the muscle belly. While the muscle fibers, which belong to the working muscles, are referred to as extrafusal muscle fibers, the term intrafusal muscle fibers is intended for the muscle fibers

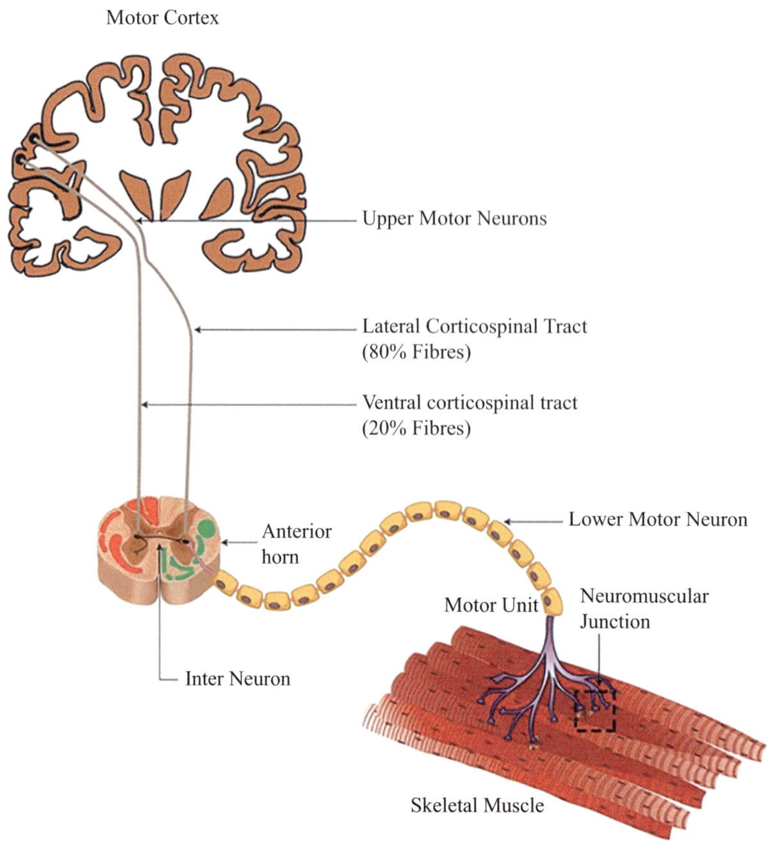

Fig. 1.11 Schematic representation of a motor unit from "Verma, S., Khurana, S., Vats, A., Sahu, B., Ganguly, N., Chakraborti, P., . . . Taneja, V. (8. January 2022). Neuromuscular Junction Dysfunction in Amyotrophic Lateral Sclerosis. Molecular Neurobiology, 59, pp. 1502–1527. doi: 10.1007/s12035-021-02658-6"—Fig. 1a

that have muscle spindles. Both extrafusal and intrafusal muscle fibers can be found in a skeletal muscle. Anatomically, muscle spindles can be divided into nuclear chain fibers and nuclear bag fibers, depending on the arrangement of the cell nuclei (Figs. 1.12 and 1.13). In nuclear chain fibers, the cell nuclei are arranged in a chain, whereas they are accumulated in one place in the nuclear bag fibers (cf. Kröger and Watkins 2021). Mechanoreceptors as well as nociceptors can be found within the connective tissue parts of the muscle (cf. Laube 2020). The receptors of the muscular connective tissue include Golgi receptors, Vater-Pacini corpuscles, Ruffini corpuscles, and free nerve endings (cf. Schleip 2003a, b).

Section 1.3.4 provides an insight into the function of the muscle spindles.

1.2.3.7 Receptor Supply of the Tendon

Afferent acting receptors in tendon tissue are focused on the musculotendinous transition (cf. O'Brien 1992). Receptors can be found both on the surface and inside the tendon. In total, four different receptors can be distinguished from each other. Type 1 receptors are Ruffini corpuscles. Type 2 receptors are represented by Vater-Paccini corpuscles. While Type 3 receptors can be recognized as Golgi tendon organs, Type 4 receptors are nociceptors (Fig. 1.14).

Section 1.3.5 provides an insight into the function of the tendon receptors.

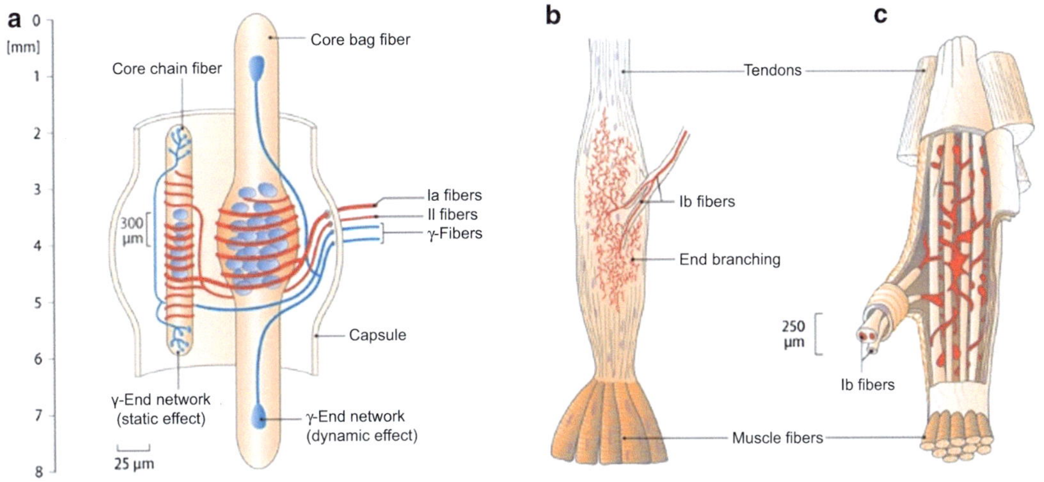

Fig. 1.12 Schematic representation of the muscle spindle from "Brandes, R., Lang, F., & Schmidt, R. (2019). Physiology of Humans. Berlin, Heidelberg: Springer-Verlag. doi: 10.1007/978-3-662-56468-4"—Fig. 4.53 a–c

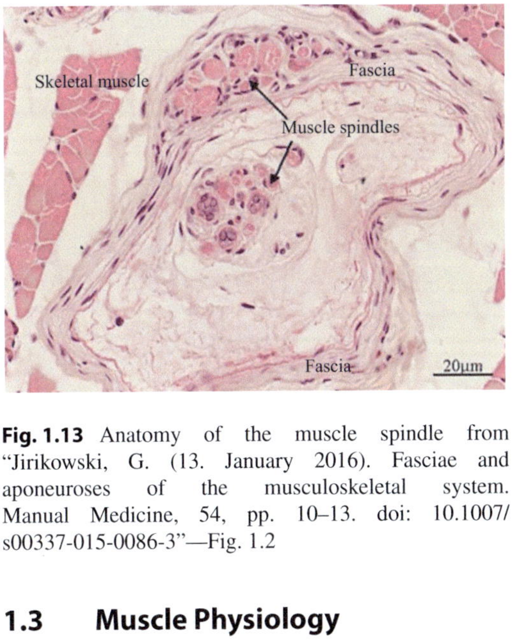

Fig. 1.13 Anatomy of the muscle spindle from "Jirikowski, G. (13. January 2016). Fasciae and aponeuroses of the musculoskeletal system. Manual Medicine, 54, pp. 10–13. doi: 10.1007/s00337-015-0086-3"—Fig. 1.2

1.3 Muscle Physiology

1.3.1 The Sensomotor System

The sensorimotor system is understood as a circular association between sensors, afferent pathways, centrally located nerve cell networks, efferent pathways, and the musculature. The creation of a motor program depends on internal or external information. This makes it clear that sensory and motor functions are not two separate systems. Rather, they should be interpreted as a cooperating system that is in constant interaction (see Baek et al. 2019). Understanding the sensorimotor system serves as a fundamental building block for medical training therapy. Fig. 1.15 visualizes the functioning and important relationships of the sensorimotor system.

1.3.1.1 Origin and Transmission of Afferent Information

Sensors can be found in the skin, joint capsules, ligaments, muscle belly, tendon, and connective tissue, among other places. The different receptors are capable of transforming information present in the periphery into action potentials. The resulting afferences are directed to the brain along different pathways, depending on the type of afference. Here, a distinction can be made between different afferent nerve fibers. Aβ fibers transmit afferent information from the muscle spindle or Golgi tendon organs at a speed of 70–120 m/s. A

fibers transmit afferences from skin receptors in relation to touch, pressure, and vibration at a speed of 30–70 m/s. Aδ fibers transmit afferent information from the skin regarding temperature and fast nociception at a speed of 12–30 m/s. C fibers transmit afferent information about

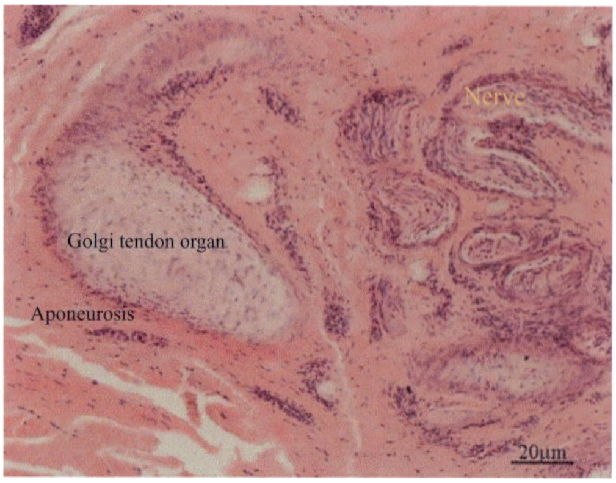

Fig. 1.14 Anatomy of the Golgi tendon organ from "Jirikowski, G. (13. January 2016). Fasciae and aponeuroses of the musculoskeletal system. Manual Medicine, 54, pp. 10–13. doi: 10.1007/s00337-015-0086-3"—Fig. 1.3

thermoreceptors and slow nociception at a speed of 0.2–0.5 m/s (see Perl 1994). The stimuli reach the spinal cord via the afferent peripheral nerve fibers. Aγ and B fibers do not play a central role in this context and are therefore not described in detail.

An afferent pathway exists via the posterior column pathway (Funiculus posterior). The tract of the spinobulbar tract is located in the area of the posterior column pathway. The spinobulbar tract is a combination of the fasciculus cuneatus and the fasciculus gracilis (Fig. 1.16). These pathways carry epicritical-sensitive afferences, which originate from the receptors of muscles, tendons, and joints, among other things. This enables fine perception in relation to touch, pressure, and vibration stimuli. While the fasciculus gracilis originates from fibers of the sacral and lumbar cord, the fibers of the fasciculus cuneatus originate from the thoracic or cervical cord (see Ayabe et al. 2005). The first sensitive neuron is located in the spinal ganglion. The switch to the second sensitive neuron then takes place in the corresponding core areas of the medulla

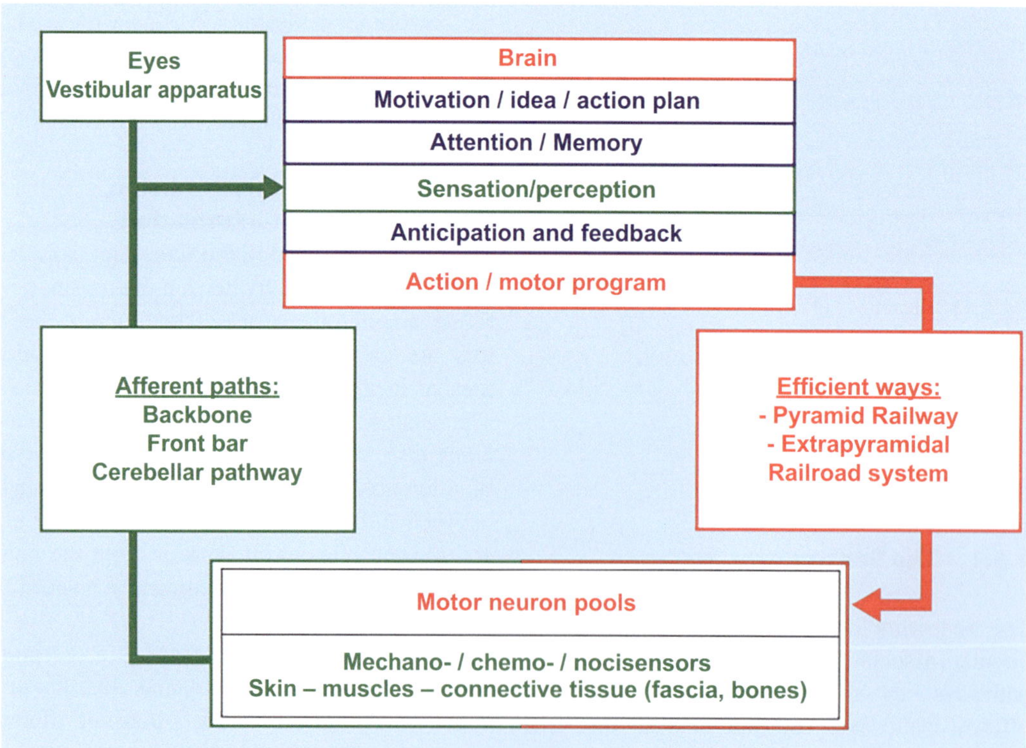

Fig. 1.15 Schematic representation of the sensorimotor system from "Laube, W. (2020). Sensorimotor and Pain: Interaction of Movement Stimuli and Pain Perception. Berlin—Heidelberg: Springer."—Fig. 2.1

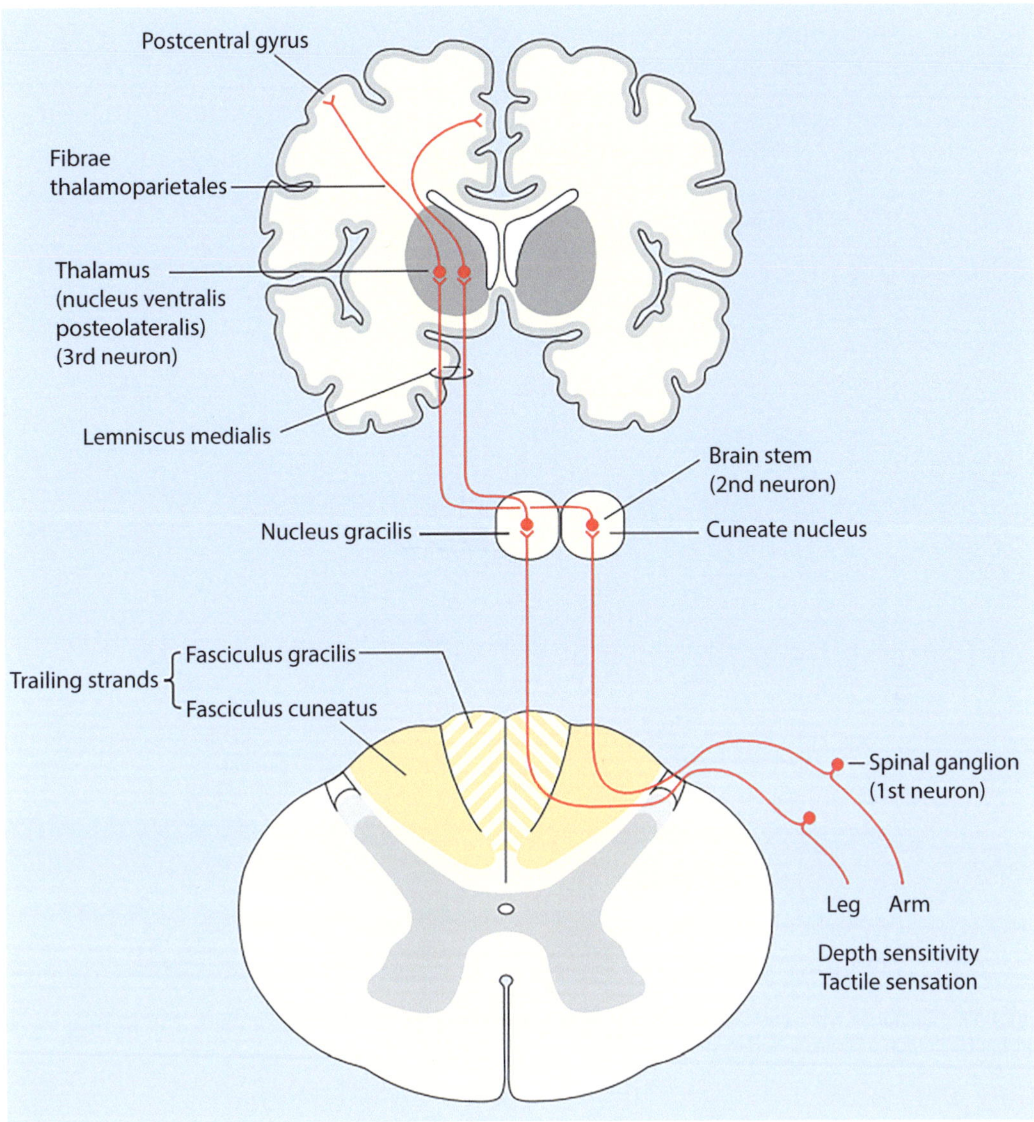

Fig. 1.16 Schematic representation of the spinobulbar tract from "Kirsch, J. (2018). Pain, let go! Berlin, Heidelberg: Springer-Verlag. doi: 10.1007/978-3-662-55358-9"—Fig. 6.3

oblongata. After the subsequent crossing to the opposite side, the fibers run through the brainstem and are switched to the third neuron in the nucleus ventralis posterior of the thalamus dorsalis. Ultimately, the fibers end up via the internal capsule at the primary somatosensory cortex in the area of the gyrus postcentralis of the telencephalon (Fig. 1.16).

The anterolateral funiculus (Funiculus anterolateralis) primarily carries protopathic-sensory information. This includes focused coarse pressure and touch stimuli as well as afferents from thermo- and nociceptors (see Bowsher, 2005). The anterolateral funiculus pathway consists of four fiber tracts. Included in the anterolateral funiculus pathway are the Tractus spinothalamicus anterior et lateralis (Figs. 1.17 and 1.18), the Tractus spinoreticularis as well as the Tractus spinotectalis. After the connection to the first sensitive pseudounipolar neuron in the

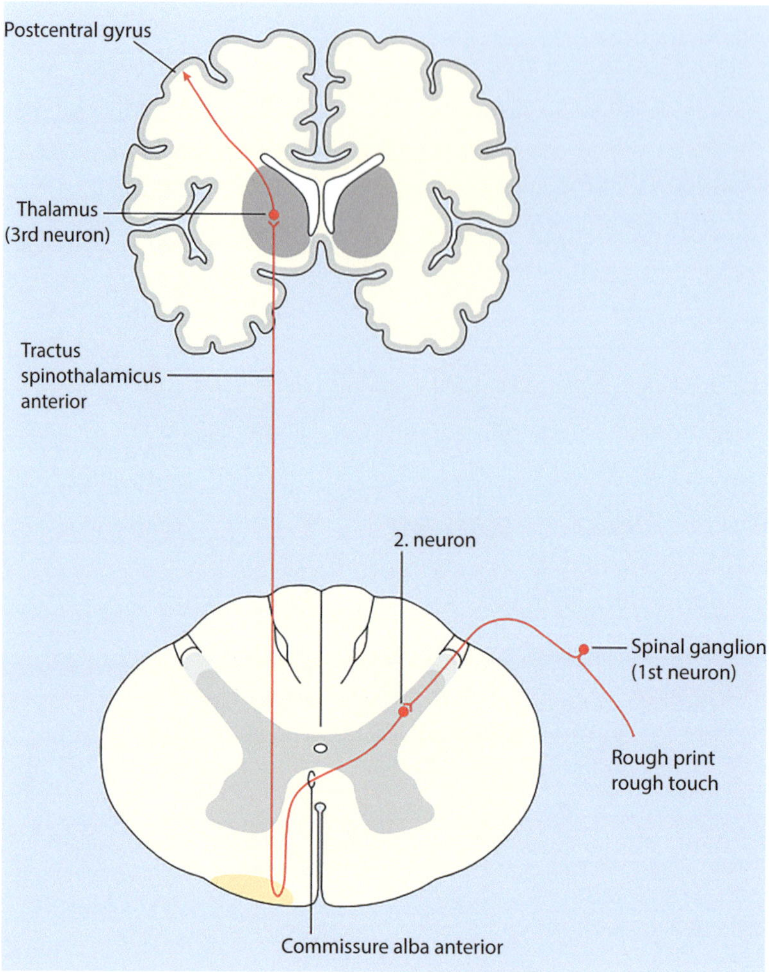

Fig. 1.17 Schematic representation of the Tractus spinothalamicus anterior from "Kirsch, J. (2018). Pain, let go! Berlin, Heidelberg: Springer-Verlag. doi: 10.1007/978-3-662-55358-9"—Fig. 6.4

spinal ganglion, the connection to the second sensitive neuron in the dorsal horn of the spinal cord takes place. Subsequently, the axons cross over the Commisura alba anterior to the opposite side. Fibers of the Tractus spinoreticularis can run crossed as well as uncrossed. The switch to the third neuron takes place depending on the fiber tract in the Thalamus dorsalis, the Formatio reticularis or the Tectum. From there, the information is projected or forwarded to the somatosensory cortex, the brainstem or the mesencephalon.

The cerebellar lateral funiculus pathway (Tractus spinocerebellaris) includes the Tractus spinocerebellaris anterior et posterior and the Tractus spinocerebellaris rostralis (see Baek et al. 2019). It serves to transmit proprioceptive information from the periphery. The switch to the first sensitive neuron takes place in the spinal ganglion. After the switch to the second sensitive neuron in the dorsal horn of the spinal cord, the Tractus spinocerebellaris anterior moves contralaterally to cranial, to then return to the ipsilateral side. The Tractus spinocerebellaris posterior and the Tractus spinocerebellaris rostralis run without crossing ipsilaterally to the cerebellum.

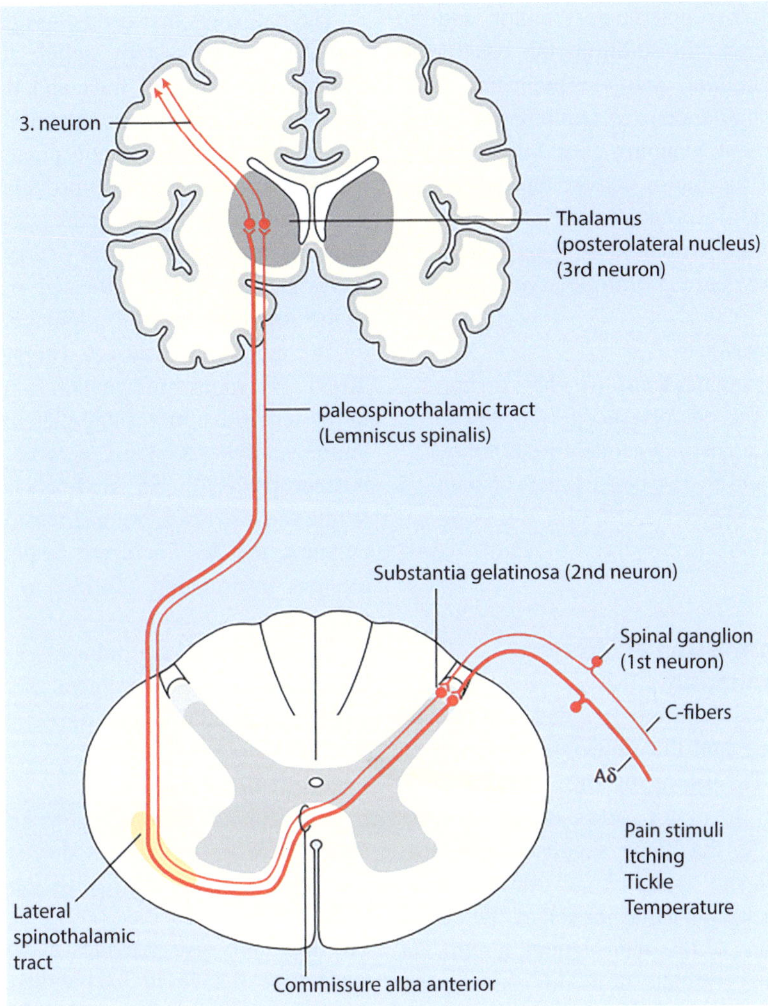

Fig. 1.18 Schematic representation of the Tractus spinothalamicus lateralis from "Kirsch, J. (2018). Pain, let go! Berlin, Heidelberg: Springer-Verlag. doi: 10.1007/978-3-662-55358-9"—Fig. 6.5

In addition to the described afferent information pathways, the brain is informed about stimuli from the visual as well as the vestibuloauditory system (see Laube 2020).

Understanding the afferent information transmission provides a basis for the control of medical training therapy.

1.3.1.2 Information Interpretation and Movement Planning in the Central Nervous System

The task of the central nervous system is to interpret incoming afferents for relevance or to weight them and, if necessary, to bring them to consciousness. In addition to the afferent information density, the brain can draw on contents stored in memory. The combination of afferents from the periphery and memory contents forms the basis for movement planning. Movement planning can be supported by motivation, ideas, attention, and anticipation. These building blocks are united in the prefrontal cortex. In addition to the integration of afferent information, the prefrontal cortex is responsible for motor control (see Chafee and Heilbronner 2022). Subordinate to the prefrontal cortex are the premotor, the supplementary motor, and the association cortex. In addition, the basal ganglia, the cerebellum, and the brainstem exert their motor influence. In combination, they ensure movement planning (see Laube 2020). In the area of the motor cortex, the first motor neuron is found. Information originating here is transmitted to the peripheral nervous system via efferent pathways of the central nervous system.

Practical Relevance

Physical training has a positive effect on cognition and the neuroplasticity of the brain. Continuous training of cardiovascular fitness can contribute to the preservation of training-induced effects (see Hötting and Röder 2013).

1.3.1.3 Transmission of Efferent Information

Efferent pathways can be classified into the lateral descending and the ventromedial descending system. The axons of the lateral system originate from the motor cortex and parts of the red nucleus. As the name suggests, the pathways of the lateral descending system primarily run in the lateral white matter of the spinal cord. The axons of the ventrolateral system, on the other hand, originate from the caudal parts of the brainstem and primarily extend in the anterior column of the spinal cord's white matter. Furthermore, the lateral system can largely be assigned to the pyramidal system, while the main parts of the ventromedial system belong to the extrapyramidal system. In general, a division into a lateral or ventromedial descending system, respectively a subdivision into a pyramidal and extrapyramidal system, can only inadequately do justice to the complexity of the real anatomy and its functionality. These divisions are therefore to be interpreted as simplifications.

Functionally, the lateral descending system is responsible for the harmonious control of the distal limb musculature. The ventromedial descending system, on the other hand, ensures activation of the proximal limb musculature and the trunk musculature.

The pathways that can be assigned to the lateral descending system include the lateral and anterior corticospinal tract and the rubrospinal tract. Components of the ventromedial descending system are the reticulospinal tract and the tectospinal tract. Fig. 1.19 provides a simplified overview of the efferent pathway systems. These transmit the information they carry to the second motor neuron, which is located in the brainstem or the anterior horn of the spinal cord depending on the motor pathway (cf. Huggenberger et al. 2019). The motor information is then passed on to the respective motor end plates of the musculature via the peripheral nervous system. This is done primarily via Aα fibers and Aγ fibers. While the Aα fibers control the extrafusal musculature, the Aγ fibers are responsible for the efferent information transfer to the intrafusal musculature.

Understanding the transmission of efferent information provides a crucial basis for controlling medical training therapy.

Practical Relevance

In patients who have undergone anterior cruciate ligament reconstruction, a decrease in volume and a reduced excitability of the corticospinal tract have been observed (cf. Lepley et al. 2020). The literature also provides evidence that pain leads to a decreased excitability of the corticospinal tract (cf. Rohel et al. 2021).

1.3.2 Process of Muscle Contraction

Starting from the motor end plate, the process of muscle contraction is described below. Action potentials arriving at the motor end plate lead to the release of acetylcholine at the synapses. This neurotransmitter pours into the synaptic cleft and is then taken up by acetylcholine receptors. These transmit the signal for the impending muscle contraction to the sarcoplasmic reticulum (Fig. 1.20). Due to these incoming stimuli, calcium is released from the sarcoplasmic reticulum. The calcium then exerts its effect in the area of the troponin or tropomyosin. This leads to a shift of these regulatory proteins with

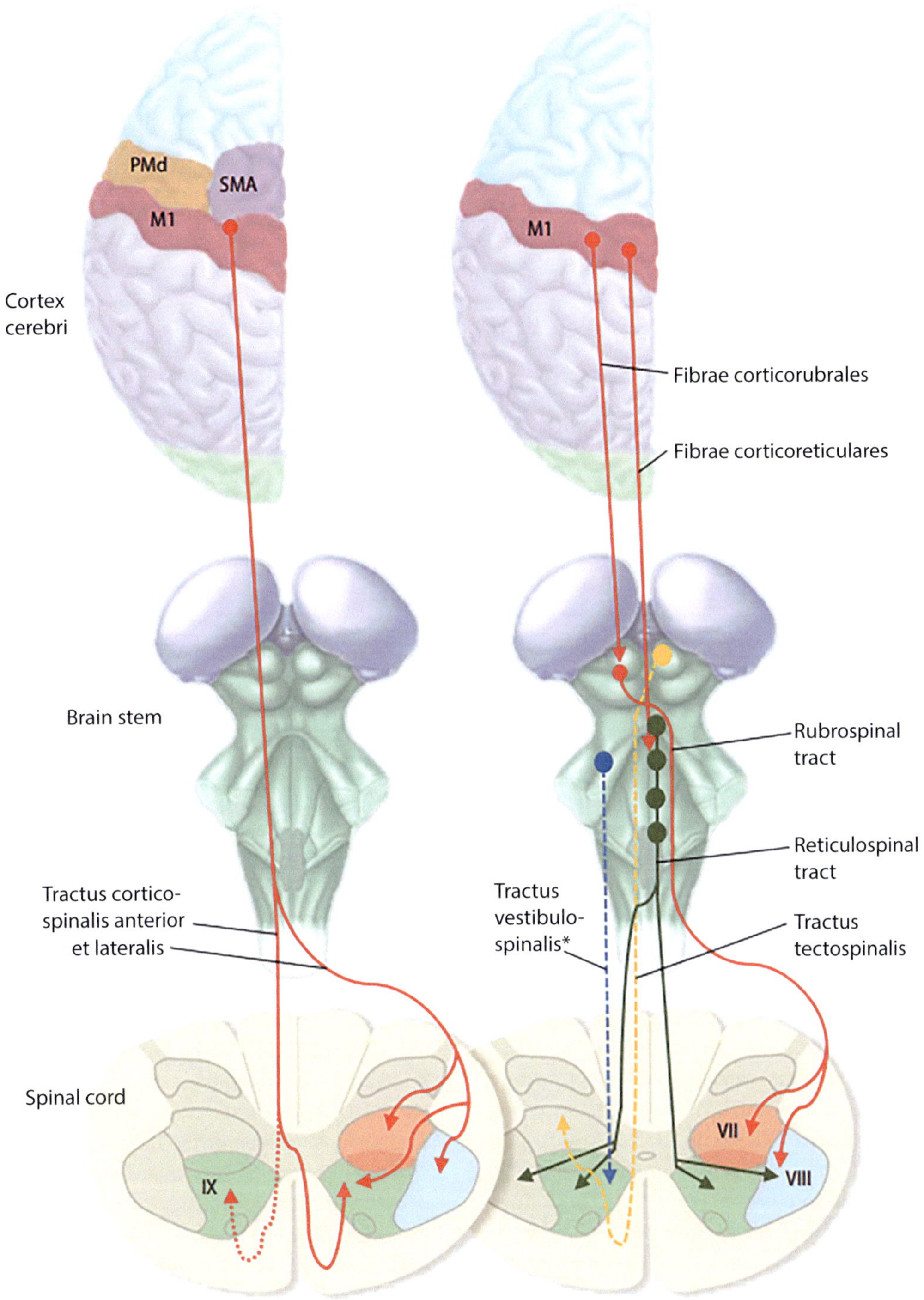

Fig. 1.19 Schematic and simplified representation of the somatomotor pathways (abbreviations: M1, primary motor cortex; PMd, dorsal premotor area; SMA, supplementary motor cortex) from "Huggenberger, S., Moser, N., Schröder, H., Cozzi, B., Granato, A., & Merighi, A. (2019). Neuroanatomy of humans. Berlin, Heidelberg: Springer-Verlag."—Fig. 5.4

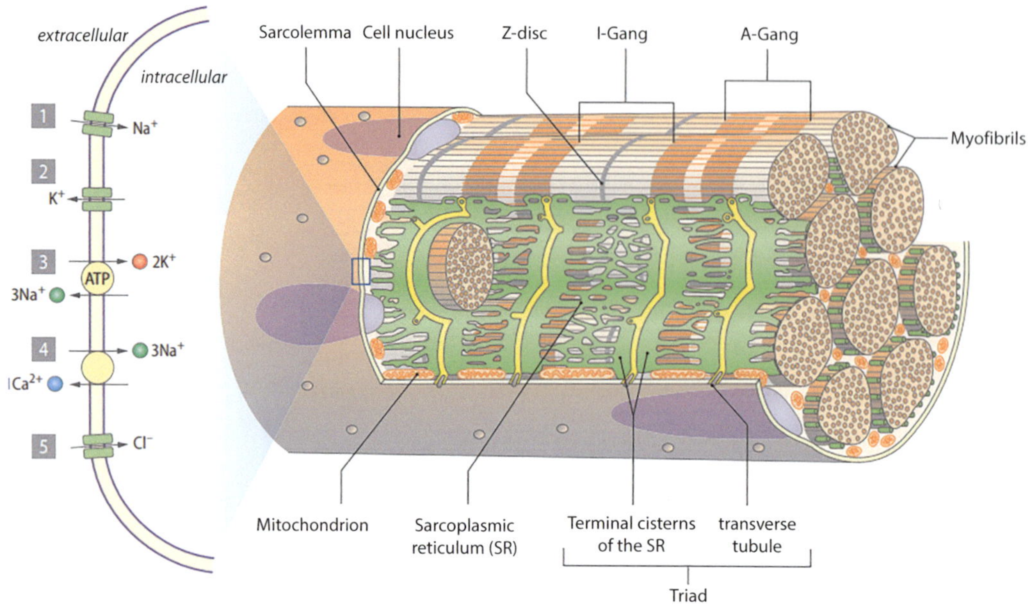

Fig. 1.20 Schematic representation of the sarcoplasmic reticulum from Brandes, R., Lang, F., & Schmidt, R. (2019). Physiology of Humans. Berlin, Heidelberg: Springer Verlag.—Fig. 13.5

the result that the binding sites of the actin are exposed (cf. Schmidt et al. 2005). In the area of the myosin head, stored adenosine triphosphate is split into adenosine diphosphate and phosphate through the process of hydrolysis. This process aligns the head part of the myosin filament so that contact with the actin becomes possible. The subsequent contact of the myosin head with the binding site of the actin is initially characterized by a slight affinity. The consumption of phosphate strengthens this affinity. With the consumption of adenosine triphosphate, there is an approximately 45-degree power stroke of the myosin head towards the center of the sarcomere. The actin filaments thus slide from both ends of the sarcomere towards the center of the sarcomere (Fig. 1.21). The following enrichment of the myosin head with adenosine triphosphate leads to a decoupling of the myosin head from the binding sites of the actin. The cross-bridge cycle then repeats itself, so that a multitude of myosin heads contribute to an approximately 20 percent shortening of the sarcomere through recurring power strokes. This causes the Z-discs to move towards each other while at the same time the I-band and the H-zone decrease in length. The summation of this process leads to a visible contraction of the skeletal muscle.

Practical Relevance

For relaxation of the skeletal muscles, the presence of adenosine triphosphate at the myosin head is essential. Energy reserves and continuous blood flow are prerequisites for the constant supply of the skeletal muscles. If this is not given, local increases in tone or muscular cramps can occur. Furthermore, after static stretching of the lower extremity muscles and thus their sarcomeres, an acute decrease in strength can occur (cf. Rubini et al. 2007). The effect of a decrease in performance with increased energy consumption was also observed in trained endurance runners (cf. Wilson et al. 2010). Leaving the acute time window after a stretch, chronic effects such as muscle hypertrophy and an increase in maximum strength can be achieved

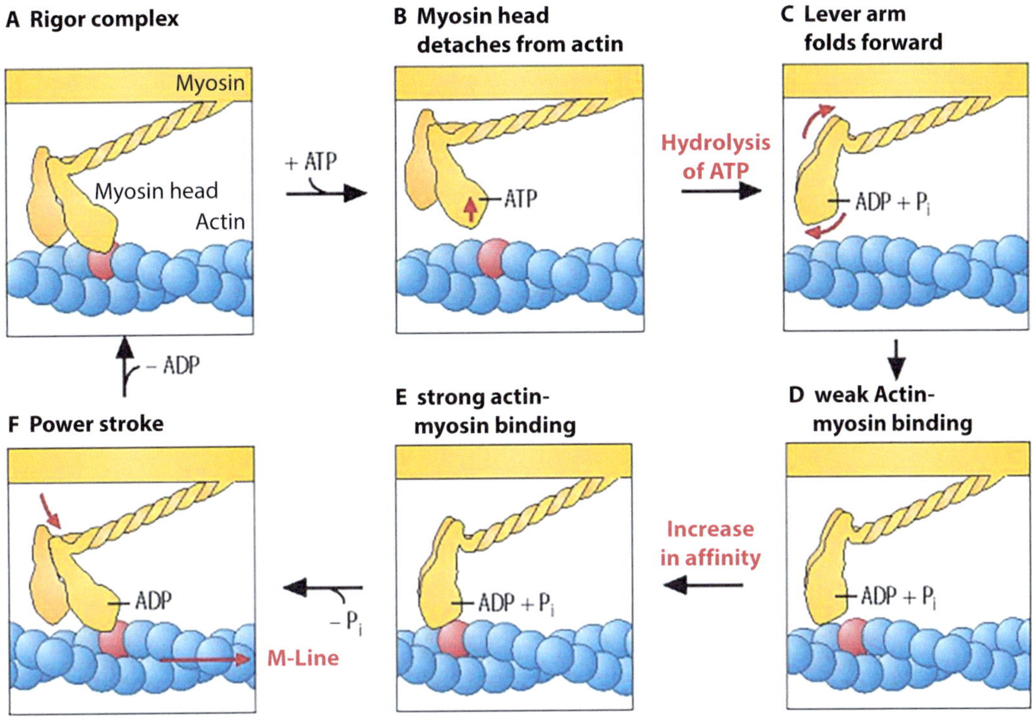

Fig. 1.21 Schematic representation of the cross-bridge cycle from "Schmidt, R., Lang, F., & Thews, G. (2005). Physiology of Humans. Berlin Heidelberg: Springer-Verlag. doi: 10.1007/b137547"—Fig. 6.3

through continuous stretching (cf. Warneke et al. 2022).

1.3.3 Energy Supply Processes of Skeletal Muscles

In order to perform muscle work, the continuous supply of adenosine triphosphate to the muscles is a prerequisite. The human body has various energy supply processes available to achieve the goal of constant adenosine triphosphate resynthesis. Fig. 1.22 schematically visualizes these processes. The individual energy supply processes do not have a hierarchical arrangement and run parallel to each other. The focus of energy supply depends on the respective physical activity. For high-intensity and short physical activities, the body relies on the hydrolysis of creatine phosphate. This metabolic process is understood as alactic and anaerobic. In addition, anaerobic glycolysis can be used for short-term, intense loads. In this process, glucose, which in turn comes from ingested carbohydrates, is processed without the consumption of oxygen. Anaerobic glycolysis is a lactic acid energy supply process. However, if activities are carried out over a longer period of time with moderate intensity, the processes of aerobic glycolysis and fatty acid oxidation come to the fore. Here, the energy derived from carbohydrates and fatty acids is obtained through the mitochondria using oxygen. These processes are largely alactic (see Brandes et al. 2019). In cases of severe malnutrition, protein, which is actually understood as a building material in the human body, can also be used as an energy carrier.

▶ **Practical Relevance**

The setting of stimuli in medical training therapy can determine which energy supply processes are primarily activated. The physical

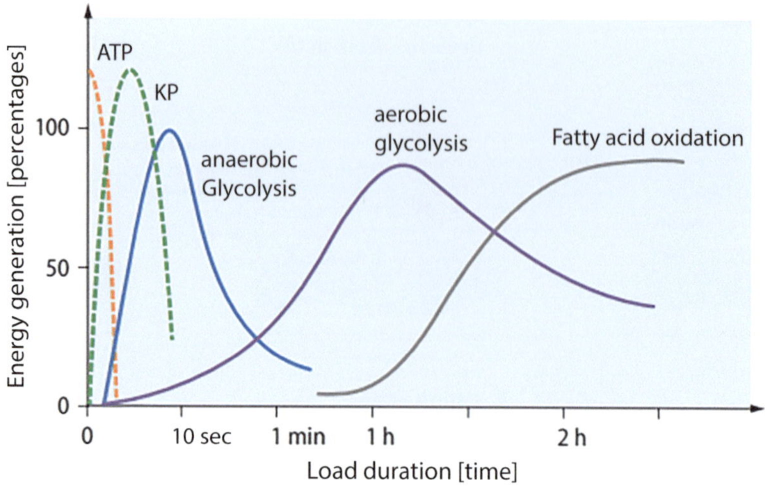

Fig. 1.22 Schematic representation of the energy supply processes (abbreviations: CP: creatine phosphate, ATP: adenosine triphosphate) from "Brandes, R., Lang, F., & Schmidt, R. (2019). Physiology of Humans. Berlin, Heidelberg: Springer Verlag."—Fig. 44.2

adaptation mechanisms differ depending on the intensity and duration of the stimulus setting.

1.3.4 Functioning of Muscle Spindles

All receptors of the myofascial system are capable of receiving individual stimuli and transcribing them into an action potential understandable for the nervous system. Muscle spindles are found in the area of the muscle belly. Muscle spindles are formed from so-called intrafusal muscle fibers and can be divided into nuclear bag fibers and nuclear chain fibers due to the arrangement of the nuclei. Furthermore, a functional subdivision into dynamic and static nuclear bag fibers can be made in the nuclear bag fibers. Muscle spindles are detectors of muscle length. They register the speed and intensity at which a change in the length of the skeletal muscle occurs (see Kröger and Watkins 2021). Dynamic nuclear bag fibers are responsible for perceiving the relative change in the length of the muscle fibers. Thus, the speed of the length change can be registered in any starting position. This function gives the skeletal muscle the ability of dynamic sensitivity (see Bewick and Banks 2015). Static nuclear bag fibers and nuclear chain fibers differ only visually due to the different arrangement of the perikarya. Functionally, both facilities are responsible for recognizing the absolute muscle length. They thus fulfill the task of static sensitivity (see Bewick and Banks 2015).

The goal of the muscle spindles is to constantly inform the central nervous system about the current or changing muscle length. By processing these afferent information, appropriate efferences can be created (see Dimitriou 2014). The goal of these efferences is a harmonious interplay between agonists and antagonists during motor activity. The described control loop can be clearly traced in practice when testing self-reflexes.

▶ **Practical Relevance**

A dynamically progressive passive stretch of the extensor digitorum muscle leads to a discharge rate of dynamic nuclear bag fibers that is about three times higher than a dynamically progressive stretch with simultaneous activation of the antagonistic flexor digitorum superficialis et profundus muscle.

In addition to a reduced discharge rate of the dynamic nuclear bag fibers during the activation of the antagonistic muscles, a reduced EMG activity can also be observed (see Dimitriou 2014). In view of these findings, simultaneous activation of the antagonistic muscles appears to be useful when stretching the agonistic muscle.

1.3.5 Functioning of Golgi (Tendon) Organs

While muscle spindles provide information about muscle length, the Golgi tendon organs are responsible for registering the tension situation (see Mileusnic and Loeb 2009). In many textbooks, the Golgi tendon organs are attributed the function of autogenic inhibition under high tension conditions. This hypothesis assumes that impending injuries can be prevented by muscular inhibition. It should be mentioned at this point that there are no corresponding findings in the field of human research for this assumption (see Chalmers 2007). Golgi tendon organs, in combination with muscle spindles, play an important role in neuromusculoskeletal dynamics. Information originating from muscle spindles or Golgi tendon organs appears to be closely interpreted in the central nervous system. Through their proprioceptive afferents, they contribute to the control of joint position, posture, and movements (see Kistemaker et al. 2013). Only about 10% of the Golgi organs are found within tendons. The remaining 90% are located in the muscular portions, the myotendinous junction, attachment zones of aponeuroses, capsules, and ligaments (see Schleip 2003a, b). In addition to registering tension states during activity, the Golgi organs are also attributed a balance-maintaining function during standing and walking (see Dietz et al. 1992).

▶ **Practical Relevance**

The stretching technique of post-isometric relaxation can contribute to significant improvements in terms of disability level, pain, mobility, and quality of life (see Khan et al. 2022). The mode of action of the technique cannot currently be satisfactorily explained by a reflex activity of the Golgi tendon organs. The explanatory model of improved perception through repeated tension and relaxation thus comes to the fore.

1.3.6 Functioning of Other Receptors of the Myofascial System

In addition to the Golgi (tendon) organs, the myofascial system contains Vater-Pacini corpuscles. These receptors are induced to produce action potentials by rapid or dynamic pressure changes or vibrations. Ruffini corpuscles are slowly adapting mechanoreceptors that respond to prolonged pressure (see Schleip 2003a, b). In summary, the receptors presented so far belong to type 1 or type 2 receptors. In addition, there are usually free nerve endings, which are either myelinated (type 3, 10%) or unmyelinated (type 4, 90%). These receptors can also be interpreted as mechanoreceptors, which can perceive low-threshold or high-threshold pressure stimuli. Through thermal, chemical, or mechanical stimuli, these receptors can be converted into nociceptors due to the release of corresponding neuropeptides. In addition, type 3 and type 4 receptors are attributed autonomous functions, such as the regulation of blood pressure and thus the fine regulation of myofascial blood flow (see Coote and Perez-Gonzalez 1970).

▶ **Practical Relevance**

Pain can be reduced through medical training therapy. This effect is also referred to as training-induced hypoalgesia. Due to mechanosensitive afferents, there is an activation of descending central opioid and cannabinoid systems (see Vaegter and Jones 2020).

1.3.7 Definition, Signaling Pathways, and Functions of Myokines

From a physiological perspective, a skeletal muscle can do much more than generate force through contraction, move joints, and generate heat. Thus, skeletal muscle fibers are capable of releasing cytokines and other peptides during activity. In summary, these substances released from the muscles can be referred to as myokines. Myokines enable communication between skeletal muscle and other organs or cells (see Severinsen and Pedersen 2020).

Myokines are capable of influencing the proliferation, differentiation, and hypertrophy of skeletal muscle, and are thus an important factor for the maintenance and training of muscle mass or muscle strength (see Lee and Jun 2019).

An organ that can also benefit from myokines on various levels is the brain (see Mattson 2012). Erickson et al (2011) were able to research that training can achieve an enlargement of the hippocampus, improved neurogenesis, increased neuroplasticity, as well as improved memory function. Existing evidence further suggests that muscular activation can positively regulate appetite (see Blundell et al. 2015). In addition, a positive influence on various sleep parameters has been demonstrated (see Kelley and Kelley 2017). A publication by Crush et al. (2017) reveals that training can also positively influence general mood. The release of myokines can also be seen as a prophylaxis of vascular dementia (see Aarsland et al. 2011). At this point, positive influences through training in relation to anxiety disorders, depression, and stress should also be mentioned (see Pedersen and Saltin 2015).

Myokines are also capable of communicating with subcutaneous or visceral fat tissue. Thus, muscular activity can stimulate the process of lipolysis. This results in a reduction of fat stores, especially visceral fat (see Nordby et al. 2012). If it is possible to reduce abdominal fat tissue through medical training therapy, this can be understood as a prophylaxis against type 2 diabetes mellitus (see Bays 2009), dementia (see Whitmer et al. 2008), cardiovascular diseases (see Haffner 2007), colon carcinomas (see Giovannucci 2007) and breast cancer (see Xue and Michels 2007). It is suspected that myokines may also play a role in the restructuring of brown into white fat tissue (see Severinsen and Pedersen 2020).

In addition, bone tissue is influenced by myokines. They exert a regulatory influence on bone formation and thus participate in bone metabolism. A reduced release of myokines can be observed with increasing age and physical inactivity and represents a risk factor for the development of osteopenia or osteoporosis (see Perrini et al. 2010).

Among other things, myokines cause the liver to produce more glucose during physical activity (see Febbraio et al. 2004). This ensures a constant blood sugar level. In addition, a hormonal feedback loop of myokines and insulin metabolism was found. Information exchange between insulin-sensitive tissues and the islets of the pancreas occurs via myokines. This allows the insulin requirement to be adapted to current needs. At the same time, a diabetic metabolism is prevented (see Ellingsgaard et al. 2011).

Research results also suggest positive effects on the vascular system. Ouchi et al. (2008) describe improved endothelial cell function through the release of myokines and mention a stimulation of revascularization.

Through signaling pathways, which are stimulated by the secretion of myokines during activity, the skin tissue can also be positively influenced. Especially through endurance training, age-associated changes can be significantly slowed down, while the ability to regenerate improves (see Crane et al. 2015).

Long-lasting intensive muscular activity is capable of exerting an immunoregulatory influence (see Pedersen and Hoffman-Götz 2000). The activated feedback loop results in an increased production of cortisol in the adrenal glands. While this can result in a reduction in the number of lymphocytes, the amount of neutrophil granulocytes increases in return (see Steensberg et al. 2003). In addition, physical activity can evoke an anti-inflammatory effect. In addition to other training-induced anti-inflammatory processes, the inhibition of tumor necrosis factor-alpha (TNF-α) is noteworthy (see Schindler et al. 1990).

The release of myokines can reduce the risk of various tumor diseases (see Christensen et al. 2018). It is suspected that this anti-oncological effect is due, among other things, to a reduction in low-grade inflammation (see Hojman et al. 2018). People who suffer from prostate, colorectal, or breast carcinomas have a higher survival rate with an active lifestyle (see Pedersen 2019).

In summary, it can be stated that the skeletal muscle communicates with other organs through the release of myokines and positively influences them. This shows that medical training therapy not only causes local adaptation mechanisms, but also makes a significant contribution to the maintenance of health or performance enhancement of other organ systems. Future research should investigate medical training interventions and the resulting specific myokine release as well as existing influencing factors more precisely. With the help of these findings, it will be possible to use training more characteristically for existing diseases or for prevention.

1.4 Muscle Fiber Types

Muscle fibers of the skeletal muscles are fundamentally similar in structure. They can be classified into different subtypes by the isoforms of heavy myosin chains (see Talbot and Maves 2016). However, there are also further differences in the ratio of the amount of myofibrils, mitochondria, and the sarcoplasm. In addition, the content of glycogen, fat, and myoglobin varies. Due to these circumstances, a functional subdivision into different muscle fiber types can be made. In addition to type 1 fibers, a distinction can be made between type 2 fibers and intermediate fibers (see Zimmer and Appell 2021).

The structure of type 1 fibers can be described as thin. Compared to other muscle fibers, type 1 fibers have a lot of sarcoplasm, which is characterized by a high proportion of fat deposits and myoglobin. Myoglobin appears as a red muscle dye. Therefore, type 1 fibers are often referred to as red muscle fibers. Between the myofibrils, there are extensively arranged mitochondria in series. Type 1 fibers are characterized by a high oxidative metabolism. From a functional point of view, type 1 fibers can optimally perform endurance activities due to slow shortening speeds. Fatigue is considered low. The first fibers to be activated during a muscular contraction are those of type 1. They are thus "the first to come and the last to go" (see Zimmer and Appell 2021).

Type 2 fibers are more powerful in their structure and have more myofibrils. Compared to type 1 fibers, there is a reduced number of mitochondria and a reduced myoglobin content. As a result, these fibers appear whitish and are accordingly referred to as white muscle fibers. Metabolic processes in the white muscle fibers predominantly occur anaerobically. Functionally, the fibers can handle short-term power or maximum strength activities. The fatigue of type 2 fibers is considered high (see Zimmer and Appell 2021).

Finally, a distinction can be made into an intermediate type, which due to its anatomy and function occupies a middle position between type 1 and type 2 fibers. Type 1 and type 2 fibers are characterized by the expression of a single heavy myosin chain isoform. In intermediate fibers (or hybrid fibers), at least two or more heavy myosin chain isoforms are found (see Pette and Staron 2000). With a proportion of 25% and higher, the intermediate muscle fibers ensure a functional continuum between the different muscle fiber types (see Medler, 2019).

A visualization of the preceding descriptions is provided in Fig. 1.23.

▶ **Practical Relevance**

By applying stimuli in medical training therapy, plastic processes of the muscle fibers can be stimulated. Thus, endurance training can increase the functionality of type 1 fibers, while the adaptation mechanisms through strength training are focused on

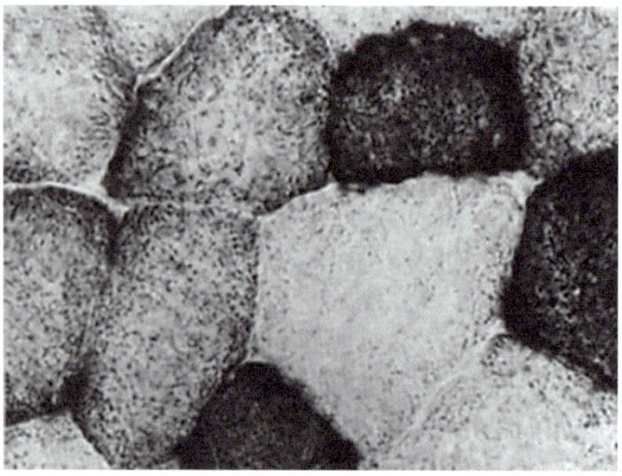

Fig. 1.23 Coloring of the mitochondria allows differentiation between the muscle fiber types in the light microscopic cross-section. Dark: Type 1 fibers, White: Type 2 fibers, Mixed form: Intermediate fibers—from Zimmer, P., & Appell, H.-J. (2021). Functional Anatomy. Berlin, Heidelberg: Springer-Verlag.—Fig. 2.4

type 2 fibers. In addition, intermediate fibers can functionally approach type 1 or type 2 fibers, depending on training stimuli, due to existing plasticity (see Qaisar et al. 2016). The preceding classification does not fully do justice to the real plasticity of the myofascial system and should therefore be interpreted as a rough division.

1.5 Forms of Muscle Work

In the forms of muscle work, holding and dynamic components can initially be distinguished from each other. The holding components represent isometric muscle work. Here, under the performance of muscular work with possible tension changes, there is no change in muscle length between origin and insertion. In the dynamic forms of muscle work, on the other hand, eccentric muscle work can be distinguished from concentric muscle work.

Eccentricity is understood as a braking form of muscle work. This means that the origin and insertion of the working muscle move away from each other during activity. In contrast, the concentric form of muscle work is characterized by the fact that the origin and insertion of the working muscle move towards each other during the performance of the muscular activity (Fig. 1.24).

In stretching and shortening cycles, eccentric and concentric muscle work can alternate (cf. Ferrauti, 2020). In the forms of work of concentric and eccentric, with constant muscular tension, one can also speak of an isotonic contraction. However, this is almost never found in everyday life. Because in addition to the muscle length, the muscular tension almost always changes as well, auxotonic contractions are to be interpreted as more practical.

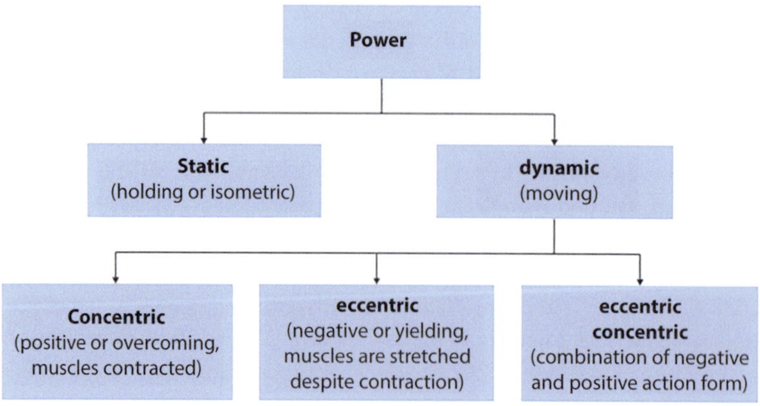

Fig. 1.24 Schematic representation of the forms of muscle work from "Ferrauti, A. (2020). Training science for sports practice. Berlin, Heidelberg: Springer-Verlag. doi: 10.1007/978-3-662-58227-5"—Fig. 4.2

Practical Relevance

Depending on the present disease pattern, the chosen form of muscle work within medical training therapy can make significant differences in terms of the success of the intervention (cf. Peterson et al. 2014). This factor should be taken into account to ensure the best current practice available. In addition, the case may occur that two different forms of muscle work lead to not significantly different results and can thus be integrated into the therapy as equivalent (cf. van Ark et al. 2016).

Due to variable pathophysiologies and symptoms, which are caused by different diseases, the question of the optimal form of muscle work also depends on the corresponding diagnosis. It should be emphasized that concentric and eccentric muscle training can be used as a single intervention but also in a combination of interventions. So there is the possibility that the combination of the eccentric and concentric approach of the respective single application is statistically significantly or clinically relevantly superior, equivalent or inferior (cf. Teissier et al. 2020). In order to make statements of this kind, scientific publications with the research question corresponding outcome measurements are a mandatory prerequisite. These statements also apply, of course, to the isometric muscle activation in addition to the concentric and eccentric forms of muscle work (cf. Stasinopoulos D. and Stasinopoulos I. 2017).

These explanations can be well illustrated using the diagnosis of patellar tendon tendinopathy. In the literature, there are comparative studies between isometric and isotonic training approaches. Rio et al. (2015) were able to induce pain relief and a reduction of muscular inhibition of the quadriceps femoris muscle in volleyball athletes with this disease pattern by applying strong isometric tension. The finding of the superiority of isometric training over the isotonic therapy approach in terms of pain intensity in existing patellar tendon tendinopathy was confirmed two years later (cf. Rio et al. 2017). Vang and Niznik (2020) point to a significant effect of both isometric and isotonic muscle activities, but highlight the superiority of the isometric training approach.

A systematic review with integrated meta-analysis from 2009 compared eccentric training in terms of muscle strength and muscle mass to a concentric training approach. Twenty randomized controlled studies were integrated into the elaboration. The evaluation of the obtained data led to the result that eccentric training at high intensity was significantly superior to concentric training in increasing total muscle strength as well as eccentric muscle strength. The eccentric approach was also superior to the concentric approach in increasing muscle mass and muscle cross-section (see Roig et al. 2009). A more recent systematic review with an additional meta-analytical evaluation focused solely on increasing muscle mass. The evaluation of data from fifteen randomized controlled studies showed that eccentric training could induce an average increase in muscle mass of 10%. In comparison, concentric training could only achieve an average increase of 6.8%. Thus, eccentric training has a higher effect size, yet no significant difference was found between the two training methods (see Schoenfeld et al. 2017).

1.6 Training-Related Biomechanics

Practical biomechanical knowledge serves for targeted training control. If the results of research, which originate from human biomechanics, are appropriately integrated into clinical everyday life, training content can be carried out in the sense of an optimal performance increase while simultaneously preventing injuries. The transfer of theoretical findings into practice forms the basis for a high-quality medical training offer.

1.6.1 Relevance of Torque in Strength Training

The torque (M) is calculated from the product of force (F) and the lever arm (a). The resulting formula M = F x a forms a cornerstone for considerations regarding the execution of strength exercises.

For a better understanding, the calculation of the torque is graphically illustrated using the example of the human elbow joint. Fig. 1.25 shows a 90° flexed elbow joint with a load in the hand, which is generated by a dumbbell. The weight of the dumbbell is 10 kilograms. Converted and rounded, 10 kilograms (kg) correspond to 100 Newton (N). The weight force of the forearm is neglected in this example, as this is not an individually variable parameter. The exact weight force is 9.81 meters per second squared. For simplification, this value was rounded to 10 meters per second squared. In the example, the pivot point corresponds to the elbow joint and the lever arm, at 90° elbow flexion, to the length of the forearm. In general, it should be noted that the lever arm is always the vertical distance from the pivot point to the line of action of the load or the force. If the length of the lever arm (a) in Fig. 1.25 is, for example, 0.3 meters (m), all relevant information for the calculation of the torque (M) is available. The calculation is therefore M = 0.3 m x 100 N. Thus, the torque (M) is to be given as 30 Newton meters (Nm).

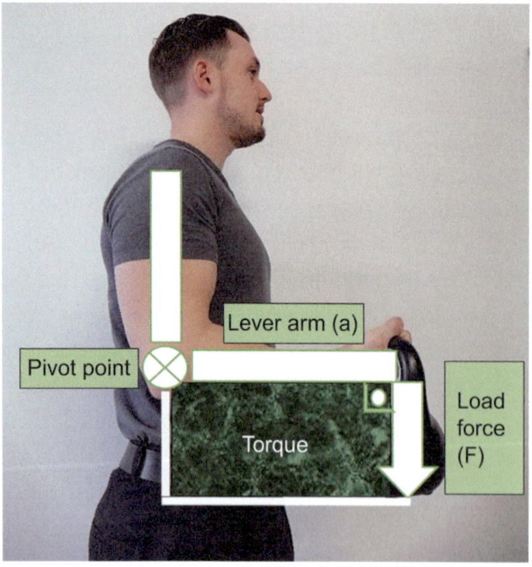

Fig. 1.25 Visual representation of torque. (Own illustration 2023)

▶ **Practical Relevance**
In Fig. 1.25, the lever arm (a), which also represents the load arm, is the longest. Thus, under these conditions, the force that must be exerted to hold the weight isometrically at 90° elbow flexion is the highest.

In Fig. 1.26, an increased flexion position of the elbow joint can be observed. This leads to a significant reduction of the lever arm (a) with an identical load of 10kg. The reduction of the lever arm (a) inevitably leads to a reduction of the torque. Thus, the force that the muscles must exert to hold the weight isometrically, despite the identical training weight, is remarkably reduced by about 38.5% compared to Fig. 1.25.

▶ **Practical Relevance**
Cable machines have extremely variable adjustment options. In addition to the training weight, the angle at which the load is to be worked with can also be adapted to the requirements.

1.6.2 Calculation of the Required Force and the Resulting Pressure on Body Structures

With the prior knowledge from Sect. 1.6.1, the question arises as to the level of force that body structures must exert during the training process. This can be specified with the following equation "Force x Force arm = Load x Load arm". In Fig. 1.27, one-legged training on the leg extension machine can be seen. The quadriceps femoris muscle has moved a weight of 10kg through the resistive movement in knee extension and now holds it in extension. Rounded, those 10 kg correspond to a load of 100 N. The pivot point is represented by the femorotibial articulation.

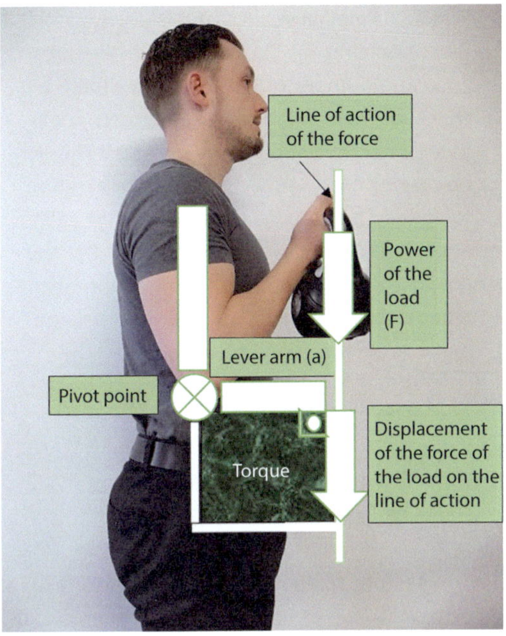

Fig. 1.26 Visual representation of the reduction of torque with flexion over 90°. (Own illustration 2023)

In knee extension, the load arm extends with a length of assumed 0.4 m in the course of the lower leg and thus forms a vertical to the force of the load, which runs to the pivot point. The force arm is formed by a vertical of the patellar ligament, which runs to the pivot point in the area of the femorotibial articulation. A length of 0.05 m is assumed for the force arm. As a result, the equation can be filled with the presented data. Force x 0.05 m = 100 N x 0.4 m. By solving the equation, the force value of the quadriceps femoris muscle or the patellar ligament can be specified as 800 N. This example shows that the patella acts as a hypomochlion.

The formula for pressure (P) is Pressure (P) = Force (F): Area (A). There is evidence that different muscular recruitment patterns are capable of modeling pressure ratios within a joint. This was demonstrated by Canals et al. (2019) on cadavers in the area of the elbow joints (see Canals et al. 2019).

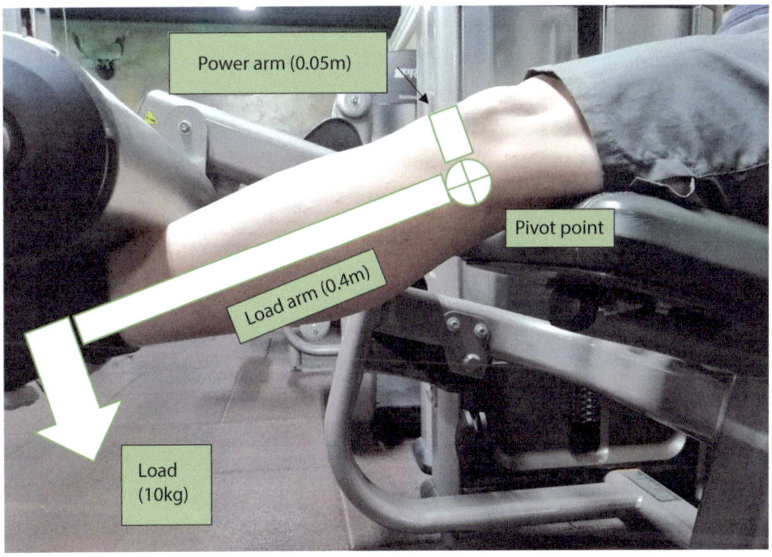

Fig. 1.27 One-legged training on the leg extension machine. (Own illustration 2023)

Practical Relevance

As early as 1993, Jensen and Graf (1993) were able to show that the injection of a saline solution into the knee joint leads to an inhibition of the quadriceps femoris muscle with simultaneous intra-articular pressure increase of the femorotibial articulation. In the presence of joint swellings, the method of medical training therapy should therefore be reconsidered (see Jensen and Graf 1993). In general, loads on body structures are to be interpreted as formative educational stimuli and thus as positive. The limit to overload is multifactorial and individually different. Therefore, before concluding a pathophysiological causality, a possibly existing correlation between load values and pathophysiological sequelae should be scientifically clarified.

1.6.3 Fixed and Loose Pulleys on the Cable Pull

Within medical training therapy practice, cable pulls are valuable training devices. Due to their manifold adjustment possibilities, countless exercise executions can be performed. Biomechanically important is the understanding of loose and fixed pulleys. If there is only a fixed pulley on a cable pull, it is to be understood as a deflection pulley. This means that with a weight of 10 kg, a force of approximately 100 N must be applied to move the weight. The resulting friction is neglected in this example. The pull path corresponds to the load path here.

However, if there is, for example, a fixed pulley and at the same time a loose pulley on the cable pull, only approximately 50 N need to be applied to move the weight of 10 kg. Here too, the influence of friction is neglected. The force that must be exerted to move the weight in the presence of a loose pulley is thus halved ($FZ=FL/2$). At the same time, the pull path doubles ($sZ=2 \times sL$). So it is not just the training weight on the cable pull that is decisive for the intensity, but also the knowledge about the number of fixed and loose pulleys.

Practical Relevance

When training on the cable pull, the presence and number of loose pulleys should be checked. With medically prescribed maximum loads in relation to the weight, it should be taken into account that the force exertion to move the load is reduced by the existence of loose pulleys. Loose pulleys offer the advantage of working against resistance over a large range of motion due to the enlargement of the pull path.

1.6.4 Biomechanical Factors in Squats

The research team led by Lorenzetti (2018) investigated the influence of foot position and stance width on mobility and the load on the hip joints or knee joints.

When both feet are positioned parallel to each other with a distance of 10% between the trochanter major and the ground, the smallest knee moments in the sagittal plane were measured. At the same time, the highest hip moments in the sagittal plane were recorded in this position. The mobility in hip and knee flexion was reduced. These results are transferable from the execution of untrained individuals, who squatted with a wooden bar, to the group which additionally moved 50% of their body weight via a barbell.

These parameters were also evaluated in a position where the participants' feet were positioned at a distance from each other, which corresponded to twice the distance between the spinae iliacae anterior superior. At the same time, the feet were rotated 42° outwards. This position led to the highest sagittal knee moments, while the sagittal hip moments were reduced to the smallest intensity. The movement excursion in hip and knee flexion also increased in both groups (cf. Lorenzetti et al. 2018).

In addition to foot position, knee position can also exert a modulating influence on force distribution. If the knee joints are behind the toes during the squat, the knee joint can be relieved. However, it is to be expected that these forces will be redistributed to the hip joint or the lower back. Therefore, it can be concluded that a slight anterior positioning of the knee joints can contribute to a harmonious load distribution between the body sections (cf. Fry et al. 2003).

These works impressively illustrate the high biomechanical importance of foot and knee positioning in the execution of squats.

With regard to the extensor moments of the ankle and knee joints, modulation can be achieved by shifting the body weight anteriorly or posteriorly. Compared to the posterior shift of body weight, a significant increase in the extensor moment of the ankle joints was registered with a simultaneous decrease in the extensor moment of the knee joints (cf. Ishida et al. 2022).

Practical Relevance

Extreme positioning of the stance width and foot rotation angle lead to both load peaks and relief peaks depending on the joint. Against this background, it becomes clear that the most "optimal" squat position is individually dependent. Lorenzetti et al. (2018) recommend a 20° foot rotation with feet positioned approximately shoulder-width apart.

From a conglomerate of individual studies, it becomes apparent that slight to moderate posterior shear forces act on the posterior cruciate ligament during the squat. In a range of motion between 0–60° knee flexion, slight anterior shear forces are also observed, which are mainly absorbed by the anterior cruciate ligament. During the exercise execution, slight to intensive compression forces were detected in the area of the femoropatellar or femorotibial joint. These increase progressively with increased flexion movement of the knee joint and reach peak values at almost full flexion. During the extension movement, there is a steady reduction of the compression forces. Shear forces and translational movements of the knee joint can be minimized by increased compression, which is generated by additional training weight (cf. Escamilla 2001).

Practical Relevance

Squats or working on a leg press in a range of 0–50° flexion is suitable in the course of rehabilitation due to the low structural stress situation. After rehabilitation, the knee joint can be moved in flexion until the thighs are parallel to the ground. Moving further from this position into increased knee flexion is not to be considered an immediate contraindication, but it should be noted here that there is an increased risk of injury to the menisci and the cruciate or collateral ligaments (cf. Escamilla 2001).

1.6.5 Biomechanical Factors of the Intervertebral Discs

An in-vivo study by Wilke et al. (1999) made it possible to measure the pressure conditions of the intervertebral disc between L4 and L5 during various everyday movements. In a selfless and heroic manner, a test subject agreed to have a pressure sensor implanted into the center of the disc between L4 and L5 under radiological control. By securing the pressure sensor located in the disc with a belt around the trunk, the test subject was instructed to perform various everyday movements. Meanwhile, measurements of the intradiscal pressure could be recorded.

The lowest measurements were caused by lying in a supine position. Here, a pressure of 0.1 megapascals (MPa) was measured.

In the initial sitting position, a value of 0.46 MPa was determined for a relaxed sitting posture without contact with the backrest. With active straightening of the trunk in the seat, the value increased to 0.55 MPa. A further increase in pressure values could be generated by maximum trunk flexion while sitting. This increased the intradiscal pressure of the intervertebral disc between L4 and L5 to 0.83 MPa. The lowest value in the initial sitting position of 0.27 MPa could be caused by a curved position while sitting. During the transfer from sitting to standing, a value of 1.10 MPa was measured.

Relaxed standing led to an intradiscal pressure of 0.5 MPa. Through trunk flexion, the pressure in the standing position could be increased to 1.10 MPa. The Valsalva maneuver performed while standing led to a pressure value of 0.92 MPa (see Wilke et al. 1999).

> **Practical Relevance**
> It was shown that the Valsalva maneuver increases intradiscal pressure. In addition, the Valsalva maneuver can increase intra-abdominal pressure (see Hackett and Chow 2013). High loads during strength training cause the Valsalva maneuver to occur reflexively and thus are able to increase trunk stability and prevent spinal injuries. This leads to hemodynamic changes in addition to an increase in trunk stability. This can pose a health risk for people who are susceptible to cardiovascular diseases, cerebrovascular pathologies, or hernias. After medical clarification, these people are recommended a Valsalva maneuver of a maximum of three seconds. Less hemodynamic differences can be observed in experienced strength athletes compared to inexperienced ones. Therefore, a tentative strength training under 80% of the one-repetition-maximum (1RM) is initially recommended. For high-performance strength sports, the Valsalva maneuver is considered relevant and not necessarily negative. Symptoms such as dizziness or fainting can occur with too long or too intense stress.

The pressure conditions during the activity of walking within the disc between L4 and L5 fluctuated between 0.53–0.65 MPa. The values remained identical when wearing tennis shoes compared to walking barefoot.

When jogging with tennis shoes, values between 0.35–0.85 MPa were measured, while wearing harder street shoes produced values between 0.35–0.95 MPa.

Climbing up one step led to values of 0.5–0.7 MPa. However, climbing up two steps at once led to values between 0.3 to 1.20 MPa. Descending one step led to a pressure of 0.38–0.6 MPa. When descending two steps at once, the value varied between 0.30–0.90 MPa.

Lifting a weight of 20 kg with a forward-leaning and flexed trunk led to a pressure of 2.3 MPa. If the flexion was eliminated during lifting, the value decreased to 1.7 MPa. The isometric holding of the 20 kilos close to the trunk evoked a pressure value of 1.1 MPa. When the distance between the 20 kg load and the trunk was increased by 60 cm, there was an increase in intradiscal pressure to 1.80 MPa.

> **Practical Relevance**
> The presented measurements provide biomechanical insights that can be transferred to medical training therapy. However, the mistake of necessarily classifying high pressure values as negative should not be made. For an appropriate metabolism, the disc material depends on a change between compression and relief. With adequate dosage, these are the formative stimuli that encourage the tissue to adapt to future loads. Important factors here are a gradual increase in load and a balance between catabolic and anabolic metabolic phases (see Kirnaz et al. 2022). If the regeneration phase between training units is too short, this, along with too intensively chosen loads, poses a risk factor for structural damage. The goal of medical training therapy is to set a suprathreshold stimulus while avoiding overload or injury.

1.6.6 Avoidance of Locked Joint Positions Under High Weight Load

A locked joint position is characterized by high tension of the capsule-ligament apparatus, little to no joint play, and high intra-articular pressure. It becomes apparent that these factors lead to a high degree of joint stabilization. At the same time, the muscular effort in the locked position is minimal.

If there is a desire within medical training therapy to strengthen muscles by means of training weight, moving into the locked position seems to bring little positive effects. Rather, there is the risk of structural damage, as the risk of injury increases proportionally with the increase in intra-articular pressure. In this regard, the femorotibial articulation and the humeroulnar articulation come to the fore.

The locked position of the femorotibial articulation is the maximum extension (cf. McGinty et al. 2000). When moved into maximum extension, the so-called terminal rotation occurs. If the extension is performed in the open system, there is a slight external rotation movement of the tibia during the last degrees of extension. However, if the knee extension is performed while standing, there is biomechanically a slight internal rotation movement in the hip joint and thus a relative external rotation in the knee joint (cf. Böhni et al. 2012).

Practical Relevance

When doing squats with weight load and when training on the leg press under high weight load, moving into maximum knee extension should be avoided due to the high intra-articular compression with simultaneously low muscular recruitment.

In the maximum extension position in the elbow joint, the humeroulnar articulation experiences the highest compression (cf. Chantelot et al. 2008). EMG measurements during the Pangorilla show the significantly reduced recruitment of the upper arm muscles during elbow extension (cf. Tuttle and Basmajian 1974).

Practical Relevance

When training on the chest press or practicing bench press, end-grade elbow extension under high weight load should be avoided due to the high intra-articular compression.

1.7 The Open and Closed System

Within medical training therapy, both the open and closed system are available for strengthening the skeletal muscles. The following presents both systems as well as their advantages and disadvantages.

1.7.1 The Open System

Training in the open system is characterized by various characteristics. First of all, it should be noted that in the open system, the distal end of the extremity to be trained is not fixed. Examples of training the lower extremity in the open system are the leg extension machine and the leg curl machine. During the execution of the exercise, it becomes clear that the foot is not fixed to the floor or the machine itself.

Furthermore, the open system offers the possibility to address skeletal muscles as isolated as possible in training therapy. Thus, with the leg extension machine, a stimulus can be focused on the quadriceps femoris muscle, while the leg curl machine allows for as isolated training of the hamstring muscles as possible.

Another characteristic of the open system is the focused movement in one joint. Using the example of the leg extension or leg curl machine, it becomes apparent that primarily the femorotibial joint is moved.

1.7.2 The Closed System

Training in the closed system is characterized by various characteristics. First of all, it should be noted that in the closed system, the distal end of the extremity to be trained is fixed. Examples of training the lower extremity in the closed system are the execution of squats or training on the leg press. During the execution of the exercise, it becomes clear that the foot is fixed to the floor or the machine.

Furthermore, the closed system offers the possibility to address skeletal muscles in chains in training therapy. Using the example of squats, the quadriceps femoris muscle, the hamstring muscles, the gluteus maximus muscle, and other skeletal muscles can be addressed simultaneously.

Another characteristic of the closed system is the simultaneous movement in several joints. Using the example of the squat, it becomes apparent that the upper ankle joint, the knee joint, and the hip joint are moved simultaneously.

1.7.3 Comparison between the Open and Closed System

The choice between training in the open or closed system depends on the status of wound healing and the underlying disease. Therefore, a concrete statement or action recommendation can only be made after an individual literature search and the finding and interpretation of research papers. Some elaborations come to the conclusion that there are no differences between the application of exercises from the category of the open or closed system (see Jewiss et al. 2017). Other studies conclude that the combination of training in the open and closed system is superior to the individual application (see Fleming et al. 2005). However, within comparative studies, a superiority of training one system over the other can also be determined (see Bakhtiary et al. 2008).

The references for decision-making, which training to favor from a scientific point of view for different diagnoses or clinical pictures, can be found in Chaps. 5 and 6.

References

Aarsland D, Sardahaee F, Anderssen S, Ballard C, Alzheimer's Society Systematic Review group (May 2010) Is physical activity a potential preventive factor for vascular dementia? A systematic review. Aging Ment Health 14(4):386–395. https://doi.org/10.1080/13607860903586136

AG Wissenschaft (2019) Egofit. https://www.egofit.de/biadata-org/. Accessed 5 Oct 2022

Ayabe S-I, Goto N, Atsumi T, Goto J, Suzuki J (August 2005) Morphometric evaluation of posterior funiculus nerve fibers in relation to aging. Okajimas Folia Anat Jpn 82(2):35–38. https://doi.org/10.2535/ofaj.82.35

Böhni U, von Heymann W, Locher H, Habring M, (22. (April 2012) Biomechanik und Dysfunktion. Man Med 50:102–116. https://doi.org/10.1007/s00337-012-0902-y

Bachl N, Löllgen H, Tschan H, Wackerhage H, Wessner B (2018) Molekulare Sport- und Leistungsphysiologie. Springer, Vienna. https://doi.org/10.1007/978-3-7091-1591-6

Baek M, Menon V, Jessell T, Hantman A, Dasen J (May2019) Molecular Logic of Spinocerebellar Tract Neuron Diversity and Connectivity. Cell Rep 27(9):2620–2635. https://doi.org/10.1016/j.celrep.2019.04.113

Bakhtiary A, Fatemi E (February 2008) Open versus closed kinetic chain exercises for patellar chondromalacia. Br J Sports Med 42(2):99–102. https://doi.org/10.1136/bjsm.2007.038109

Barrett E, Eggleston E, Inyard A, Wang H, Li G, Chai W, Liu Z, (13 March 2009) The vascular actions of insulin control its delivery to muscle and regulate the rate-limiting step in skeletal muscle insulin action. Diabetologia 52:752–764. https://doi.org/doi.org/10.1007/s00125-009-1313-z

Bays H (January 2009) „Sick fat," metabolic disease, and atherosclerosis. Am J Med 122(1 Suppl):26–37. https://doi.org/10.1016/j.amjmed.2008.10.015

Benjamin M, Ralphs J (2000) The cell and developmental biology of tendons and ligaments. Int Rev Cytol 196:85–130. https://doi.org/10.1016/s0074-7696(00)96003-0

Bewick G, Banks R (January 2015) Mechanotransduction in the muscle spindle. Pflugers Arch 467(1):175–190. https://doi.org/10.1007/s00424-014-1536-9

Blundell J, Gibbons C, Caudwell P, Finlayson G, Hopkins M (February 2015) Appetite control and energy balance: impact of exercise. Obes Rev 16(Suppl 1):67–76. https://doi.org/10.1111/obr.12257

Bowsher D (2005) Representation of somatosensory modalities in pathways ascending from the spinal anterolateral funiculus to the thalamus demonstrated by lesions in man. Eur Neurol 54(1):14–22. https://doi.org/10.1159/000086884

Brandes R, Lang F, Schmidt R (2019) Physiologie des Menschen. Springer, Berlin. https://doi.org/10.1007/978-3-662-56468-4

Canals X, Claramunt A, Jou M, Abad M, Muñoz D, Baeza A (3 December 2019) Study of intraarticular pressures in the elbow joints. J Biomech 97:109378. https://doi.org/10.1016/j.jbiomech.2019.109378

Canty E, Kadler K (December 2002) Collagen fibril biosynthesis in tendon: a review and recent insights. Comp Biochem Physiol A Mol Integr Physiol 133(4):979–985. https://doi.org/10.1016/s1095-6433(02)00212-x

Causey L, Cowin S, Weinbaum S (June2012) Quantitative model for predicting lymph formation and muscle compressibility in skeletal muscle during contraction and stretch. Proc Natl Acad Sci U S A 109(23):9185–9190. https://doi.org/10.1073/pnas.1206398109

Chafee M, Heilbronner S (April 2022) Prefrontal cortex. Curr Biol 32(8):R346–R351. https://doi.org/10.1016/j.cub.2022.02.071

Chalmers G, (20 July 2007) Strength training Do Golgi tendon organs really inhibit muscle activity at high force levels to save muscles from injury, and adapt with strength training? Sports Biomechanics 1(2):239–249. https://doi.org/10.1080/14763140208522800

Chantelot C, Wavreille G, Remedios C, Landejerit B, Fontaine C, Hildebrand H (March 2008) Intra-articular compressive stress of the elbow joint in extension: an experimental study using Fuji films. Surg Radiol Anat 30(2):103–111. https://doi.org/10.1007/s00276-007-0297-y

Cheng A, Jude B, Lanner J (August 2020) Intramuscular mechanisms of overtraining. Redox Biol 35:101480. https://doi.org/10.1016/j.redox.2020.101480

Christensen J, Simonsen C, Hojman P (13 December 2018) Exercise Training in Cancer Control and Treatment. Compr Physiol 9(1):165–205. https://doi.org/10.1002/cphy.c180016

Coote J, Perez-Gonzalez J (June 1970) The response of some sympathetic neurones to volleys in various afferent nerves. J Physiol 208(2):261–278. https://doi.org/10.1113/jphysiol.1970.sp009118

Crane J, MacNeil L, Lally J, Ford R, Bujak A, Brar I, Tarnopolsky M (August 2015) Exercise-stimulated interleukin-15 is controlled by AMPK and regulates skin metabolism and aging. Aging Cell 14(4):625–634. https://doi.org/10.1111/acel.12341

Crush E, Frith E, Loprinzi P (15 March 2018) Experimental effects of acute exercise duration and exercise recovery on mood state. J Affect Disord 229:282–287. https://doi.org/10.1016/j.jad.2017.12.092

Dayal A, Medvedeva N, Nekrasova T, Duhalin S, Surin A, Minin A (30 October 2020) Desmin Interacts Directly with Mitochondria. Int J Mol Sci 21(21):8122. https://doi.org/10.3390/ijms21218122

Dietz V, Gollhofer A, Kleiber M, Trippel M (1992) Regulation of bipedal stance: dependency on „load“ receptors. Exp Brain Res 89(1):229–231. https://doi.org/10.1007/BF00229020

Dimitriou M (18 October 2014) Human Muscle Spindle Sensitivity Reflects the Balance of Activity between Antagonistic Muscles. J Neurosci 34(41):13644–13655. https://doi.org/10.1523/JNEUROSCI.2611-14.2014

Ellingsgaard H, Hauselmann I, Schuler B, Habib A, Baggio L, Meier D, Donath M (30. (October 2011) Interleukin-6 enhances insulin secretion by increasing glucagon-like peptide-1 secretion from L cells and alpha cells. Nat Med 17(11):1481–1489. https://doi.org/10.1038/nm.2513

Erickson K, Voss M, Prakash R, Basak C, Szabo A, Chaddock L, Kramer A (15 February 2011) Exercise training increases size of hippocampus and improves memory. Proc Natl Acad Sci U S A 108(7):3017–3022. https://doi.org/10.1073/pnas.1015950108

Escamilla R (January 2001) Knee biomechanics of the dynamic squat exercise. Med Sci Sports Exerc 33(1):127–141. https://doi.org/10.1097/00005768-200101000-00020

Febbraio M, Hiscock N, Sacchetti M, Fischer C, Pedersen B (July 2004) Interleukin-6 is a novel factor mediating glucose homeostasis during skeletal muscle contraction. Diabetes 53(7):1643–1648. https://doi.org/10.2337/diabetes.53.7.1643

Ferrauti A (2020) Trainingswissenschaft für die Sportpraxis. Springer, Berlin. https://doi.org/10.1007/978-3-662-58227-5

Fleming B, Oksendahl H, Beynnon B (July 2005) Open- or closed-kinetic chain exercises after anterior cruciate ligament reconstruction? Exerc Sport Sci Rev 33(3):134–140. https://doi.org/10.1097/00003677-200507000-00006

Fry AC, Smith JC, Schilling BK. Effect of knee position on hip and knee torques during the barbell squat. J Strength Cond Res. 2003 Nov;17(4):629–33. https://doi.org/10.1519/1533-4287(2003)017<0629:eokpoh>2.0.co;2. PMID: 14636100.

Gartlehner G, Wild C, Mad P (February 2008) Systematische Übersichtsarbeiten und Meta-Analysen. Wien Med Wochenschr 158:127–133. https://doi.org/10.1007/s10354-007-0499-2

Giovannucci E (September 2007) Metabolic syndrome, hyperinsulinemia, and colon cancer: a review. Am J Clin Nutr 86(3):836–842. https://doi.org/10.1093/ajcn/86.3.836S

Hötting K, Röder B (November 2013) Beneficial effects of physical exercise on neuroplasticity and cognition. Neurosci Biobehav Rev 37(9 Pt B):2243–57. https://doi.org/10.1016/j.neubiorev.2013.04.005

Hackett D, Chow C-M (August 2013) The valsalva maneuver its effect on intra-abdominal pressure and safety issues during resistance exercise. J Strength Cond Res 27(8):2338–2345. https://doi.org/10.1519/JSC.0b013e31827de07d

Haffner S (September 2007) Abdominal adiposity and cardiometabolic risk: do we have all the answers? Am J Med 120(9 Suppl 1):10–16. https://doi.org/10.1016/j.amjmed.2007.06.006

Heckman C, Enoka R (October 2012) Motor unit. Compr Physiol 4:2629–2682. https://doi.org/10.1002/cphy.c100087

Henderson C, Gomez C, Novak S, Mi-Mi L, Gregorio C, (18. (June 2017) Overview of the muscle cytoskeleton. Compr Physiol 7(3):891–944. https://doi.org/10.1002/cphy.c160033

Hojman P, Gehl J, Christensen J, Pedersen B (9 January 2018) Molecular mechanisms linking exercise to cancer prevention and treatment. Cell Metab 27(1):10–21. https://doi.org/10.1016/j.cmet.2017.09.015

Huggenberger S, Moser N, Schröder H, Cozzi B, Granato A, Merighi A (2019) Neuroanatomie des Menschen. Springer, Berlin

Ishida T, Samukawa M, Endo D, Kasahara S, Tohyama H (September 2022) Effects of changing center of pressure position on knee and ankle extensor moments during double-leg squatting. J Sports Sci Med 21(3):341–346. https://doi.org/10.52082/jssm.2022.341

Jensen K, Graf B (1993) The effects of knee effusion on quadriceps strength and knee intraarticular pressure.

Arthroscopy 9(1):52–56. https://doi.org/10.1016/s0749-8063(05)80343-3

Jewiss D, Ostman C, Smart N (2017) Open versus closed kinetic chain exercises following an anterior cruciate ligament reconstruction: a systematic review and meta-analysis. J Sports Med (Hindawi Publ Corp):1–10. https://doi.org/10.1155/2017/4721548

Jirikowski G (13 January 2016) Faszien und Aponeurosen des Bewegungsapparats. Man Med 54:10–13. https://doi.org/10.1007/s00337-015-0086-3

Kellermayer D, Smith J 3rd, Granzier H (May 2019) Titin mutations and muscle disease. Pflugers Arch 471(5):673–682. https://doi.org/10.1007/s00424-019-02272-5

Kelley G, Kelley K (February 2017) Exercise and sleep: a systematic review of previous meta-analyses. J Evid Based Med 10(1):26–36. https://doi.org/10.1111/jebm.12236

Khan Z, Ahmed S, Baig A., Farooqui W (13. June 2022) Effect of post-isometric relaxation versus myofascial release therapy on pain, functional disability, rom and qol in the management of non-specific neck pain: a randomized controlled trial. BMC Musculoskelet Disord 23(1):567. https://doi.org/10.1186/s12891-022-05516-1

Kirnaz S, Capadona C, Wong T, Goldberg J, Medary B, Sommer F, Härtl R (January 2022) Fundamentals of intervertebral disc degeneration. World Neurosurg 157:264–273. https://doi.org/10.1016/j.wneu.2021.09.066

Kirsch J (2018) Schmerz, lass' nach! Springer, Berlin. https://doi.org/10.1007/978-3-662-55358-9

Kistemaker D, Van Soest A, Wong J, Kurtzer I, Gribble P (February 2013) Control of position and movement is simplified by combined muscle spindle and Golgi tendon organ feedback. J Neurophysiol 109(4):1126–1139. https://doi.org/10.1152/jn.00751.2012

Kröger S, Watkins B (7 January 2021) Muscle spindle function in healthy and diseased muscle. Skelet Muscle 11(1):3. https://doi.org/10.1186/s13395-020-00258-x

Lacour J-R (December 2011) Muscle activity and energy expenditure. Rev Mal Respir 28(10):1278–1292. https://doi.org/10.1016/j.rmr.2011.06.014

Lange S, Pinotsis N, Agarkova I, Ehler E (March 2020) The M-band: the underestimated part of the sarcomere. Biochim Biophys Acta Mol Cell Res 1867(3):118440. https://doi.org/10.1016/j.bbamcr.2019.02.003

Latroche C, Gitiaux C, Chrétien F, Desguerre I, Mounier R, Chazaud B (November 2015) Skeletal muscle microvasculature: a highly dynamic lifeline. Physiology (Bethesda) 30(6):417–427. https://doi.org/10.1152/physiol.00026.2015

Laube W (2020) Sensomotorik und Schmerz: wechselwirkung von Bewegungsreizen und Schmerzempfinden. Springer, Berlin.

Lee J, Jun H-S (30. January 2019) Role of myokines in regulating skeletal muscle mass and function. Front Physiol 10:42. https://doi.org/10.3389/fphys.2019.00042

Lepley A., Ly M, Grooms D, Kinsella-Shaw J, Lepley L (2020) Corticospinal tract structure and excitability in patients with anterior cruciate ligament reconstruction: A DTI and TMS study. Neuroimage Clin 25:102157. https://doi.org/10.1016/j.nicl.2019.102157

Lorenzetti S, Ostermann M, Zeidler F, Zimmer P, Jentsch L, List R, Schellenberg F (17. July 2018) How to squat? Effects of various stance widths, foot placement angles and level of experience on knee, hip and trunk motion and loading. BMC Sports Sci Med Rehabil 10:14. https://doi.org/10.1186/s13102-018-0103-7

Müller-Wohlfahrt H-W, Ueblacker P, Hänsel L (2010) Muskelverletzungen im Sport. Georg Thieme Verlag KG, Stuttgart

Mad P, Felder-Puig R, Gartlehner G (May2008) Randomisiert kontrollierte Studien. Wien Med Wochenschr 158:234–239. https://doi.org/10.1007/s10354-008-0526-y

Mattson M (12. December 2012) Energy intake and exercise as determinants of brain health and vulnerability to injury and disease. Cell Metab 16(6):706–722. https://doi.org/10.1016/j.cmet.2012.08.012

McGinty G, Irrgang J, Pezzullo D (March 2000) Biomechanical considerations for rehabilitation of the knee. Clin Biomech (Bristol, Avon) 15(3):160–166. https://doi.org/10.1016/s0268-0033(99)00061-3

Medler S (29. November 2019) Mixing it up: the biological significance of hybrid skeletal muscle fibers. J Exp Biol, 222(Pt 23):jeb200832. https://doi.org/10.1242/jeb.200832

Mileusnic M, Loeb G (June 2009) Force estimation from ensembles of Golgi tendon organs. J Neural Eng 6(3):036001. https://doi.org/10.1088/1741-2560/6/3/036001

Murad M, Asi N, Alsawas M, Alahdab F (August 2016) New evidence pyramid. Evid Based Med 21(4):125–127. https://doi.org/10.1136/ebmed-2016-110401

Murrant C, Fletcher N, Fitzpatrick E, Gee K (May2021) Do skeletal muscle motor units and microvascular units align to help match blood flow to metabolic demand? Eur J Appl Physiol 121(5):1241–1254. https://doi.org/10.1007/s00421-021-04598-4

Nishimune H, Shigemoto K (May2018) Practical Anatomy of the Neuromuscular Junction in Health and Disease. Neurol Clin 36(2):231–240. https://doi.org/10.1016/j.ncl.2018.01.009

Nordby P, Auerbach P, Rosenkilde M, Kristiansen L, Thomasen J, Rygaard L, Stallknecht B (November 2012) Endurance training per se increases metabolic health in young, moderately overweight men. Obesity (Silver Spring) 20(11):2202–2212. https://doi.org/10.1038/oby.2012.70

O'Brien M (July 1992) Functional anatomy and physiology of tendons. Clin Sports Med 11(3):505–520

O'Brien M (April 1997) Structure and metabolism of tendons. Scand J Med Sci Sports 7(2):55–61. https://doi.org/10.1111/j.1600-0838.1997.tb00119.x

O'Brien M (June 2005) The anatomy of the achilles tendon. Foot Ankle Clin 10(2):225–238. https://doi.org/10.1016/j.fcl.2005.01.011

Ojima K (July 2019) Myosin: formation and maintenance of thick filaments. Anim Sci J 90(7):801–807. https://doi.org/10.1111/asj.13226

Ouchi N, Oshima Y, Ohashi K, Higuchi A, Ikegami C, Izumiya Y, Walsh K, (21. (November 2008) Follistatin-like 1, a secreted muscle protein, promotes endothelial cell function and revascularization in ischemic tissue through a nitric-oxide synthase-dependent mechanism. J Biol Chem 283(47):32802–32811. https://doi.org/10.1074/jbc.M803440200

Ovalie W (1987) The human muscle-tendon junction. Anat Embryol 176:281–294. https://doi.org/10.1007/BF00310184

Pedersen B, (10. February 2019) The physiology of optimizing health with a focus on exercise as medicine. Annu Rev Physiol 81:607–627. https://doi.org/10.1146/annurev-physiol-020518-114339

Pedersen B, Hoffman-Goetz L (July 2000) Exercise and the immune system: regulation, integration, and adaptation. Physiol Rev 80(3):1055–1081. https://doi.org/10.1152/physrev.2000.80.3.1055

Pedersen B, Saltin B (December 2015) Exercise as medicine—evidence for prescribing exercise as therapy in 26 different chronic diseases. Scand J Med Sci Sports 25(Suppl 3):1–72. https://doi.org/10.1111/sms.12581

Perl E (July 1994) The 1944 nobel prize to erlanger and gasser. FASEB J 8(10):782–783. https://doi.org/10.1096/fasebj.8.10.8050679

Perrini S, Laviola L, Carreira M, Cignarelli A, Natalicchio A, Giorgino F (June 2010) The GH/IGF1 axis and signaling pathways in the muscle and bone: mechanisms underlying age-related skeletal muscle wasting and osteoporosis. J Endocrinol 205(3):201–210. https://doi.org/10.1677/JOE-09-0431

Petersen W, Bobka T, Stein V, Tillmann B (April 2000) Blood supply of the peroneal tendons: injection and immunohistochemical studies of cadaver tendons. Acta Orthop Scand 71(2):168–174. https://doi.org/10.1080/000164700317413148

Peterson, M., Butler , S., Eriksson, M., & Svärdsudd, K. (September 2014) A randomized controlled trial of eccentric vs. concentric graded exercise in chronic tennis elbow (lateral elbow tendinopathy). Clin Rehabil 28(9):862–872. https://doi.org/10.1177/0269215514527595

Pette D, Staron R, (15. September 2000) Myosin isoforms, muscle fiber types, and transitions. Microsc Res Tech 50(6):500–509. https://doi.org/10.1002/1097-0029(20000915)50:6<500::AID-JEMT7>3.0.CO;2-7

Prabhat S (20. February 2011) differencebetween.net. http://www.differencebetween.net/science/health/difference-between-cardiac-and-skeletal-muscle/. Accessed 5 Oct 2022

Qaisar R, Bhaskaran S, Remmen H (September 2016) Muscle fiber type diversification during exercise and regeneration. Free Radic Biol Med 98:56–67. https://doi.org/10.1016/j.freeradbiomed.2016.03.025

Rassier D (August 2017) Sarcomere mechanics in striated muscles: from molecules to sarcomeres to cells. Am J Physiol Cell Physiol 313(2):134–145. https://doi.org/10.1152/ajpcell.00050.2017

Rio E, Kidgell D, Purdam C, Gaida J, Moseley G, Pearce A, Cook J (October 2015) Isometric exercise induces analgesia and reduces inhibition in patellar tendinopathy. Br J Sports Med 49(19):1277–1283. https://doi.org/10.1136/bjsports-2014-094386

Rio E, van Ark M, Docking S, Moseley G, Kidgell D, Gaida J, Cook J (May2017) Isometric Contractions Are More Analgesic Than Isotonic Contractions for Patellar Tendon Pain: An In-Season Randomized Clinical Trial. Clin J Sport Med 27(3):253–259. https://doi.org/10.1097/JSM.0000000000000364

Rohel A, Bouffard J, Patricio P, Mavromatis N, Billot M, Roy J-S, Masse-Alarie H (July2021) The effect of experimental pain on the excitability of the corticospinal tract in humans: A systematic review and meta-analysis. Eur J Pain 25(6):1209–1226. https://doi.org/10.1002/ejp.1746

Roig M, O'Brien K, Kirk G, Murray R, McKinnon P, Shadgan B, Reid W (August 2009) The effects of eccentric versus concentric resistance training on muscle strength and mass in healthy adults: a systematic review with meta-analysis. Br J Sports Med 43(8):556–568. https://doi.org/10.1136/bjsm.2008.051417

Rosenthal R, DiMatteo M (February 2001) Meta-Analysis: recent developments in quantitative methods for literature reviews. Annu Rev Psychol 52(59–82):59–82. https://doi.org/10.1146/annurev.psych.52.1.59

Rubini E, Costa A, Gomes P (2007) The effects of stretching on strength performance. Sports Med 37(3):213–224. https://doi.org/10.2165/00007256-200737030-00003

Schindler R, Mancilla J, Endres S, Ghorbani R, Clark S, Dinarello C (1. (January 1990) Correlations and interactions in the production of interleukin-6 (IL-6), IL-1, and tumor necrosis factor (TNF) in human blood mononuclear cells: IL-6 suppresses IL-1 and TNF. Blood 75(1):40–47

Schleip R (April 2003a) Fascial plasticity—a new neurobiological explanation Part 2. J Bodyw Mov Ther 7(2):104–116. https://doi.org/10.1016/S1360-8592(02)00076-1

Schleip R (2003b) Fascial plasticity—a new neurobiological explanation: part 1. J Bodyw Mov Ther 7(1):11–19. https://doi.org/10.1016/S1360-8592(02)00067-0

Schmidt R, Lang F, Thews G (2005) Physiologie des Menschen. Springer, Berlin. https://doi.org/10.1007/b137547

Schoenfeld B, Ogborn D, Vigotsky A, Franchi M, Krieger J (September 2017) Hypertrophic effects of concentric vs. eccentric muscle actions: a systematic review and meta-analysis. J Strength Cond Res 31(9):2599–2608. https://doi.org/10.1519/JSC.0000000000001983

Severinsen M, Pedersen B (August 2020) Muscle-organ crosstalk: the emerging roles of myokines. Endocr Rev 41(4):594–609. https://doi.org/10.1210/endrev/bnaa016

Silver F, Freeman J, Seehra G (October 2003) Collagen self-assembly and the development of tendon mechanical properties. J Biomech 36(10):1529–1553. https://doi.org/10.1016/s0021-9290(03)00135-0

Stasinopoulos D, Stasinopoulos I (January-March 2017) Comparison of effects of eccentric training, eccentric-concentric training, and eccentric-concentric training combined with isometric contraction in the treatment of lateral elbow tendinopathy. J Hand Ther 30(1):13–19. https://doi.org/10.1016/j.jht.2016.09.001

Steensberg A, Fischer C, Keller C, Møller K, Pedersen B (August 2003) IL-6 enhances plasma IL-1ra, IL-10, and cortisol in humans. Am J Physiol Endocrinol Metab 285(2):E433–E437. https://doi.org/10.1152/ajpendo.00074.2003

Talbot J, Maves L (July2016) Skeletal muscle fiber type: using insights from muscle developmental biology to dissect targets for susceptibility and resistance to muscle disease. Wiley Interdiscip Rev Dev Biol 5(4):518–534. https://doi.org/10.1002/wdev.230

Teissier V, Leclercq R, Schiano-Lomoriello S, Nizard R, Portier H (June 2020) Does eccentric-concentric resistance training improve early functional outcomes compared to concentric resistance training after total knee arthroplasty? Gait Posture 79:145–151. https://doi.org/10.1016/j.gaitpost.2020.04.020

Tuttle R, Basmajian J (July 1974) Electromyography of brachial muscles in Pan gorilla and hominoid evolution. Am J Phys Anthropol 41(1):71–90. https://doi.org/10.1002/ajpa.1330410110

Vaegter H, Jones M (23 September 2020) Exercise-induced hypoalgesia after acute and regular exercise: experimental and clinical manifestations and possible mechanisms in individuals with and without pain. Pain Rep 5(5):e823. https://doi.org/10.1097/PR9.0000000000000823

van Ark M, Cook J, Docking S, Zwerver J, Gaida J, van den Akker-Scheek I, Rio E (September 2016) Do isometric and isotonic exercise programs reduce pain in athletes with patellar tendinopathy in-season? A randomised clinical trial. J Sci Med Sport 19(9):702–706. https://doi.org/10.1016/j.jsams.2015.11.006

Vang C, Niznik A (October 2020) The Effectiveness of Isometric Contractions Compared With Isotonic Contractions in Reducing Pain For In-Season Athletes With Patellar Tendinopathy. J Sport Rehabil 30(3):512–515. https://doi.org/10.1123/jsr.2019-0376

Verma S, Khurana S, Vats A, Sahu B, Ganguly N, Chakraborti P, Taneja V (8. (January 2022) Neuromuscular Junction Dysfunction in Amyotrophic Lateral Sclerosis. Mol Neurobiol 59:1502–1527. https://doi.org/10.1007/s12035-021-02658-6

Walters B, Read C, Estes A (September 2018) The effects of resistance training, overtraining, and early specialization on youth athlete injury and development. J Sports Med Phys Fitness 58(9):1339–1348. https://doi.org/10.23736/S0022-4707.17.07409-6

Warneke K, Brinkmann A, Hillebrecht M, Schiemann S (25. May 2022) Influence of long-lasting static stretching on maximal strength, muscle thickness and flexibility. Front Physiol, 13:878955. https://doi.org/10.3389/fphys.2022.878955

Whitmer R, Gustafson D, Barrett-Connor E, Haan M, Gunderson E, Yaffe K (30. September 2008) Central obesity and increased risk of dementia more than three decades later. Neurology 71(14):1057–1064. https://doi.org/10.1212/01.wnl.0000306313.89165.ef

Wilke H, Neef P, Caimi M, Hoogland T, Claes L (April 1999) New in vivo measurements of pressures in the intervertebral disc in daily life. Spine (Phila Pa 1976), 24(8):755-62. https://doi.org/10.1097/00007632-199904150-00005

Wilson J, Hornbuckle L, Kim J-S, Ugrinowitsch C, Lee S-R, Zourdos M, Panton L (September 2010) Effects of static stretching on energy cost and running endurance performance. J Strength Cond Res 24(9):2274–2279. https://doi.org/10.1519/JSC.0b013e3181b22ad6

Xue F, Michels K (September 2007) Diabetes, metabolic syndrome, and breast cancer: a review of the current evidence. Am J Clin Nutr 86(3):823–835. https://doi.org/10.1093/ajcn/86.3.823S

Yin L, Li N, Jia W, Wang N, Liang M, Yang X, Du G (October 2021) Skeletal muscle atrophy: from mechanisms to treatments. Pharmacol Res 172:105807. https://doi.org/10.1016/j.phrs.2021.105807

Zeng X, Zhang Y, Kwong J, Zhang C, Li S, Sun F, Du L (February 2015) The methodological quality assessment tools for preclinical and clinical studies, systematic review and meta-analysis, and clinical practice guideline: a systematic review. J Evid Based Med 8(1):2–10. https://doi.org/10.1111/jebm.12141

Zilles K, Tillmann B (2010) Anatomie. Springer, Berlin. https://doi.org/10.1007/978-3-540-69483-0

Zimmer P, Appell H-J (2021) Funktionelle Anatomie. Springer, Berlin

Zschäbitz A (2005) Anatomie und Verhalten von Sehnen und Bändern. Orthopade 34:516–525. https://doi.org/10.1007/s00132-005-0799-4

Subareas of Medical Exercise Therapy

2

Contents

Trailer

Discover the diversity and depth of medical training therapy in this enlightening second chapter, which illuminates the core elements of physical fitness. From muscle endurance to peak strength, this chapter covers the entire spectrum and provides profound knowledge based on the latest research findings.

Begin your journey with an insight into strength endurance training, where you will learn about the crucial parameters and the impressive benefits of this form of training.

S. Wolfram and R. Bauer, *Evidence-Based Medical Exercise Therapy*,
https://doi.org/10.1007/978-3-662-70774-6_2

Dive into current research results that expand the understanding and applications of strength endurance training.

Next, we move on to maximal strength—the zenith of physical strength. Learn how you can safely extend your strength limits and what scientific findings underpin the effectiveness of maximal strength training.

The chapter then introduces you to the world of power, a crucial component for explosive movements. Understand the basics of power training and how current studies illuminate the methods and results of this training area.

Learn more about reactive power, an often overlooked but essential ability for dynamic and reactive movements. Penetrate the definitions, parameters, and the latest research findings that highlight the importance of reactive power training.

Endurance training is presented in all its breadth, from the basics to specific training methods and load zones. A particular focus is on the latest scientific findings that show how endurance affects health and performance.

Proprioceptive training, a key element for improving body perception and injury prevention, is explained in detail. Discover the principles and benefits of this form of training and how research shapes practice.

Finally, the chapter sheds light on flexibility training, a fundamental aspect for the overall functionality of the body. Learn more about the causes of limited joint mobility and innovative methods for their improvement, such as stretching and the use of the fascia roller.

This chapter is a must for anyone who wants to gain a deep and broad understanding of the various aspects of medical training therapy. With profound knowledge and the latest insights from research, it offers an invaluable resource for practitioners, students, and enthusiasts alike. Get ready to deepen your knowledge and revolutionize your training approaches.

This chapter first introduces the different types of strength. Depending on the type of strength, different physiological reactions of the human body occur. These are presented for each type of strength and serve as an important theoretical foundation for the selection of the required training method. Subsequently, repetition and set numbers as well as break times, load intensities, and contraction speeds are discussed for each type of strength. Other components include endurance training, proprioceptive training, and flexibility training.

2.1 Strength Endurance

2.1.1 Definition and Parameters of Endurance Strength Training

There are diverging definitions for the term endurance strength. The definition established by Schmidtbleicher (1989) includes both qualitative and quantitative information (cf. Fröhlich et al. 2001). Literally, Schmidtbleicher describes endurance strength as "… the abilities of the neuromuscular system to produce as large a pulse sum as possible in a defined period (at most 2 min at maximum load) against higher loads (more than 30% of maximum strength) and to keep the reduction of the produced pulses as low as possible during the load" (Schmidtbleicher 1989, p. 13). The type of strength in endurance strength can be divided into two components. On the one hand, there is the intensity of the individual force impulse. On the other hand, the ability to keep the reduction of the force impulse sum as low as possible or to increase fatigue resistance (cf. Güllich and Schmidtbleicher 1999). The components that significantly determine the intensity of the individual force impulse are the deployable maximum or explosive strength. In addition to high neuronal fatigue resistance, a pronounced buffering capacity with regard to lactate concentration also contributes to the slow reduction of the force impulse sum (cf. Bigland-Ritchie 1981; cf. Hultman et al. 1981). Sports that require endurance strength performance include swimming, wrestling, and canoe racing (cf. Schnabel et al. 1997).

Ehlenz et al. (1998) distinguish between three forms of endurance strength training in terms of stimulus intensity. They refer to endurance strength training with a stimulus intensity of over 75% of maximum strength as maximum strength endurance. Submaximal strength endurance is characterized between 75% and 50% of maximum strength. If the training is carried out with a stimulus intensity between 50% and 30% of maximum strength, it can also be referred to as aerobic strength endurance training (cf. Ehlenz et al. 1998). The number of repetitions is given by Güllich and Schmidtbleicher (1999) with a range between 20 and 40 at a slow to brisk execution speed. If a consistent number of repetitions is prescribed from series to series in endurance strength training, it is necessary to reduce the training weight over time (cf. Fröhlich et al. 2001). Between the 6–8 series, break times between 30 s and one minute should be observed (cf. Güllich and Schmidtbleicher 1999). The recovery time can be stated with a duration of 24–48 h. This results in 2–3 therapy units per week (cf. Haas and Fox 2005). Figure 2.1 provides an overview of the described parameters of endurance strength training.

2.1.2 Research Findings on Endurance Strength Training

A publication from 2004 by Fröhlich et al. deals with the metabolic and cardiovascular reactions caused by endurance strength training. With the sport as a basis, wrestlers, athletes, and recreational athletes were divided into three different groups. The endurance strength training was carried out in 6 series with a repetition number of 20 on a multipress in the sense of bench pressing. An outcome measurement was the physical work. This is calculated from the product of performed repetitions, the mastered load, and the stroke height. At this point, it should be noted that the performance of physical work across groups only significantly reduced from the first to the second series. In terms of the performance of physical work, sets 3–6 did not differ from each other (cf. Fröhlich et al. 2004).

▶ **Practical Relevance**
If a fixed number of repetitions is prescribed during endurance training, focus should be placed on an adequate adjustment of the training weight between the first and second series.

The lactate production significantly increased during series 1–3 in all three groups. Between the 4th (6.4 ± 1.0 mmol l·1–^{1}) and the 5th (6.7

Stimulus intensity (cf. Ehlenz et al., 1998)	> 75% = maximum strength endurance 75%-50% = submaximal strength endurance 50%-30% = aerobic strength endurance
Number of repetitions (cf. Güllich & Schmidtbleicher, 1999)	20-40
Series (cf. Güllich & Schmidtbleicher, 1999)	6-8
Break time (cf. Güllich & Schmidtbleicher, 1999)	30 seconds – 1 minute
Speed of implementation (cf. Güllich & Schmidtbleicher, 1999)	Slow to fast
Regeneration time (cf. Haas & Fox, 2005)	24-48 hours
Therapy units per week (cf. Haas & Fox, 2005)	2-3

Fig. 2.1 Overview of the parameters of endurance strength training. (Own illustration 2023)

± 1.0 mmol l·l^{-1}) series, no significant difference was observed. Similarly, no difference was found between the 5th and 6th (6.7 ± 1.0 mmol l·l−^{1}) series (see Fröhlich et al. 2004).

The heart rate during the 6 series was approximately 144 beats per minute. In a similar study, which also examined strength endurance training using the bench press exercise, an average heart rate of 121 ± 20 beats per minute was observed at 15 ± 3 repetitions (see Buskies 1999). The systolic blood pressure, except for an increase from the first (124.6 ± 14.5) to the fourth series (133.9 ± 17.1), with a p-value less than 0.05, showed no significant changes between the series. The myocardial oxygen demand increased across groups between the individual series (see Fröhlich et al. 2004).

Practical Relevance

For both recreational and competitive athletes, strength endurance training seems to have no negative health consequences. Even in normotensive heart patients, under appropriate supervision, strength endurance training can positively contribute to the rehabilitation process (see Urhausen et al. 2000). The increase in blood pressure during training is the most important measure for estimating potential risk. In practice, an acceptable increase in blood pressure was observed during strength endurance training with 40–60% of maximum strength at 15–20 repetitions. This is comparable to the blood pressure increase during aerobic endurance training (see Bjarnason-Wehrens et al. 2004).

A comparative study by Hillebrecht et al. (2012) examined the effect of hypertrophy training and strength endurance training in individuals diagnosed with type 2 diabetes mellitus. After a six-month training period, a significant antidiabetic effect was demonstrated with both training methods. In a follow-up measurement after another six months, the antidiabetic effect of strength endurance training was highly significant (p>0.003) superior to hypertrophy training (see Hillebrecht et al. 2012). Accordingly, positive effects on the metabolic syndrome through strength endurance training were demonstrated. Specifically, an improvement in glucose metabolism and a significant improvement in performance were demonstrated through a ten-week strength endurance intervention (see Lehmann et al. 2011).

If women over the age of 65 perform strength endurance training 2 to 3 times a week at an intensity of 40% of maximum strength, this has positive consequences for the immune system after a six-week period. Specifically, a training-induced inhibitory effect on the senescence of T cells was observed (see Dinh et al. 2019).

Thiele et al. (2020) examined the effect of strength endurance training in rowing athletes. Over a period of nine weeks, a strength endurance training that covered the entire body was conducted. Through 4 series, 30 repetitions, and an intensity of 50–60% of maximum strength, a significant improvement in sport-specific performance was achieved (see Thiele et al. 2020). This is due to an improved blood circulation situation and an associated improved metabolism as well as hypertrophy of the ST muscle fibers. For the optimal exploitation of hypertrophy effects, an intensity of strength endurance training of 65–80% is recommended (see Haas and Fox 2005).

In summary, it can be stated that strength endurance training has an interaction with other types of strength. Furthermore, trainees can benefit from antidiabetic and myokine-induced effects in terms of metabolism. This form of training is also recommended to increase specific strength endurance performance in activity or sport. Under appropriate conditions, heart patients can also have an indication for strength endurance training. The deliberately induced structural damage to the muscles, which is caused by maximum strength training, seems to be more of an inevitable consequence of training than a stimulus for hypertrophy (see Gonzalez 2016).

2.2 Maximum Strength

2.2.1 Definition and Parameters of Maximum Strength Training

Maximum strength can be understood as the ability of the neuromuscular system to exert maximum force against an external resistance (cf. Hollmann and Hettinger, 2000). This results in a maximum contraction of the activated skeletal muscles (cf. Thompson et al. 2019). Within maximum strength training, a distinction can be made between targeted training of intramuscular coordination and hypertrophy training.

The training of intramuscular coordination aims to increase the number of simultaneously activated motor units within a muscle during force exertion. This goal is achieved by improving the neuronal control of the muscle to be trained (cf. Holzgreve et al. 2022).

In hypertrophy training, on the other hand, the focus is on the increase in volume and the increase in the number of myofibrils of the skeletal muscle. These adaptation mechanisms are largely achieved by the incorporation of sarcomere proteins such as myosin, actin, and titin filaments (cf. Raeder et al. 2020).

The parameters of intramuscular coordination training and hypertrophy training differ in some respects. Hypertrophy training can be performed with a load intensity between 60–90% of dynamic maximum strength (cf. Fry 2004). The number of repetitions is given as 6–15 repetitions (cf. Schoenfeld 2020). It should be noted that due to the fatigue situation after the last repetition, no further repetition should be possible. Schoenfeld (2020) recommends a series number of 3–6. Regarding the rest periods between the series, different time periods can be found depending on the publication. While Fröhlich (2011) defines a rest period of 1.5–2 min, Raeder et al. (2020) specify a time span of 2–5 min. It can be added to this topic that the innervation ability of the muscle to be trained improves with increasing rest time (cf. Wirth and Schmidtbleicher 2002). Shorter rest periods focus on the targeted fatigue of the skeletal muscle. Longer rest periods, on the other hand, focus on maximum force development during exercise execution.

A regeneration time of 48 to 72 hours between the stimuli results in 2–3 weekly therapy units (cf. Haas and Fox 2005). Figure 2.2 provides an overview of the described parameters of hypertrophy training.

The parameters of intramuscular coordination training differ in part from those of hypertrophy training. Thus, Haas and Fox (2005) advocate a training intensity of 90–100% of the One-Repetition Maximum. This results in repetition numbers of 1–3 per series. The execution speed should be as explosive as possible. Rest periods of 6–10 min should be observed between the 3–5 series. Once a training session regarding intramuscular coordination has been completed, a rest period of approx. 72 hours is recommended. This results in 2 to a maximum of 3 training sessions per week (cf. Haas and Fox 2005). It should be added that the regeneration

Stimulus intensity (cf. Fry, 2004)	60-90%
Number of repetitions (see Schoenfeld, 2020)	6-15
Series (see Schoenfeld, 2020)	3-6
Break time (see Fröhlich, 2011 / Raeder et al., 2020)	1.5-2 minutes / 2-5 minutes
Speed of implementation (see Ferrauti & Remmert, 2020)	Slow to fast
Regeneration time (cf. Haas & Fox, 2005)	48-72 hours
Therapy units per week (cf. Haas & Fox, 2005)	2-3

Fig. 2.2 Overview of the parameters of hypertrophy training. (Own illustration 2023)

Stimulus intensity (cf. Haas & Fox, 2005)	90-100%
Number of repetitions (cf. Haas & Fox, 2005)	1-3
Series (cf. Haas & Fox, 2005)	3-5
Break time (cf. Haas & Fox, 2005)	6-10 minutes
Speed of implementation (cf. Haas & Fox, 2005)	as explosive as possible
Regeneration time (cf. Haas & Fox, 2005)	72 hours
Therapy units per week (cf. Haas & Fox, 2005)	2-3

Fig. 2.3 Overview of the parameters of intramuscular coordination training. (Own illustration 2023)

time only refers to the trained muscle groups. If the general condition allows, another muscle group can be trained during the regeneration time of one muscle group. This principle is transferable to all types of strength. Figure 2.3 provides an overview of the parameters of intramuscular coordination training.

2.2.2 Research Findings on Maximum Strength Training

In the study by Staniszewski et al. (2020), the approach of hypertrophy training was compared with the approach of intramuscular coordination training. Specifically, the biceps brachii muscle was trained. After an eight-week training period, an increase in the one-repetition maximum of over 20% could be determined for both forms of training. No significant differences could be calculated in a group comparison in this regard. While the upper arm circumference significantly increased after the eight-week training period in the hypertrophy group, no significant increase in circumference could be detected in the group practicing intramuscular coordination training. In the participants of the intramuscular training group, a more significant reduction in skinfold thickness over the biceps brachii and triceps brachii muscles could be measured compared to the hypertrophy group.

The scientists around Nicholson et al. (2016) examined the differences between intramuscular coordination training and hypertrophy training using the barbell squat with additional weight. In addition to increased time under tension and impulse generation, the one-repetition maximum could be significantly improved through intramuscular coordination training compared to hypertrophy training.

Compared to intramuscular coordination training, hypertrophy training leads to a significantly higher release of anabolic hormones (see Crewther et al. 2008). These include growth hormones (see Smilios et al. 2003), testosterone (see McCaulley et al. 2009), and the anti-inflammatory cortisol (see Uchida et al. 2009). This temporary increased release of the listed hormones leads to positive effects on the overall organism, but does not seem to stimulate muscular protein synthesis (see Gonzalez et al. 2016). The hypoxia generated within the muscles during training is the result of a severely restricted arterial blood supply. This lasts significantly longer in hypertrophy training than in intramuscular coordination training. Therefore, the hypothesis of metabolic stress, generated by prolonged hypoxia and higher lactate levels compared to intramuscular coordination, as a driver of muscular hypertrophy seems justified. Further research is needed to identify the exact mechanisms (see Schoenfeld 2013).

2.3 Power

2.3.1 Definition and Parameters of Power Training

Power is defined as the ability of the neuromuscular system to perform a high force impulse within the shortest possible time span (cf. Güllich and Schmidtbleicher 1999). Within power development, a distinction can be made between starting strength and explosive strength. Starting strength focuses on the highest possible increase in force at the beginning of a movement (cf. Werchoshanskij 1972). Regarding the defined duration of starting strength after the onset of contraction, divergent time specifications can be found in the literature. Bührle et al. (1983) define the value of starting strength as the force development that was unfolded 30 ms after the onset of contraction. Müller (1987), on the other hand, considers the force value that can be measured 50 ms after the onset of contraction as starting strength. Explosive strength is understood as the greatest increase in the force-time curve following the starting strength (Bührle et al. 1983).

If a skeletal muscle can rely on many fast-contracting muscle fibers, it is capable of realizing a more intense power development than a muscle that has relatively more slow-contracting muscle fibers.

For optimal power development, as many motor units as possible should be recruited simultaneously by the central nervous system. In this context, the motor neurons, which can generate action potentials at different frequencies, play a crucial role. Small motor units, which contain ST fibers, are driven at an action potential frequency of up to 20 Hz. The innervation of larger motor units, which contain FT fibers, on the other hand, occurs at a frequency of up to 50 Hz (cf. Haas and Fox 2005).

The intensity of power training should be set high at 90–100 %. The number of repetitions ranges between 1–3. The number of series is given as 3–5. A rest period of 6–10 min is recommended between individual sets. The execution speed during the exercise should be explosive. From an approximate recovery time of 72 h between individual training sessions, 2–3 training sessions per week result. Figure 2.4 provides an overview of the described parameters of power training.

2.3.2 Research Findings on Power Training

In a randomized controlled study, Hendrey et al. (2018) compared power training in a six-week intervention period with a conventional exercise program in patients with subacute stroke. The power training of the lower extremity significantly improved comfortable walking speed, maximum jump height, and fastest walking speed.

A meta-analysis by Tschopp and Sattelmayer (2011) examined the effectiveness of power training compared to conventional strength training. It became clear that power training of the lower extremity with an intensity of approx. 20% benefits older people in terms of improving mobility and balance.

Stengel et al. (2005) were able to demonstrate in women in the postmenopausal stage that power training is superior to conventional strength training in terms of the change in training-induced bone mineral density in the area

Stimulus intensity (cf. Haas & Fox, 2005)	90-100%
Number of repetitions (cf. Haas & Fox, 2005)	1-3
Series (cf. Haas & Fox, 2005)	3-5
Break time (cf. Haas & Fox, 2005)	6-10 minutes
Speed of implementation (cf. Haas & Fox, 2005)	explosive
Regeneration time (cf. Haas & Fox, 2005)	72 hours
Therapy units per week (cf. Haas & Fox, 2005)	2-3

Fig. 2.4 Overview of the parameters of power training. (Own illustration 2023)

of the lumbar spine and the proximal femur. During the examination period, no increase in pain could be detected due to the influence of power training.

2.4 Reactive Strength

2.4.1 Definition and Parameters of Reactive Strength

Reactive strength is understood as a force impulse, which is generated within a rapid cycle of stretching and shortening (cf. Bührle 1989). The stretch-shortening cycle describes a combination of eccentric muscle activity followed shortly by concentric muscle activity. When an activated muscle is stretched or a muscle is passively stretched, the myofascial system is capable of storing a certain amount of energy. This energy is released in the subsequent concentric activation of the skeletal muscle, thus providing a performance-enhancing contribution to muscle work. An example of a stretch-shortening cycle is a jump from a standing position into a bilateral squat and back again. When jumping into the squat, the activated skeletal muscles perform eccentric work and additionally store energy. If the muscles are activated concentrically towards knee extension shortly afterwards, the stored energy can be released and support the concentric force development.

Targeted reactive strength training leads to a reduction in inhibition while simultaneously promoting the reflexes of the trained skeletal muscles. In addition, the functionality of the connective tissue is optimized so that forces can be better stored during the eccentric phase and subsequently released. On the side of neural adaptation, as with speed strength training, the recruitment of motor units, the frequency of motor neurons, and the synchronization of motor units are improved (cf. Haas and Fox 2005).

The intensity of reactive strength training should be adapted to the performance capacity of the person to be trained. The range of repetitions is to be given as 10–12. Rest periods of 6–10 minutes are recommended between the 3–5 sets. The characteristic of the execution is described as explosive. A recovery phase of approximately 72 hours should follow the training session. This results in 2–3 feasible training sessions per week. Figure 2.5 provides an overview of the described parameters of reactive strength training.

2.4.2 Research Findings on Reactive Strength Training

Büsch et al. (2015) investigated the influence of reactive strength training of the lower extremity in young elite athletes in the field of handball aged between 16–18 years. A training execution on a stable surface was compared to the realization of the exercises on an unstable surface. Despite 100–150 jumps per training session during the intervention period, no training-related injuries occurred. Both groups were able to achieve significant improvements in jump height and speed in sprints. The unstable surface did not lead to any additional positive

Stimulus intensity (cf. Haas & Fox, 2005)	adapted
Number of repetitions (cf. Haas & Fox, 2005)	10-12
Series (cf. Haas & Fox, 2005)	3-5
Break time (cf. Haas & Fox, 2005)	6-10 minutes
Speed of implementation (cf. Haas & Fox, 2005)	as explosive as possible
Regeneration time (cf. Haas & Fox, 2005)	72 hours
Therapy units per week (cf. Haas & Fox, 2005)	2-3

Fig. 2.5 Overview of the parameters of reactive strength training. (Own illustration 2023)

results, which is why training on a stable surface is recommended.

This confirmed the results of Matavulj et al. (2001). They researched the influence of plyometric training of the lower extremity in young basketball players. In this work too, the vertical jump height improved significantly through reactive strength training. In addition, it was found in this work that the effects between a jump height of 50 cm and 100 cm do not differ.

A meta-analysis from 2016 examined the effect of different jump executions in relation to a change in the skill of changing direction during locomotion. A significant improvement was researched after a seven-week training period with two weekly units. In this regard, a moderate intensity with 100 jumps per training session is propagated. Correct exercise execution, the variation of different jump executions, and a good fitness level are factors that can increase the effectiveness of plyometric training (cf. Asadi et al. 2016).

In a review by Grgic et al. (2021), the question is pursued whether there are differences between conventional strength training and plyometric training in terms of muscular hypertrophy. In summary, it can be stated that similar and significant effects can be induced in both methods in terms of muscle hypertrophy in a training period of less than 12 weeks. This statement refers to the skeletal muscles of the lower extremity in untrained people and recreational athletes.

2.5 Endurance

2.5.1 Definition of Endurance Training

Endurance ability is defined as the function of myocytes to resynthesize ATP to an appropriate extent during active muscle contraction (see Haber and Tomasits 2006). When examining endurance training more closely, it can be further specified by the information of the percentage measure of the muscle mass used, the energy supply, and the working method of the muscles. If during endurance performance about 15% of the total skeletal muscle mass is used, it can be referred to as local endurance training. On the other hand, if more than about 15% of the skeletal muscle is integrated into the endurance training through activation, it can be referred to as general endurance training. Regarding the training adaptation processes, local endurance training leads to a focused adaptation of the working muscles used. Thus, the skeletal muscle is locally able to adapt the myoglobin content and the capillarization of the working muscles to enhance performance. In addition, training-induced increases in glycogen and creatine phosphate stores as well as the enzyme set can be induced (see Ferrauti 2020). While local endurance only slightly influences the heart rate in terms of an increase, more significant increases can be found in general endurance stress.

Practical Relevance

The knowledge about the different reactions of the cardiopulmonary system to local and general endurance stress can be used in terms of load control. Local endurance training puts less strain on the cardiopulmonary system. General endurance training, on the other hand, is capable of initiating both a local performance increase of the working muscles and adaptation mechanisms of the cardiopulmonary system.

In terms of energy supply, the aerobic metabolism can be distinguished from the anaerobic metabolism. Various energy suppliers are available to the skeletal muscle for the resynthesis of ATP. In addition to creatine phosphate, glucose and free fatty acids can be used. If the intensity of the load is so high that the energy can be obtained through the oxidation of nutrients, it is referred to as aerobic metabolism. If the intensity of the load during endurance training exceeds the level of maximum oxygen uptake, the anaerobic metabolism is used primarily for energy production.

Practical Relevance

By increasing the maximum oxygen uptake (VO2max) that can be absorbed by the human body during exhaustion through training-induced means, the transition from aerobic to anaerobic metabolism can be delayed. An increase in VO2max is associated with an increase in mitochondrial volume (see Hoppeler 2018).

In the muscle work methods of endurance training, a distinction can be made between static and dynamic stress. It should be noted that the supply of oxygen is reduced due to the permanently increased intramuscular pressure in the static muscle work form. During dynamic contractions and the associated alternation between tension and relaxation, arterial supply and venous-lymphatic disposal are comparatively simplified. More information on practice is provided in Chaps. 5 and 6.

Depending on the duration of the endurance activity, a distinction can be made between short-term endurance, medium-term endurance, and long-term endurance. Short-term endurance is limited to a time span of 35 seconds—2 minutes. Medium-term endurance follows with a time span of 2–10 minutes. From 10 minutes onwards, the endurance training is attributed to long-term endurance. Within long-term endurance, a further subdivision into further subcategories is possible (see Zintl and Eisenhut 2009). Detailed information on the individual control of long-term endurance can be found in disease-specific Chaps. 5 and 6.

2.5.2 Stress Zones of Endurance Training

In terms of stress, endurance training can be divided into four zones. The phase with the lowest intensity is the regeneration or compensation phase. Characteristic of this form of training is a low intensity and a short training duration. The exhausted percentage of VO2max lies in a range of 45–65%. The production of lactate varies between a range of 0.8–1.5 mmol/l. The maximum heart rate is exhausted to 55–75% (see Ferrauti 2020).

Practical Relevance

The regeneration or compensation phase can be performed after intense stress or between training intervals within a unit with the aim of lightly stimulating the metabolism or active recovery.

The next higher intensity level is titled basic endurance 1. The intensity is low to moderately strenuous with a medium to high training duration. The VO2max is used between 66–80%. The lactate value fluctuates in a range of 1.5–2.5 mmol/l. The maximum heart rate is utilized to 75–85% (see Seiler and Tönnessen 2009).

Practical Relevance

When training in the area of basic endurance 1, aerobic performance can be increased. The local adaptations of the muscles mainly relate to the skeletal muscles, which do most of the work. For example, the entire cardiopulmonary system benefits from cycling, while the local adaptation processes focus on the lower extremity.

Following the training methodology of basic endurance 1, basic endurance 2 is introduced. The intensity is moderate to high with a medium duration. Here, an exhaustion of the VO2max of 81–87% is defined. The lactate value moves in a range of 2.5–4 mmol/l. The maximum heart rate is utilized to 85–90% (see Seiler and Tönnessen 2009).

Practical Relevance

In basic endurance 2, the focus is on training the interplay between aerobic and anaerobic metabolism.

As the most intense form of endurance training, Seiler and Tönnessen (2009) define competition-specific endurance training. With a low to medium duration, this method is trained with high intensity. Regarding the exhaustion of VO2max, values of 88–100% are trained. The lactate value is between about 4–10 mmol/l. The maximum heart rate is used to 90–100%.

Practical Relevance
Competition-specific endurance training can lead to an improvement in endurance ability in the anaerobic metabolism.

2.5.3 Methods of Endurance Training

In the methods of endurance training, the continuous method can be distinguished from the interval method.

2.5.3.1 Continuous Methods

The continuous method is characterized by a continuous endurance load, which is mainly performed in the aerobic metabolism (see Adler et al. 2016). Within the continuous method, extensive endurance training can be distinguished from intensive and variable endurance training.

The extensive continuous method is characterized by an exhaustion of the maximum heart rate of 50–80%. The lactate value of about 2 mmol/l is not exceeded. From a short duration of load, which is useful for example in regeneration, work can be done in fat metabolism for several hours. In addition to improving and consolidating basic endurance 1, the extensive continuous method leads to improved capillarization of the working muscles and gives the mitochondria of these more volume. Furthermore, fat metabolism is stimulated (see Ferrauti 2020).

The intensive continuous method is similar to the extensive continuous method, but differs in the training intensity. Thus, the maximum heart rate, depending on individual performance level, is utilized to 70–90%. The lactate value moves in a range between 2.5 and 4 mmol/l. This variant of endurance training trains the metabolism between aerobic and anaerobic energy supply. In addition to improved capillarization and an increase in mitochondrial volume of the working muscles, the maximum oxygen uptake (VO2max) and basic endurance 2 are improved.

The variable continuous method is understood as a mixture of the extensive and intensive continuous method. Here, the intensity during endurance training varies in relation to the maximum heart rate between 60–90%. The blood lactate values fluctuate in a range of about 3–6 mmol/l. The physiological training-induced effects of the extensive and intensive continuous method mix. With the variable continuous method, it is possible to accentuate the adaptability of the energy supply processes (see Ferrauti 2020).

2.5.3.2 Interval Methods

In the endurance training form of interval methods, fixed load phases alternate with relief phases. During the relief phases, there is not a complete cessation of training, but so-called "rewarding breaks", which are characterized by a degree of lower load (see De Marées 2002). The planned alternation between phases of higher and lower load leads to the heart rate repeatedly increasing, only to fall again in the phases of rewarding breaks. A central goal of the interval method is the improvement of fatigue resistance (see Ferrauti and Remmert, 2020). Through the variables of load intensity or load duration, the interval training method can be differentiated into an extensive, intensive and high-intensity form.

In the extensive interval method, the maximum heart rate is utilized in a relatively long range between 60–80%. The blood lactate value should remain below 6 mmol/l. The objectives of the extensive interval method include consolidation and further development of basic endurance 2, optimization of the aerobic or anaerobic mixed metabolism, training of the metabolic conversion in relation to the energy supply processes, and increasing the maximum oxygen uptake (see Ferrauti 2020).

In the intensive interval method, which is practiced in a short to moderate range, the intensity related to the maximum heart rate increases to 80–90% with simultaneous blood lactate values between 4–6 mmol/l. This leads to an optimization of the anaerobic metabolism with a simultaneous faster breakdown of lactate and an increase in the tolerability of increased lactate values (see Ferrauti 2020).

The effects of the intensive interval method can be further expanded with the high-intensity interval method. Here, the maximum heart rate is exhausted to 80–90% and the blood lactate concentration is kept between 4–10 mmol/l over a 30-45 minute period (see Ferrauti 2020).

2.5.4 Research Findings on Endurance Training

In a publication by König and Berg (2012), it was shown that both isolated endurance training and the combination of endurance and strength training can contribute to the therapy and prevention of type 2 diabetes mellitus. With appropriate medical indication, high-intensity interval training can also be successful in people with type 2 diabetes mellitus (see Brinkmann 2019). Francesconi et al. (2016) mention that reducing insulin resistance and improving insulin production while reducing the risk of cardiovascular diseases requires a minimum weekly activity of 150 minutes of strength or intense endurance activity. These training-induced effects can only be maintained through continuous physical activity.

A good insight into the effects of endurance training on the cardiovascular system is provided by the meta-analysis of Lopes et al. (2021). It was shown that endurance training in people with hypertension leads to a reduction in arterial stiffness. In addition, in people with high blood pressure, ambulatory blood pressure can be lowered by practicing aerobic endurance training (see Saco-Ledo et al. 2020).

In a meta-analysis from 2022, Pearce et al. (2022) point to the significantly positive effect of physical activity on the psyche. Furthermore, the antidepressant effect of physical activity and regular training can be confirmed (see Kandola et al. 2019).

Another meta-analysis from 2021 examined the optimal training form for obese individuals in terms of changing the health-promoting body composition and optimizing cardiopulmonary performance based on 45 primary studies with a total population number of 3566. After statistical evaluation of the data sets, regular high-intensity endurance training along with continuous resistance training at high intensity is recommended as the optimal training strategy (see O'Donoghue et al. 2021). In addition, in a meta-analysis by García-Hermoso et al. (2018) on morbidly obese adolescents, the combination of endurance and strength training was also explored as the optimal training form. In addition to improved body composition, a significant improvement in metabolic status and an anti-inflammatory effect were demonstrated. The same effects were observed in a randomized controlled study in adults. In this context, Dâmaso et al. (2014) mention the significant effect of the combination of strength and endurance training on the reduction of visceral fat tissue.

Using the example of chronic nonspecific back pain, it was shown that both progressive strength and endurance training are capable of significantly reducing pain intensity (see Wewege and Booth 2018). García-Correa et al. (2021) confirm these results and add a positive effect on quality of life and an improvement in aerobic capacity through endurance training. Similar effects can be observed in the diagnosis of fibromyalgia (see Bidonde et al. 2017).

Chapters 5 and 6 provide disease-specific insights into the use of endurance training.

2.6 Proprioceptive Training

2.6.1 Definition and Parameters of Proprioceptive Training

If the goal of training therapy is to improve sensorimotor skills in relation to prevention, rehabilitation, and physical performance, it can be referred to as the proprioceptive training approach (cf. Pfeifer et al. 2009). Risberg et al. (2001) mention that the terms sensorimotor or neuromuscular training can be used synonymously with the term proprioceptive training. Taube et al. (2008) add the terms balance and balance training as synonymous. Sensorimotor training aims to optimize neuromuscular recruitment. In addition, the motor skills of movement and posture control should be optimized. Sensorimotor training leads to peripheral stimulation of receptors. Proprioceptors include muscle spindles, Golgi tendon organs, and Ruffini and Vater-Pacini corpuscles. While muscle spindles are capable of detecting muscle length, Golgi tendon apparatuses are capable of transcribing the information of muscle tension into an afferent action potential. Ruffini corpuscles and Vater-Pacini corpuscles are located in the skin, in ligamentous structures, and the joint capsule and are responsible for the perception of joint position or joint movement (cf. Riemann and Lephart 2002). The brain receives information from the proprioceptors, all other peripheral receptors, the visual system, and the vestibular system via afferents. This information is transmitted to the brain via the spinal cord and brainstem and interpreted by the responsible neurons. From this interpretation of afferent information, the brain generates motor movement patterns during proprioceptive training. These are transmitted efferently from the brain via the spinal cord and the peripheral nervous system to the target musculature. The target musculature, as the effector, executes the movement pattern, thus closing the constantly running sensorimotor cycle (cf. Steib et al. 2014).

Sensorimotor training is realized through balance exercises. These specifically include exercise selections that aim at active joint stabilization. A combination of these exercises with strengthening or plyometric training components is common practice. Agility exercises also represent a suitable combination variant (cf. Granacher et al. 2011; Hübscher et al. 2010; Zech et al. 2009).

Regarding the exploration of optimal training parameters of proprioceptive training, currently little high-quality literature is available. A guideline for the choice of load control is provided by the recommendation of the American College of Sports Medicine (cf. Garber et al. 2011). The following statements, which concern the control of proprioceptive training, refer to the publication by Steib et al. (2014). Sensorimotor training should begin with about a ten-minute warm-up. Regarding the stimulus duration, a time span of 20–40 seconds is recommended. The rest periods between the individual sets are given as 20–40 seconds. The rest time between the individual exercises diverges between 30 seconds and five minutes. The total volume of training comprises 2–10 exercises with 1–10 repetitions each. Two to three training sessions per week are advised. The duration of a training session should be between 15–45 minutes. The stimulus intensity should be chosen so that it is challenging for the person to be trained. Figure 2.6 provides an overview of the described parameters of proprioceptive training.

2.6.2 Research Findings on Proprioceptive Training

A systematic review followed by an upgrade to a meta-analysis concluded that proprioceptive training is a therapy component for total knee arthroplasty to improve balance and functionality (see Domínguez-Navarro et al. 2018). These results were confirmed in 2020 in another meta-analysis, which is based on seven randomized controlled studies (see Zhang and Xiao 2020). Preoperative proprioceptive training before the insertion of a total knee arthroplasty also leads to a significant improvement in standing balance six weeks after the operation (see Gstoettner et al. 2011). Regardless of surgery, individuals with knee osteoarthritis can benefit from proprioceptive training in terms of pain and everyday functionality (see Jeong et al. 2019).

Proprioceptive training can reduce the risk of supination trauma of the ankle in athletes. This is especially true for individuals who have suffered supination traumas in the past (see Schiftan et al. 2015). In addition to reducing the frequency of supination traumas in athletes, proprioceptive training can train neuromuscular control and reduce postural sway. Additionally, the sense of joint position of the upper ankle

Warming (see Steib et al., 2014)	10 minutes
Stimulus duration (see Steib et al., 2014)	20-40 seconds
Stimulus density (see Steib et al., 2014)	20-40 seconds between series / 30 seconds to five minutes between exercises
Stimulus range (see Steib et al., 2014)	2-10 exercises /1-10 repetitions
Stimulus intensity (see Steib et al., 2014)	individually demanding
Duration of a training session (see Steib et al., 2014)	15-45 minutes
Therapy units per week (see Steib et al., 2014)	2-3

Fig. 2.6 Overview of the parameters of proprioceptive training. (Own illustration 2023)

can be refined (see Souza de Vasconcelos et al. 2018).

Older healthy individuals can improve their static and dynamic balance through proprioceptive training. The individuals studied also performed better on balance test batteries (see Lesinski et al. 2015). Similar effects were also observed in older people with diabetic peripheral neuropathy (see Ahmad et al. 2019). After a twelve-week proprioceptive training, improved postural control, improved static and dynamic balance, and better walking ability were observed in older people. It is noteworthy that in this context, a reduced risk of falls was achieved in older people aged 65 and over (see Martínez-Amat et al. 2013). In addition to older people, children from the age of six can also benefit from proprioceptive training (see Wälchli et al. 2018).

2.7 Training of Mobility

2.7.1 Causes of Restricted Joint Mobility

The restriction of mobility can bring with it multifaceted causes. In addition to structural changes in the myofascial, capsuloligamentous, and neuromeningeal systems, the cortical processing of afferents from the musculoskeletal system also appears to modulate the achievable range of motion. Here, nociceptive and proprioceptive afferents seem to play a crucial role. In addition to these structural and functional changes, the influence of personal and environmental factors should not be overlooked. If the phenomenon of kinesiophobia is generated by intrinsic psychological processes of the affected person or by external persons through communication, this can lead to a premature limitation of the movement excursion alone. Therefore, if the goal is to train or increase mobility, the existing influencing factors should be clarified as precisely as possible within the examination.

Myofascial structures should be subjected to palpation as well as stretch and resistance tests. Ligaments should also be subjected to palpation and targeted tension increase. The joint capsule can be subjected to a holistic solution or tightening or stretching through targeted traction, at least in theory. If only specific capsular components are to be put under increased tension, the application of glide tests from the field of manual therapy is recommended. The possible influence of increased tension absorption in the neuromeningeal system on a mobility restriction can be clarified by nerve tension tests.

If these tests do not provide any information about the causes of hypomobility, a closer look should be taken at the joint architecture. The question of the condition of the hyaline joint cartilage and possible osteophytes or tumors in the area of the joint space, if it still exists, should be clarified as well as the presence of possible free joint bodies (cf. Venbrocks et al. 1988). Swelling, which occurs in a classic inflammatory reaction, can have a major influence on the reduction of joint mobility. Special caution is required when signs of inflammation do not subside or reappear after the actual inflammation phase. These conditions are found, for example, in the complex regional pain syndrome or infection of the affected joint (cf. Shim et al. 2019; Rohde 2014).

Another contributing factor is the shape and alignment of the joint surfaces and neighboring joints, the tension state of ligamentous plastics, and the position of osteosynthesis material or endoprostheses in the bone.

It is clear from the last two paragraphs that medical training therapy is not directly or at all indicated for hypomobility. Therefore, a clarification of the relevance and prerequisites for mobility-promoting training is absolutely necessary.

2.7.2 Mobility Enhancing Instruments of Medical Training Therapy

2.7.2.1 Stretching

A proven means of exerting a mobility-promoting influence on the myofascial system is muscular stretching (see Diemer 2018). With the goal of increasing mobility and its long-term maintenance, McHugh and Cosgrave (2010) recommend a stretching duration of 4 minutes per muscle group. The stretching method does not seem to be of great importance in this regard. In addition to static and dynamic stretching methods, post-isometric variations or the effect of reciprocal inhibition can also be used. To maintain the mobility-promoting effect, the stretching intervention of the myofascial target structures should be performed at least twice a week.

If the stretching is to serve as preparation for a subsequent main training, the stretching time per muscle group should not exceed 1–2 minutes. The execution of the stretching should be dynamic (see Opplert and Babault 2018).

If the intervention of stretching is aimed at injury prevention, Behm et al (2016) recommend a stretching duration of 5 minutes for the muscle group to be treated. The type of stretching can be static or can also be performed with post-isometric relaxation or the effect of reciprocal inhibition. The type of application can reduce the risk of injury by approximately 54% (see Behm et al. 2016).

In general, it is recommended that not the person who is leading the training performs the stretches, but rather instructs the person to be trained to perform the stretching themselves. This enables the person to be trained to perform the corresponding exercises at any time and independently.

2.7.2.2 Foam Roller

Another instrument to achieve a mobility-enhancing effect through myofascial stimulation is the foam roller (see Wiewelhove et al. 2019). The cited meta-analysis concludes that the use of the foam roller is particularly suitable during warm-up to increase flexibility in this phase. A regenerative accelerating effect could not be determined. In the elaboration by Konrad et al. (July 2022), it is found that there is no difference in terms of acute improvement of joint mobility between the use of a foam roller and a stretching intervention. Both means are equally capable of increasing joint mobility. According to current evidence, training with the foam roller for more than four weeks is recommended to induce long-term mobility extensions. The mobility-promoting effect also seems to depend on the muscle group to be treated. While rolling in the area of the quadriceps femoris muscle and in the area of the ischiocrural muscles was able to increase mobility, the use of the foam roller in the area of the triceps surae muscle did not produce any detectable extension of the range of motion (see Konrad et al. October 2022).

Cheatham and Stull (2018a, b) recommend an active movement of the joint during rolling, at which the range of motion is to be increased. Grooved foam rollers seem to have a better effect on the acute increase in knee joint excursion than foam rollers with a smooth surface (see Cheatham and Stull 2019). An examination, which investigated three different hardness levels of foam rollers, found a significant mobility-promoting effect at each hardness level. No significant differences could be calculated between the individual hardness levels. This suggests that the hardness level does not play a significant therapeutic role in terms of mobility improvement (see Cheatham and Stull 2018a, b). In terms of mobility in the knee and hip joint, the use of a vibrating foam roller was superior to a non-vibrating foam roller (see Park et al. 2021).

References

Adler S, Glöckl R, Jarosch I, Kenn K (2016) Effekte eines Laufbandtrainings nach der Intervall- versus Dauermethode bei COPD-Patienten – eine randomisierte, kontrollierte Pilotstudie. Pneumol 70:145 https://doi.org/10.1055/s-0036-1572179

Ahmad I, Noohu M, Verma S, Singla D, Hussain M (October 2019) Effect of sensorimotor training on balance measures and proprioception among middle and older age adults with diabetic peripheral neuropathy. Gait Posture 74:114–120 https://doi.org/10.1016/j.gaitpost.2019.08.018

Asadi A, Arazi H, Young W, de Villarreal E (July 2016) The effects of plyometric training on change-of-direction ability: a meta-analysis. Int J Sports Physiol Perform 11(5):563–573 https://doi.org/10.1123/ijspp.2015-0694

Bührle M (1989) Maximalkraft – Schnellkraft – Reaktivkraft. Sportwissenschaft 19(3):311–325

Bührle M, Schmidtbleicher D, Ressel H (1983) Die spezielle Diagnose der einzelnen Kraftkomponenten im Hochleistungssport. Leistungssport 13:11–16

Büsch D, Pabst J, Mühlbauer T, Ehrhardt P, Granacher U (2015) Effects of plyometric training using unstable surfaces on jump and sprint performance in young sub-elite handball players. Sports Orthop Traumatol 31(4):299–308 https://doi.org/10.1016/j.orthtr.2015.07.007

Behm D, Blazevich A, Kay A, McHugh M (January 2016) Acute effects of muscle stretching on physical performance, range of motion, and injury incidence in healthy active individuals: a systematic review. Appl Physiol Nutr Metab 41(1):1–11 https://doi.org/10.1139/apnm-2015-0235

Bidonde J, Busch A, Schachter C, Overend T, Kim S, Góes S, Foulds H (21 June 2017) Aerobic exercise training for adults with fibromyalgia. Cochrane Database Syst Rev 6(6):CD012700 https://doi.org/10.1002/14651858.CD012700

Bigland-Ritchie B (1981) EMG and fatigue of human voluntary and stimulated contractions. In: Porter R, Whelan J (eds) Human muscle fatigue: physiological mechanisms. Novartis Foundation Symposia, London, S 130–148 https://doi.org/10.1002/9780470715420.ch9

Bjarnason-Wehrens B, Mayer-Berger W, Meister E, Baum K, Hambrecht R, Gielen S (2004) Einsatz von Kraftausdauertraining und Muskelaufbautraining in der kardiologischen Rehabilitation. Z Kardiol 93(5):357–370 https://doi.org/10.1007/s00392-004-0063-7

Brinkmann C (2019) Hochintensives Intervalltraining (HIIT) und Typ-2-Diabetes mellitus. Bewegungstherapie und Gesundheitssport 35(02):62–65. https://doi.org/10.1055/a-0860-1300

Buskies W (1999) Sanftes Krafttraining. Sport und Buch Strauß, Köln

Cheatham S, Stull K (June 2018) Comparison of three different density type foam rollers on knee range of motion and pressure pain threshold: a randomized controlled trial. Int J Sports Phys Ther 13(3):474–482

Cheatham S, Stull K (July 2018) Comparison of a foam rolling session with active joint motion and without joint motion: a randomized controlled trial. J Bodyw Mov Ther 22(3):707–712 https://doi.org/10.1016/j.jbmt.2018.01.011

Cheatham S, Stull K (July 2019) Roller massage: comparison of three different surface type pattern foam rollers on passive knee range of motion and pain perception. J Bodyw Mov Ther 23(3):555–560 https://doi.org/10.1016/j.jbmt.2019.05.002

Crewther B, Cronin J, Keogh J, Cook C (January 2008) The salivary testosterone and cortisol response to three loading schemes. J Strength Cond Res 22(1):250–255 https://doi.org/10.1519/JSC.0b013e31815f5f91

Dâmaso A, da Silveira CR, Caranti D, de Piano A, Fisberg M, Foschini D, de Mello M (2014) Aerobic plus resistance training was more effective in improving the visceral adiposity, metabolic profile and inflammatory markers than aerobic training in obese adolescents. J Sports Sci 32(15):1435–1445 https://doi.org/10.1080/02640414.2014.900692

De Marées H (2002) Sportphysiologie. Sport & Buch Strauss, Köln

Diemer F (2018) Evidenz-Update Dehnen – Dehnen – oder nicht? Physiopraxis 16(03):22–25 https://doi.org/10.1055/s-0043-121837

Dinh H, Njemini R, Onyema O, Beyer I, Liberman K, Dobbeleer L, Bautmans I (13 November 2019) Strength endurance training but not intensive strength training reduces senescence-prone T cells in peripheral blood in community-dwelling elderly women. J Gerontol 74(12):1870–1878 https://doi.org/10.1093/gerona/gly229

Domínguez-Navarro F, Igual-Camacho C, Silvestre-Muñoz A, Roig-Casasús S, Blasco J (May 2018) Effects of balance and proprioceptive training on total hip and knee replacement rehabilitation: a systematic review and meta-analysis. Gait Posture 62:68–74 https://doi.org/10.1016/j.gaitpost.2018.03.003

Ehlenz H, Grosser M, Zimmermann E (1998) Krafttraining.Grundlagen, Methoden, Übungen, Leistungssteuerung, Trainingsprogramme. BLV-Verlagsgesellschaft Münchenn

Ferrauti A, Remmert H (2020) Grundlagenwissen zum sportlichen Training. In: Ferrauti A (ed)

Trainingswissenschaft für die Sportpraxis. Springer, Berlin, S 21–65 https://doi.org/10.1007/978-3-662-58227-5_2

Ferrauti A (2020) Trainingswissenschaft für die Sportpraxis. Springer, Berlin. https://doi.org/10.1007/978-3-662-58227-5

Fröhlich M (2011) Methodik des Krafttrainings-Stand der Dinge. Die Säule 21(4):2

Fröhlich M, Klein M, Emrich E, Schmidtbleicher D (January 2001) Arbeit als Bruttokriterium der Belastung im Kraftausdauertraining. Leistungssport 2(01)

Fröhlich M, Schmidtbleicher D, Emrich E (2004) Metabolische und kardiovaskuläre Beanspruchung im Kraftausdauertraining. Sportverletz Sportschaden 18(3):136–141. https://doi.org/10.1055/s-2004-813050

Francesconi C, Lackinger C, Weitgasser R, Haber P, Niebauer J (April 2016) Körperliche Aktivität und Training in der Prävention und Therapie des Typ 2 Diabetes mellitus. Wien Klin Wochenschr 128:141–145

Fry A (2004) The role of resistance exercise intensity on muscle fibre adaptations. Sports Med 34(10):663–679. https://doi.org/10.2165/00007256-200434100-00004

Güllich A, Schmidtbleicher D (1999) Struktur der Kraftfähigkeiten und ihrer Trainingsmethoden. Dtsch Z Sportmed 50(7+8):223–234

Garber C, Blissmer B, Deschenes M, Franklin B, Lamonte M, Lee I-M, American College of Sports Medicine (July 2011) American college of sports medicine position stand. Quantity and quality of exercise for developing and maintaining cardiorespiratory, musculoskeletal, and neuromotor fitness in apparently healthy adults: guidance for prescribing exercise. Med Sci Sports Exerc 43(7):1334–59 https://doi.org/10.1249/MSS.0b013e318213fefb

García-Correa H, Sánchez-Montoya L, Daza-Arana J, Ordoñez-Mora L (5 August 2021) Aerobic physical exercise for pain intensity, aerobic capacity, and quality of life in patients with chronic pain: a systematic review and meta-analysis. J Phys Act Health 18(9):1126–1142 https://doi.org/10.1123/jpah.2020-0806

García-Hermoso A, Ramírez-Vélez R, Ramírez-Campillo R, Peterson M, Martínez-Vizcaíno V (February 2018) Concurrent aerobic plus resistance exercise versus aerobic exercise alone to improve health outcomes in paediatric obesity: a systematic review and meta-analysis. Br J Sports Med 52(3):161–166. https://doi.org/10.1136/bjsports-2016-096605

Gonzalez A (October 2016) Acute anabolic response and muscular adaptation after hypertrophy-style and strength-style resistance exercise. J Strength Cond Res 30(10):2959–2964. https://doi.org/10.1519/JSC.0000000000001378

Gonzalez A, Hoffman J, Stout J, Fukuda D, Willoughby D (May 2016) Intramuscular anabolic signaling and endocrine response following resistance exercise: implications for muscle hypertrophy. Sports Med 46(5):671–685 https://doi.org/10.1007/s40279-015-0450-4

Granacher U, Muehlbauer T, Zahner L, Gollhofer A, Kressig R (1 May 2011) Comparison of traditional and recent approaches in the promotion of balance and strength in older adults. Sports Med 41(5):377–400 https://doi.org/10.2165/11539920-000000000-00000

Grgic J, Schoenfeld B, Mikulic P (September 2021) Effects of plyometric vs. resistance training on skeletal muscle hypertrophy: a review. J Sport Health Sci 10(5):530–536 https://doi.org/10.1016/j.jshs.2020.06.010

Gstoettner M, Raschner C, Dirnberger E, Leimser H, Krismer M (August 2011) Preoperative proprioceptive training in patients with total knee arthroplasty. Knee 18(4):265–270 https://doi.org/10.1016/j.knee.2010.05.012

Hübscher M, Zech A, Pfeifer K, Hänsel F, Vogt L, Banzer W (March 2010) Neuromuscular training for sports injury prevention: a systematic review. Med Sci Sports Exerc 42(3):413–421 https://doi.org/10.1249/MSS.0b013e3181b88d37

Haas H-J, Fox T (2005) Muskelaufbau Schritt für Schritt. Physiopraxis 3(1):26–28 https://doi.org/10.1055/s-0032-1307863

Haber P, Tomasits J (2006) Medizinische Trainingsberatung Anleitung für die Praxis. Springe, Wien

Hendrey G, Clark R, Holland A, Mentiplay B, Davis C, Windfeld-Lund C, Williams G (December 2018) Feasibility of ballistic strength training in subacute stroke: a randomized, controlled, assessor-blinded pilot study. Arch Phys Med Rehabil 99(12):2430–2446 https://doi.org/10.1016/j.apmr.2018.04.032

Hillebrecht A, Zeißler S, Frech T, Rechner M, Haas U, Mooren F, Hamar D (2012) Vergleich der Effekte von zwei Krafttrainingsmethoden als spezifische Trainingsintervention bei Patienten mit Diabetes mellitus Typ 2– Hypertrophiekrafttraining versus Kraftausdauertraining. Diabetol Stoffwechs 7:128 https://doi.org/10.1055/s-0032-1314625

Hollmann W, Hettinger T (2000) Sportmedizin. Grundlagen für Arbeit, Training und Präventivmedizin. Schattauer, Stuttgart

Holzgreve F, Schulte L, Germann U, Wanke E (11 August 2022) Krafttraining als Verhaltenspräventionsmaßnahme bei berufsbedingten muskuloskeletalen Beschwerden. Zentralblatt für Arbeitsmedizin, Arbeitsschutz und Ergonomie 72:236–240 https://doi.org/10.1007/s40664-022-00476-8

Hoppeler H (2018) Anpassung an Ausdauertraining. Bachl N, Löllgen H, Tschan H, Wackerhage H, Wessner B (eds) Molekulare Sport- und Leistungsphysiologie. Springer, Wien, S 291–304

Hultman E, Sjöholm H, Sahlin K, Edström L (1981) Glycolytic and oxidative energy metabolism and contraction characteristics of intact human muscle. In: Porter R, Whelan J (eds) Human muscle fatigue: physiological mechanisms. Novartis Foundation Symposia, London, S 19–35 https://doi.org/10.1002/9780470715420.ch9

Jeong H, Lee S-C, Jee H, Song J, Chang H, Lee S (April 2019) Proprioceptive training and outcomes of patients with knee osteoarthritis: a meta-analysis of randomized controlled trials. J Athl Train 54(4):418–428 https://doi.org/10.4085/1062-6050-329-17

König D, Berg A (2012) Bewegung als Therapie bei diabetes mellitus Typ 2. Der Internist 53(6):678–687 https://doi.org/10.1007/s00108-011-2936-y

Kandola A, Ashdown-Franks G, Hendrikse J, Sabiston C (December 2019) Physical activity and depression: towards understanding the antidepressant mechanisms of physical activity. Neurosci Biobehav Rev 107:525–539 https://doi.org/10.1016/j.neubiorev.2019.09.040

Konrad A, Nakamura M, Tilp M, Donti O, Behm D (October 2022) Foam rolling training effects on range of motion: a systematic review and meta-analysis. Sports Med 52(10):2523–2535 https://doi.org/10.1007/s40279-022-01699-8

Konrad A, Nakamura M, Paternoster F, Tilp M, Behm D (July 2022) A comparison of a single bout of stretching or foam rolling on range of motion in healthy adults. Eur J Appl Physiol 122(7):1545–1557 https://doi.org/10.1007/s00421-022-04927-1

Lehmann S, Blüher M, Peschel P, Kugler J, Oberbach A (2011) Kombinierter Präventionskurs zur nachhaltigen Risikominimierung des Metabolischen Syndroms? Effekte von Kraft und Kraftausdauer im Follow-up. Diabetol Stoffwechs 6:261 https://doi.org/10.1055/s-0031-1277532

Lesinski M, Hortobágyi T, Muehlbauer T, Gollhofer A, Granacher U (December 2015) Effects of balance training on balance performance in healthy older adults: a systematic review and meta-analysis. Sports Med 45(12):1721–1738 https://doi.org/10.1007/s40279-015-0375-y

Lopes S, Afreixo V, Teixeira M, Garcia C, Leitão C, Gouveia M, Ribeiro F (February 2021) Exercise training reduces arterial stiffness in adults with hypertension: a systematic review and meta-analysis. J Hypertens 39(2):214–222 https://doi.org/10.1097/HJH.0000000000002619

Müller K-J (1987) Statische und dynamische Muskelkraft: Beiträge zur Sportwissenschaft, Bd 7. Verlag Harri Deutsch, Frankfurt a. M., S 151

Martínez-Amat A, Hita-Contreras F, Lomas-Vega R, Caballero-Martínez I, Alvarez P, Martínez-López E (August 2013) Effects of 12-week proprioception training program on postural stability, gait, and balance in older adults: a controlled clinical trial. J Strength Cond Res 27(8):2180–2188 https://doi.org/10.1519/JSC.0b013e31827da35f

Matavulj D, Kukolj M, Ugarkovic D, Tihanyi J, Jaric S (June 2001) Effects of plyometric training on jumping performance in junior basketball players. J Sports Med Phys Fitness 41(2):159–164

McCaulley G, McBride J, Cormie P, Hudson M, Nuzzo J, Quindry J, Triplett N (March 2009) Acute hormonal and neuromuscular responses to hypertrophy, strength and power type resistance exercise. Eur J Appl Physiol 105(5):695–704 https://doi.org/10.1007/s00421-008-0951-z

McHugh M, Cosgrave C (April 2010) To stretch or not to stretch: the role of stretching in injury prevention and performance. Scand J Med Sci Sports 20(2):169–181 https://doi.org/10.1111/j.1600-0838.2009.01058.x

Nicholson G, Ispoglou T, Bissas A (October 2016) The impact of repetition mechanics on the adaptations resulting from strength-, hypertrophy- and cluster-type resistance training. Eur J Appl Physiol 116(10):1875–1888 https://doi.org/10.1007/s00421-016-3439-2

O'Donoghue G, Blake C, Cunningham C, Lennon O, Perrotta C (February 2021) What exercise prescription is optimal to improve body composition and cardiorespiratory fitness in adults living with obesity? A network meta-analysis. Obes Rev 22(2):e13137 https://doi.org/10.1111/obr.13137

Opplert J, Babault N (February 2018) Acute effects of dynamic stretching on muscle flexibility and performance: an analysis of the current literature. Sports Med 48(2):299–325 https://doi.org/10.1007/s40279-017-0797-9

Park S-J, Lee S-I, Jeong H-J, Kim B-G (23 August 2021) Effect of vibration foam rolling on the range of motion in healthy adults: a systematic review and meta-analysis. J Exerc Rehabil 17(4):226–233 https://doi.org/10.12965/jer.2142322.161

Pearce M, Garcia L, Abbas A, Strain T, Schuch F, Golubic R, Woodcock J (1 June 2022) Association between physical activity and risk of depression: a systematic review and meta-analysis. JAMA Psychiat 79(6):550–559 https://doi.org/10.1001/jamapsychiatry.2022.0609

Pfeifer K, Banzer W, Hänsel F, Hübscher M, Vogt L, Zech A (2009) Wissenschaftliche Expertise "Sensomotorisches Training-Propriozeptives Training". Sportverlag Strauß, Köln

Raeder C, Vuong J-L, Ferrauti A (2020) Trainingswissenschaft für die Sportpraxis. Springer, Berlin. https://doi.org/10.1007/978-3-662-58227-5_4

Riemann B, Lephart S (January 2002) The sensorimotor system, part I: the physiologic basis of functional joint stability. J Athl Train 37(1):71–79

Risberg M, Mork M, Jenssen H, Holm I (2001) Design and implementation of a neuromuscular training program following anterior cruciate ligament reconstruction. J Orthop Sports Phys Ther 31(11):620–663

Rohde H (2014) Freund und Feind: Hautbakterien als Erreger von Krankenhausinfektionen. In: Fischer M (ed) Neue und alte Infektionskrankheiten. Springer

Spektrum, Wiesbaden, S 79–105 https://doi.org/10.1007/978-3-658-04124-3_4

Saco-Ledo G, Valenzuela P, Ruiz-Hurtado G, Ruilope L, Lucia A (15 December 2020) Exercise reduces ambulatory blood pressure in patients With hypertension: a systematic review and meta-analysis of randomized controlled trials. J Am Heart Assoc 9(24):e018487 https://doi.org/10.1161/JAHA.120.018487

Schiftan G, Ross L, Hahne A (May 2015) The effectiveness of proprioceptive training in preventing ankle sprains in sporting populations: a systematic review and meta-analysis. J Sci Med Sport 18(3):238–244 https://doi.org/10.1016/j.jsams.2014.04.005

Schmidtbleicher D (1989) Zum Problem der Definition des Begriffs Kraftausdauer. In: Carl K, Starischka S, Storck H-M (eds) Kraftausdauer. Sport und Buch Strauß, Köln, S 10–30

Schnabel G, Harre D, Borde A (1997) Trainingswissenschaft. Leistung – Training – Wettkampf. Sportverlag, Berlin

Schoenfeld B (2020) Science and development of muscle hypertrophy. Human Kinetics Champaign, Illinois, USA

Schoenfeld B (March 2013) Potential mechanisms for a role of metabolic stress in hypertrophic adaptations to resistance training. Sports Med 43(3):179–194 https://doi.org/10.1007/s40279-013-0017-1

Seiler S, Tönnessen E (2009) Intervals, thresholds, and long slow distance: The role of intensity and duration in endurance training. Sportscience 13:32–53

Shim H, Rose J, Halle S, Shekane P (August 2019) Complex regional pain syndrome: a narrative review for the practising clinician. Br J Anaesth 123(2):e424–e433 https://doi.org/10.1016/j.bja.2019.03.030

Smilios I, Pilianidis T, Karamouzis M, Tokmakidis S (April 2003) Hormonal responses after various resistance exercise protocols. Med Sci Sports Exerc 35(4):644–654 https://doi.org/10.1249/01.MSS.0000058366.04460.5F

Souza de Vasconcelos G, Cini A, Sbruzzi G, Lima C (December 2018) Effects of proprioceptive training on the incidence of ankle sprain in athletes: systematic review and meta-analysis. Clin Rehabil 32(12):1581–1590 https://doi.org/10.1177/0269215518788683

Staniszewski M, Mastalerz A, Urbanik C (7 February 2020) Effect of a strength or hypertrophy training protocol, each performed using two different modes of resistance, on biomechanical, biochemical and anthropometric parameters. Biol Sport 37(1):85–91 https://doi.org/10.5114/biolsport.2020.92517

Steib S, Pfeifer K, Zech A (2014) Sensomotorisches Training. In: Kempf H-D (ed) Funktionelles Training mit Hand- und Kleingeräten. Springer, Berlin, S 13–19

Stengel S, Kemmler W, Pintag R, Beeskow C, Weineck J, Lauber D, Engelke K (2005) Power training is more effective than strength training for maintaining bone mineral density in postmenopausal women. J Appl Physiol 99(1):181–188 https://doi.org/10.1152/japplphysiol.01260.2004

Taube W, Gruber M, Gollhofer A (June 2008) Spinal and supraspinal adaptations associated with balance training and their functional relevance. Acta Physiol (Oxf) 193(2):101–116 https://doi.org/10.1111/j.1748-1716.2008.01850.x

Thiele D, Prieske O, Lesinski M, Granacher U (21 July 2020) Effects of equal volume heavy-resistance strength training versus strength endurance training on physical fitness and sport-specific performance in young elite female rowers. Front Physiol 11:888 https://doi.org/10.3389/fphys.2020.00888

Thompson S, Rogerson D, Ruddock A, Barnes A (11 December 2019) The effectiveness of two methods of prescribing load on maximal strength development: a systematic review. Sports Med 50:919–938 https://doi.org/10.1007/s40279-019-01241-3

Tschopp M, Sattelmayer M (September 2011) Is power training or conventional resistance training better for function in elderly persons? A meta-analysis. Age Ageing 40(5):549–556 https://doi.org/10.1093/ageing/afr005

Uchida M, Crewther B, Ugrinowitsch C, Bacurau R, Moriscot A, Aoki M (1 October 2009) Hormonal responses to different resistance exercise schemes of similar total volume. J Strength Cond Res 23(7):2003–2008 https://doi.org/10.1519/jsc.0b013e3181b73bf7

Urhausen A, Schwarz M, Stefan S, Schwarz L, Gabriel H, Kindermann W (2000) Kardiovaskuläre und metabolische Beanspruchung durch einen Kraftausdauerzirkel in der ambulanten Herztherapie. Dtsch Z Sportmed 51(4):130–136

Venbrocks R, Münzenberg K, Kempis V (January-February 1988) Comparison and evaluation of conservative and surgical therapeutic possibilities in osteochondrosis dissecans of the knee joint. Z Orthop Ihre Grenzgeb 121(1):30–33 https://doi.org/10.1055/s-2008-1044863

Wälchli M, Ruffieux J, Mouthon A, Keller M, Taube W (1 February 2018) Is young age a limiting factor when training balance? Effects of child-oriented balance training in children and adolescents. Pediatr Exerc Sci 30(1):176–184 https://doi.org/10.1123/pes.2017-0061

Werchoshanskij J (1972) Grundlagen des speziellen Krafttrainings. In: Adam K, Werchoshanskij J (eds) Modernes Krafttraining im Sport. Bartels & Wernitz KG, Berlin, S 37–148

Wewege M, Booth J (2018) Aerobic vs. resistance exercise for chronic non-specific low back pain: A systematic review and meta-analysis. J Back Musculoskelet Rehabil 31(5):889–899 https://doi.org/10.3233/BMR-170920

Wiewelhove T, Döweling A, Schneider C, Hottenrott L, Meyer T, Kellmann M, Ferrauti A (9 April 2019) A Meta-Analysis of the Effects of Foam Rolling on

Performance and Recovery. Front Physiol 10:376 https://doi.org/10.3389/fphys.2019.00376
Wirth K, Schmidtbleicher D (2002) Trainingshäufigkeit beim Hypertrophietraining unter Berücksichtigung des Leistungsniveaus. Bundesinstitut für Sportwissenschaften Bonn, Deutschland
Zech A, Hübscher M, Vogt L, Banzer W, Hänsel F, Pfeifer K (October 2009) Neuromuscular training for rehabilitation of sports injuries: a systematic review. Med Sci Sports Exerc 41(10):1831–1841 https://doi.org/10.1249/MSS.0b013e3181a3cf0d
Zhang W-C, Xiao D (3 November 2020) Efficacy of proprioceptive training on the recovery of total joint arthroplasty patients: a meta-analysis. J Orthop Surg Res 15(1):505 https://doi.org/10.1186/s13018-020-01970-6
Zintl F, Eisenhut A (2009) Ausdauertraining. Grundlagen, Methoden, Trainingssteuerung BLV Sportwissen, 7., überarb. edn., Neuausg Ausg. BLV, München

3 Age-Dependent or Disease-Associated Changes in Organ Systems and the Effect of Medical Exercise Therapy

Contents

S. Wolfram and R. Bauer, *Evidence-Based Medical Exercise Therapy*,
https://doi.org/10.1007/978-3-662-70774-6_3

Trailer

In this enlightening third chapter, a comprehensive analysis unfolds on how aging and diseases affect our vital organ systems and how targeted medical exercise therapy can act as a potent counterplayer. Explore the fascinating interactions between physical activity and the well-being of our organs, from the heart and lungs to muscles and the nervous system.

Starting with the cardiovascular system, the engine of life, this chapter reveals how age- and disease-related changes impair this central system and how exercise therapies can contribute to its revitalization and strengthening. A deep look into the blood and immune system shows how exercise not only strengthens our defenses but can also improve the quality of our blood.

The lymphatic and respiratory systems are also examined, highlighting the crucial role of exercise therapy in promoting lymphatic and respiratory health. By understanding how movement can improve the flow properties of the lymphatic system and increase breathing efficiency, new doors open for disease prevention and management.

The analysis extends to the muscular system, where you will learn how age-related muscle atrophy can be reversed and muscle strength maintained or even increased through targeted training. The importance of exercise therapy also extends to the central and peripheral nervous system, promoting neuroplasticity and contributing to the preservation of cognitive functions.

This chapter also illuminates how medical exercise therapy impacts the digestive and excretory systems, the reproductive system, as well as skin and hormone balance. Each section carefully connects the dots between age- or disease-related changes and the positive effects of regular, targeted physical activity.

Finally, this chapter invites you to explore the transformative power of medical exercise therapy in the prevention, treatment, and management of age- and disease-related conditions. It offers a source of hope and action for all those who wish to improve their health through conscious movement. Prepare to be inspired and discover the diverse ways in which evidence-based medical exercise therapy can change lives.

3.1 Cardiovascular System

3.1.1 Age-Dependent or Disease-Associated Changes in the Cardiovascular System

The aging process leads to morphological changes in the heart. With increasing age, an increase in the thickness of the myocardium can be observed. This is focused in the area of the left ventricle (see Marcomichelakis et al. 1983). The main cause of myocardial hypertrophy of the left ventricle is considered to be the continuously increasing systolic blood pressure with age. In addition, activation of the sympathetic nervous system and the renin-angiotensin-aldosterone system, as well as possible insulin resistance, can be considered as influencing factors (see Tsunoda et al. 1986). From a functional perspective, the myocardium experiences a slowed contraction speed during systole and delayed relaxation during diastolic heart activity. Wei et al. (1984) attribute this condition to a deteriorated calcium-myosin-ATPase reaction of the sarcoplasmic reticulum.

Another age-related change in the heart is the decline of pacemaker cells in the excitation formation or conduction system. Starting from the second decade of life, the number of pacemaker cells decreases by up to 90% by the eighth decade of life (see James 1964; Lev 1954). The functional consequences of this morphological change are manifested in a reduction of heart rate variability and a continuous decrease in maximum heart rate during stress situations (see Lakatta 1986).

Further age-related changes in the myocardium lead to a reduced ejection fraction of the heart chambers. This restricts the cardiac output, thereby reducing the maximum oxygen transport capacity of the cardiovascular system in stress situations (see Rogers et al. 1990).

On the side of the arterial vascular system, there is a continuous thickening of the intima (innermost vascular layer). The endothelial cells of the intima show changes in size, shape, and arrangement with increasing age. In addition to hypertrophic processes, an uneven arrangement and thus a no longer smooth surface texture exist. In addition, there are increased subendothelial deposits of phospholipids, calcium, and cholesterol (see Wei 1992). With increasing age, there is a reduction of elastic fibers within the arterial blood vessels. Arteries of the elastic type are mainly affected by this process (see Huonker et al. 2014). In addition, there are increased collagen and calcium deposits (see Kitzman et al. 1990). Arteries of the muscular type, on the other hand, are characterized in the aging process primarily by an increase in smooth muscle. In summary, it can be stated that there is a deterioration in vascular elasticity (see Gaballa et al. 1998). This manifests itself in an increase in systolic resting blood pressure, blood pressure amplitude, and a limited ability to adjust the affected blood vessels into vasodilation during a stress situation (see Huonker et al. 2014).

3.1.2 Effects of Medical Exercise Therapy on the Cardiovascular System

In a study by Levy et al. (1993), the influence of aerobic endurance training on the cardiovascular system was investigated. The intervention group consisted of heart-healthy older men aged between 60 and 82 years. The control group was represented by younger men with an age range of 24 to 32 years. Both groups completed aerobic endurance training in four to five units per week. After a six-month intervention period, an increased passive left ventricular filling could be measured in the older intervention group. At the same time, a decrease in active late diastolic filling during rest and stress situations could be explored. The training increased heart rate variability by 68% and the VO2max from 28.8 ± 1.3 ml· kg$-^{1}$ to 35.1 ± 1.0 ml· kg^{-1}. The resting heart rate dropped by nine beats per minute after the intervention period.

McKenzie (2012) distinguishes between structural and functional changes in the adaptation reactions of the cardiovascular system. Structural changes include an enlargement of the left ventricular cavity, a thickening of the left ventricular myocardial layer, an enlargement of the heart mass, improved left ventricular flexibility, and an enlargement of the left atrium. On a functional level, improved myocardial contractility, increased stroke volume, higher cardiac output, improved diastolic function, reduction of peripheral resistance, and improved venous return can be observed.

In a comparative study, Vaitkevicius (1993) was able to evaluate that older trained people have less wall stiffness in the area of the aorta or the common carotid artery than untrained people of the same age. In addition, the pulse wave velocity was measurably slower in the trained individuals (see Vaitkevicius et al. 1993). In measurements of the dilation capability of the brachial artery comparing older endurance-trained individuals to untrained older people, a significantly improved vasoreactivity in favor of the trained population was recognized (see Rywik et al. 1999). Beere et al. (1999) found an increase in maximum leg blood flow during a stress situation after a three-month aerobic endurance training, which was practiced three times a week using the bicycle ergometer. This increase was 50% and was researched in older healthy men.

In the area of peripheral arterial occlusive disease (PAOD), medical exercise therapy is an essential therapeutic component. McDermott (2018) highlights in her meta-analysis the importance of walking and treadmill training for those affected in the area of the lower extremity.

In a systematic Cochrane Review with subsequent meta-analysis, it becomes clear that activity-oriented rehabilitation after myocardial infarction, revascularization, angina pectoris, or coronary heart disease brings significant advantages. In addition to a reduction in the mortality rate and the number of hospital admissions, training can contribute to an improvement in quality of life (see Anderson et al. 2016).

The effect of medical exercise therapy is not only evident in existing diseases of the cardiovascular system. Rather, regular physical training can produce a cardio-protective effect. This highlights the relevance of medical exercise therapy within prevention (see Valenzuela et al. 2023; Fiuza-Luces et al. 2018).

> **Practical Relevance**
> Continuous training of the cardiovascular system is capable of significantly slowing down aging processes, reducing pathophysiological changes, and producing preventive health-promoting effects.

3.2 Blood and Immune System

3.2.1 Age-Dependent or Disease-Associated Changes in the Blood and Immune System

With increasing age, the functionality of the human immune system reduces. External barriers such as the skin and mucous membranes decrease their ability to prevent pathogens from penetrating into the body due to structural and functional changes. This change can be accelerated by chronic stress, as the antibody production in the area of the mucous membranes is downregulated (see Freese and Proschinger 2020). This includes not only the mucous membranes of the urogenital system but also particularly the mucous membranes of the digestive system. The cause is that the barrier function of the epithelium decreases and at the same time changes in the pH value on the surface as well as the lipid composition and a reduced hydration of the stratum corneum are observed. These factors increase the risk of infections. In addition, the non-specific immune system is no longer as capable of responding to the chronic low-grade inflammation of the body that continues to increase with age. Thus, pathogens that have penetrated the body are less effectively combated by granulocytes, macrophages, dendritic cells or humoral mechanisms such as the complement system. On the side of the specific immune system, there is a reduced formation of naive T lymphocytes, B lymphocytes as well as a deteriorated diversity of the cells and the antibodies produced by these blood cells (see Großkopf and Simm 2022). This is primarily due to the reduction of the hematopoietic tissue in the bone marrow (see Djukic et al. 2014). The described changes can be summarized under the term immunosenescence.

3.2.2 Effects of Medical Training Therapy on the Blood and Immune System

Freese and Proschinger (2020) mention that the blood and immune system can be trained at any age. The prerequisite is adequate stress in the area of endurance and coordination training. A well-controlled high-intensity interval training (HIIT) can also achieve the desired effect. In particular, the form of interval training seems to have a positive influence on the immune system. The person performing the training should be stressed according to their fitness level. At the same time, regeneration phases (see Chap. 2), adapted to the intensity of the training, should be strictly adhered to. This can counteract the processes of immune senescence. Bloch (2019) adds in this context that regular physical stress can shift the release of pro-inflammatory cytokines towards an increased production of anti-inflammatory cytokines. Thus, the systematic low-grade inflammation that intensifies with age can be elegantly curbed. In addition to various organ systems and structures such as vessels, muscles, connective tissue, and heart, the brain in particular benefits from reduced neurodegeneration due to the positive immunological influence (cf. Bloch 2019).

In relation to altitude training, Gatterer and Faulhaber (2019) add that intermittent hypoxia is a suitable means to increase the number of erythrocytes and thus the oxygen transport capacity. For this purpose, a passive hypoxia exposure of 4–12 h at a (simulated altitude) of 2000–3000 m or higher is recommended. The training approach follows the philosophy of "live high—train low". The temporal approach of the intervention lasts several weeks and takes place on individual days to daily. McKenzie (2012) adds both a training-induced increase in plasma volume and total blood volume.

Zimmer et al. (2016) researched the effect of running a half marathon in women who were in rehabilitation after breast cancer. A healthy population acted as a control group. It was shown that the stress in the form of a half marathon in both groups leads to an increased number of T-killer cells and T-memory cells. Since these cells are capable of identifying and eliminating or recognizing tumor cells, improved endurance performance can be attributed to a more effective immune defense. In addition, further anti-inflammatory effects could be measured through the training. Otto and Ebner (2016) add in this context a reduction of the C-reactive protein, which could be caused by a six-week high-intensity endurance training.

However, the increase in T-killer cells does not necessarily require the half marathon distance. A 15-week training on the bicycle ergometer also resulted in an increase in the number of T-killer cells in postmenopausal breast cancer patients in aftercare. The intensity was set at 70–75% of maximum oxygen consumption. In the first three weeks, training was carried out three times a week for 15 min each. The training time was increased by 5 min every three weeks. Thus, the training time in weeks 13–15 was 35 min each (cf. Fairey et al. 2005).

In the guidelines of the American College of Sports Medicine, survivors of a cancer diagnosis are recommended to have 3–5 units of moderate physical activity of more than 30 min each week. Intense stresses of more than 20 min are also advocated three days a week (cf. Schmitz et al. 2010).

3.3 Lymphatic System

3.3.1 Age-Related or Disease-Associated Changes in the Lymphatic System

The most obvious symptom of a dysfunctional lymphatic system is lymphedema. Here, a distinction can be made between the primary and secondary forms. In the primary form, genetic factors lead to a suboptimal development of the lymphatic system. In addition to insufficient lymphatic valves, lymphatic vessels can show hyper- or hypoplastic changes, depending on the cause. Secondary lymphedemas, on the other hand, arise due to a blockage of lymphatic vessels. Obstructions can be triggered by progressive degenerative processes or poor quality nutrition, as well as by surgeries, radiation, or infections (see Cueni and Detmar 2008).

Diseases of the lymphatic system are also strongly associated with obesity. Obesity, in turn, represents a significant risk factor for the development of metabolic syndrome up to type 2 diabetes mellitus. The risk for cardiovascular diseases also increases significantly (see Jiang et al. 2019). The existence of the lymphatic system enables both the absorption of fats from food and the peripheral breakdown of cholesterol. The transport is largely ensured by the autonomously controlled smooth muscle of the lymphangions.

The lymphatic system is thus the integral link between the small intestine and the rest of the body in terms of the absorption and transport of lipids. There are indications that the morphology of the lymph capillaries in the area of the small intestine could have an influence on the development of obesity (see McDonald 2018). Furthermore, in areas of the body where there is damage to the lymphatic system, the accumulation of fat in the area of the lymphedema can often be observed (see Jiang et al. 2018). The accumulation of lymph fluid in the area of dysfunctional lymph vessels significantly reduces the accumulation of immunological cells. Thus, a reduced immune function in the area of lymphedemas can be assumed (see Chakraborty et al. 2019). If there is a diabetic metabolism, the lymphatic system may react with lymphangiogenesis and accelerated lymph transport due to the increased interstitial pressure (see Mottillo et al. 2010; Haemmerle et al. 2013). In summary, it can be stated that a dysfunctional lymphatic system is a risk factor for the development of overweight and at the same time overweight further restricts the functionality of the lymphatic system.

3.3.2 Effects of Medical Exercise Therapy on the Lymphatic System

Neudecker and Baumann (2016) recommend the implementation of dynamic strength training for women in rehabilitation after breast cancer. The practice of strength training can prevent the deterioration of an existing lymphedema (see Schmitz et al. 2009). In addition, strength training leads to a 70% reduction in the risk of developing a secondary lymphedema after resection of at least five lymph nodes (see Schmitz et al. 2010). During strength training, large muscle groups should be dynamically addressed to maximize the effect of the muscle pump (see Nelson 2016). Regarding intensity, 8–12 repetitions should be chosen at two to three sets and 60–80% load (see Neudecker and Baumann 2016).

In addition to the demonstrated effect of the muscle pump on extremities, conscious breathing can also have a reflux-promoting influence on the lymphatic system. Crucial here is a deep inhalation with as high an activation of the respiratory diaphragm and the inspiratory auxiliary muscles as possible (see Moriondo et al. 2005).

3.4 Respiratory System

3.4.1 Age-Dependent or Disease-Associated Changes in the Respiratory System

Age-related changes in the respiratory system extend across both the upper and lower respiratory tracts. In the area of the pharynx, muscular support recedes. This can lead to obstruction (see Berry et al. 1987). Furthermore, a decrease in reflex activity during coughing and swallowing can be observed. This is likely due to a reduction in afferents from the area of the pharynx as well as reduced central reflex activity. This circumstance increases the risk of aspiration (see Pontoppidan and Beecher 1960).

The lung tissue experiences a gradual decline in capillary supply, which can increase arterial blood pressure in the remaining capillaries by up to 30%, while pulmonary vascular resistance increases by up to 80% (see Davidson and Fee 1990). With regard to the alveolar surface, a reduction of about 30% is expected between the ages of 20 and 70 (see Kenney 1989). The bronchial tree and the alveolar ducts dilate with increasing age. These changes are referred to as ductectasia (see Ryan et al. 1965). The lung parenchyma gradually loses its support function, causing the air spaces to widen. This change can also be described as "senile emphysema" (see Sharma and Goodwin 2006). Sobin et al. (1988) add that the proportion of collagen tissue in the lungs of older people increases. An increasing proteolysis of elastin leads to a reduction of cross-links and a changed quantity and composition of lung surfactant.

In the area of the thorax, in addition to increasing stiffness due to the calcification of rib joints, muscular atrophy of the respiratory muscles can also be observed (see Turner et al. 1968). The respiratory diaphragm loses performance in the aging process (see Tolep et al. 1995). Furthermore, the intervertebral discs of the thoracic spine show an age-related height reduction, which can be accompanied by an increasing kyphosis (see Sharma and Goodwin 2006). The reduced mobility of the thorax in conjunction with an increasingly limited extension ability of the thoracic spine lead to a progressive deterioration of the expansion ability of the lung wings during inspiration.

The mentioned structural changes lead to a reduced diffusion capacity, an increase in anatomical and physiological dead space, an increased risk of tracheobronchial instability with premature closure of smaller airways, the development of a barrel chest, altered lung volumes as well as a mismatch between ventilation and perfusion with a progressive reduction in arterial oxygen supply. Normally, however, there is no arterial oxygen undersupply (see Grinton 1994). While the arterial oxygen supply continues to decrease with increasing age, the release of carbon dioxide remains possible (see Raine and Bishop 1963). While the residual volume and the functional residual volume increase with increasing age, the inspiratory and expiratory reserve volume decrease at the same time (see Zaugg and Lucchinetti 2000). The peak of maximum oxygen uptake (VO2max) is located in the third decade of life. After the age of thirty, about one percent of the VO2max is lost per year. It should be noted that the VO2max value is highly dependent on individual training status. McClaran et al. (1995) examined the change in VO2max in 18 very well-trained men over a period of six years. The average starting age was 67 years. The average VO2max value was 45 ml.kg−1.min−1. This value is approximately double the normal value for this age. Over the six-year period, this average fell by 11.2 ± 3.4%.

3.4.2 Effects of Medical Training Therapy on the Respiratory System

When considering minute ventilation, it can increase up to twentyfold during intense physical exertion. Thus, even in untrained individuals, the respiratory system has a very high adaptability to physical challenges. This characteristic distinguishes the respiratory system significantly from the cardiovascular system and the muscular system. Due to the naturally high tolerance to stress of the respiratory system, it is not surprising that the respiratory system hardly reacts structurally to training stimuli (see McKenzie 2012).

Functionally, endurance training can improve the endurance capacity of the respiratory muscles. In addition, training can lead to an increase in the force exerted by the respiratory muscles. These muscular adaptations, along with improved ventilation in conjunction with the cardiovascular system, the blood and immune system, and the muscular system, contribute to an improved maximum oxygen uptake (see McKenzie 2012).

Souza et al. (2014) investigated the effect of an eight-week strength training program in older women aged between 60 and 80 years.

The training was carried out twice daily over the two-month intervention period using a Threshold-IMT breathing trainer. The intensity was set at approximately 40%. The training increased the inspiratory pressure by 37%, while the expiratory pressure improved by 13%. The thickness of the respiratory diaphragm increased by 11%. In addition, the mobility of the respiratory diaphragm increased by 9%. Compared to the control group, the values generated by the intervention group were significantly superior. Similar effects can also be observed in people in their third decade of life when the intensity is increased to 80% (see Enright et al. 2006).

Langer et al. (2018) found that targeted training of the inspiratory respiratory muscles can reduce dyspnea in people with COPD during physical training.

3.5 Muscular System

3.5.1 Age-Dependent or Disease-Associated Changes in the Muscular System

Changes and maladaptations of muscular tissue during the aging process can be summarized under the term sarcopenia. This is a geriatric syndrome characterized by a reduction in muscle mass accompanied by a simultaneous decline in function (see Ferrari and Drey 2020). A main cause of muscular degeneration is physical inactivity, which often increases with advancing age. In addition, both metabolic and endocrinological changes in old age have their impact (see Seefried and Genest 2017). Kemmler et al. (2018) add that genetic and epigenetic factors, malnutrition and undernutrition, chronic inflammation, and an expansion of inhibitory factors of tissue regeneration also contribute to an increasing prevalence of sarcopenia with advancing age.

In a time span from the 20th to the 80th year of life, the number of muscle fibers in a human decreases by about 50% (see Drey 2011). Focused in the time after the 60th year of life, this process accelerates, mainly affecting the fast-twitch type 2 fibers compared to the slow-twitch type 1 fibers (see Verdijk et al. 2010). This morphological transformation of skeletal muscle into fat and connective tissue is causally related to a reduction in muscular performance. When comparing the muscle strength of 70-year-olds with that of 20-year-olds, a decrease in muscle strength of 20–40% can be measured. This loss of performance increases to 50% in the ninth decade of life (see Goodpaster et al. 2006). Regarding the functional deterioration of the muscular system, muscle power should be differentiated from muscle strength. Muscle power is understood as the combination of exerted muscle strength and its speed. In the process of sarcopenia, type II fibers are primarily affected, which primarily reduces muscle power (see Metter et al. 1997). In the everyday life of older people, a reduced muscle power primarily leads to restrictions of the physical system (see Bean et al. 2003).

From a structural perspective, changes in mitochondria can be observed in the aging process. The number of mitochondrial proteins decreases, while at the same time the activity of the remaining mitochondrial proteins decreases (see Rooyackers et al. 1997). Over time, these changes lead to a 50% reduction in oxidative capacity and thus a 50% loss of ATP supply to the skeletal muscles. An age-dependent reduction in aerobic capacity is the logical consequence (see Short et al. 2005).

Changes in the nervous system in aging humans also contribute to the development of sarcopenia. This is primarily due to a gradual decline of spinal motor neurons and a consequent reduction of motor units (see Roubenoff 2001). Up to the age of 60, the spinal motor nerve cells do not undergo any significant changes in terms of number. However, a massive decline of neurons in the anterior horn can be observed during the seventh decade of life (see Ling et al. 2009). The death of neurons mainly affects neurons that innervate fast-twitching type 2 fibers. This explains the atrophy of muscle mass. In part, type 2 muscle fibers are reinnervated by a slow-twitching neuron after the death of the originally supplying neuron. This process, referred to in English as "motor unit remodeling," maintains some residual function, but at the same time explains the progressive loss of precise movements, force development, and the slowing of motor skills (see Roth 2000). In addition to the spinal motor neurons, the motor end plate also undergoes age-related morphological changes. These primarily affect the postsynaptic membrane (see Wokke et al. 1990).

Another influencing factor that has a relationship to the development of sarcopenia is the hormone system. While the levels of anabolic hormones decrease in older people, the levels of catabolic hormones increase at the same time. The most important anabolic hormones in this context are testosterone and estrogen (see Wang et al. 2008). Age-related reduced levels of both hormones, in both males and females, drive the process of sarcopenia forward.

In addition to its own production of myokines, skeletal muscle also responds to cytokines. Here, a distinction can be made between catabolic and anabolic cytokines. In young years and a generally healthy lifestyle, these signaling substances maintain a stimulus-adapted physiological balance within the various organ systems. In the course of the aging process, pro-inflammatory cytokines gain the upper hand. This leads, in relation to the whole body, to an increase in low-grade inflammation (see Roubenoff et al. 1998; Harris et al. 1997; Payette et al. 2003). These factors lead to a decreased muscular performance and additionally significantly increase the risk of mortality (see Roubenoff et al. 2003).

In addition to physical inactivity, a lack of vitamin D and a deficient intake of proteins are factors that promote the process of sarcopenia (see Drey 2011).

Severe sarcopenia leads to a gradual loss of function in everyday activities, an increased risk of falls, an increased risk of fractures, a dwindling independence, and an increased risk of mortality (see Lauretani et al. 2003; Rolland et al. 2008).

3.5.2 Effects of Medical Training Therapy on the Muscular System

Regular training of the muscular system can enhance quality of life. In addition, it can reduce hospitalization rates and health problems. Also, due to the possibility of increasing individual lifespan, training of the muscular system should be an integral part of the therapy or prevention of sarcopenia (see Musumeci 2017).

Primarily, high-intensity resistance training is recommended. In addition to isometric training, dynamic forms of training should also be used (see Nicastro et al. 2011). Resistance training releases myokines from the activated muscles, which have a strengthening effect on the immune system and at the same time possess an anti-inflammatory effect. In addition, growth factors are released, which stimulate the proliferation of satellite cells and muscle fiber hypertrophy (see Spiering et al. 2008). In this context, it is possible to stimulate hypertrophy processes and simultaneously increase muscle strength by specifically addressing type II fibers (see Johnston et al. 2008).

The effects of strength training can be supplemented by aerobic endurance training (see Koopman et al. 2011). The effects of aerobic endurance training include an increase in the number of mitochondria with simultaneous improvement in bioenergetics, an improvement in protein synthesis and insulin sensitivity, as well as a reduction in oxidative stress and inflammatory processes (see Short et al. 2004). Endurance training is also capable of suppressing the expression of catabolic genes (see Erlich et al. 2016). In addition to suppressing the process of apoptosis in the muscles, endurance training can stimulate the process of autophagy (see Yan et al. 2012). Endurance training also slows down the expression of the extracellular cytokine myostatin, which is attributed to accelerating the process of sarcopenia (see Ko et al. 2014). In summary, it can be concluded that endurance training is capable of slowing down or preventing mitochondrial changes while simultaneously increasing muscle hypertrophy and muscle strength (see Yoo et al. 2018).

The regular combination of strength and endurance training is an essential component for the prevention and therapy of sarcopenia (see Yoo et al. 2018). The intensity should be as challenging as possible for the person performing both forms of training. Beckwée et al. (2019) recommend 80% intensity for strength training based on the individual's one-repetition maximum. Musumeci (2017) also mentions the potential of high-intensity endurance training in relation to endurance training.

3.6 Central and Peripheral Nervous System

3.6.1 Age-Dependent or Disease-Associated Changes in the Central and Peripheral Nervous System

Günnewig et al. (2022) explain that about 65% of functional limitations in people aged 65 and over are due to changes in the nervous system. These limitations manifest themselves in a deteriorating auditory, optical, thermal, and tactile stimulus reception, in mobility restrictions, gait uncertainty, and balance problems (see Verdú et al. 2000). The age-dependent changes affect both the central and peripheral nervous system.

The brain can show a weight reduction of 10–20% in old age (see Svennerholm et al. 1997). Low physical activity and high inflammation levels are drivers of volume reduction (see Braskie et al. 2014). The changes in the central nervous system extend to both white and gray matter. From about the age of 20, the brain loses an estimated 1,000–100,000 nerve cells daily. The decline in total neurons amounts to about a third by the age of 80. In addition to cell death, which is caused by pre-programmed apoptosis or other influences such as trauma, aging neurons show a decrease in volume, which can be associated with functional limitations. The process of nerve cell shrinkage is reversible compared to cell death (see Klimaschewski 2021). This change affects the brain and, from a motor perspective, particularly the anterior horn of the spinal cord (see Roubenoff 2001). The death of neurons mainly affects neurons that innervate fast-twitching type 2 fibers. This explains the atrophy of muscle mass. In part, type 2 muscle fibers are reinnervated by a slow-twitching neuron after the death of the originally supplying neuron (see Roth 2000). A similar takeover of functions is also found in brain neurons. Thus, functions can be maintained into old age through neuroplastic processes, even with a gradually dwindling number of nerve cells (see Svennerholm et al. 1997).

At the same time, the blood supply to the approximately 80 billion nerve cells, which are supplied via a network of over 600 km, also changes in the aging brain. In addition to arteriosclerotic changes, changes are found in the blood-brain barrier. The supply of glucose and water-soluble molecules is reduced. Proteins, which cannot pass the blood-brain barrier in young years, reach the neurons in the aged brain and stimulate inflammatory processes there (see Klimaschewski 2021).

The white matter of the central and peripheral nervous system also shows structural changes with increasing age. In particular, a decrease in myelination should be mentioned here. The diameter of the nerve fiber is smaller and less circularly shaped. This leads to a reduction in conduction speed (see Günnewig et al. 2022).

An age-dependent reduction of peripheral receptors, such as Pacini and Meissner receptors, leads to a gradually deteriorating afferent information supply to the central nervous system (see Ebenbichler and Kerschan-Schindl 2009).

3.6.2 Effects of Medical Training Therapy on the Central and Peripheral Nervous System

Cotman et al. (2007) report that physical activity is capable of making a significant contribution to maintaining brain health. Training is able to improve the uptake and storage of information in memory. In addition, it can benefit from a protective effect against neurodegenerative changes and an antidepressant effect. Neuroplastic processes can be stimulated by physical activity. In addition to synaptic plasticity, the process of neurogenesis is also stimulated (see Cotman et al. 2007).

To best stimulate neurogenesis in the hippocampus, Curlik 2nd and Shors (2013) recommend combining physical and mental training. Firth et al. (2018) were able to show in the publication of a meta-analysis that aerobic endurance training can contribute a protective effect to the preservation of the left hippocampus volume. Even in people in their eighth decade of life, a significant increase in the volume of the left hippocampus can be observed through 24 months of physical training at moderate intensity (see Rosano et al. 2017).

Essentially, forms of training such as dancing, which require intensive collaboration between the brain and muscles, can contribute positively to improved cognitive functions. In addition, positive effects on executive function, delayed recall ability, verbal fluency, working memory function, and attention in older people with mild cognitive impairments can be observed (see Biazus-Sehn et al. 2020). General strength and endurance training can also have a positive effect on cognition (see Landrigan et al. 2020; Guadagni et al. 2020).

The morphology of the basal ganglia also correlates with the level of physical fitness. The volume of the basal ganglia can provide insights into motor performance and executive control. Similar to the hippocampus, the basal ganglia also respond to regular training with a structural change. A twelve-month coordination training was able to induce a volume increase of the caudate nucleus and the globus pallidus (see Niemann et al. 2014).

However, the mentioned positive effects of medical training therapy cannot be explained solely by an increase in volume of individual brain areas. Gogniat et al. (2021) found in a meta-analysis that training in people aged 60 and over does not significantly increase brain volume. In contrast to this are the research results of Colcombe et al. (2006), who were able to detect a volume increase of both gray and white matter through a six-month aerobic endurance training in people aged 60–79 years.

Endurance training also has the property of increasing the blood flow to the brain. Compared to the resting state, the blood flow to the brain can be increased by about 20% during endurance stress with an intensity of about 50%–80%. This represents the highest level of brain blood flow. If the intensity of 80% is exceeded, the brain blood flow decreases compared to 50%–80% intensity from about 20% to about 10% increased blood flow (see Smith and Ainslie 2017).

Medical training therapy is also capable of preventing depression. This effect can be observed at low and high intensities of training (see Hu et al. 2020). In addition, physical activity represents a promising therapy option for existing depression (see Philippot et al. 2022). Both regular endurance and strength training, or a combination of both, can lead to the desired antidepressant effect (see Zhao et al. 2020).

The described training-induced changes can mainly be explained by the influence on neurotrophic factors. The growth factor BDNF plays a fundamental role in synaptic plasticity, the survival and growth of neurons, neurogenesis, and memory function (see Cowansage et al. 2010). The BDNF gene and protein expression is increased by physical training in the area of the hippocampus and maintains the increased level for a period of two weeks after training (see Berchtold et al. 2010). Another neurotrophic factor, which interacts closely with BDNF, is IGF-1 (see Gomez-Pinilla et al. 2008). Both IGF-1 and the neurotrophic factor VEGF participate in the training-induced remodeling of blood vessels, particularly the endothelial cells, and the angiogenesis of the brain-supplying vessels (see Lopez-Lopez et al. 2004; Ding et al. 2004). Medical training therapy is thus capable of stimulating or increasing both neurogenesis and cerebral blood volume (see van der Borght et al. 2009).

3.7 Digestive System

3.7.1 Age-Dependent or Disease-Associated Changes in the Digestive System

The aging process globally impairs the functions of the digestive system. This includes processes such as motility, hormone and enzyme secretion, and digestion and absorption processes (see Dumic et al. 2019).

In the area of the oral cavity, there is an age-related reduction in saliva mass and its function due to a changed saliva composition. This circumstance can lead to oral-sensory symptoms (see Nagler and Hershkovich 2005). In addition, the swallowing reflex can be impaired due to deteriorated neuromuscular control (see Durazzo et al. 2017).

Some studies have found that the peristalsis of the esophagus is more susceptible to faulty contractions in old age and that the transport of food within the esophagus takes longer (see Ferriolli et al. 1996). The altered motility of the esophagus could not always be confirmed in similar studies and therefore does not seem to be transferable to every older population (see Robson and Glick 2003). The occurrence of these symptoms suggests a decline in intrinsic neurons (see Saffrey 2013).

The aging stomach is characterized by altered gastric microbiota, a reduced protective function of the gastric mucosa, and a decrease in blood flow. The latter complicates repair processes in the stomach area (see Parsons et al. 2017). Regarding the motility of the stomach in older people, research results diverge. While Madsen and Graff (2004) could not detect any change in motility in relation to age and BMI, Shimamoto et al. (2002) were able to identify a reduced contractility of the stomach muscles. This was particularly evident in older inactive people. Similar to the motility of the esophagus, the death of enteric neurons also seems to be a main cause for the altered muscular control in the stomach area.

In the area of the small intestine, no impairments of the absorption function can be detected in older people. The hormonal secretion is also unchanged compared to younger people (see D'Souza 2007). Due to a higher proliferation and differentiation of enterocytes, the intestinal architecture can be maintained even at an advanced age (see Ciccocioppo 2002). With increasing age, the risk of angiodysplasias in the area of the small intestine also increases. These are acquired changes in arterial and venous capillaries as well as larger arteries and veins. Angiodysplasias are characterized by an increasing thinness of the vessel wall, convolutions, and an expansion of the blood vessels. This increases the risk of bleeding (see Lewis 2000). Another age-dependent condition is the bacterial overgrowth of the small intestine. This is predominant when the small intestine aspirate per milliliter shows a presence of bacteria over 10^5–10^6 (see Dukowicz 2007). It has been shown that bacterial overgrowth of the small intestine occurs significantly more frequently in older people than in younger people (see Parlesak et al. 2003). Clinically, bacterial overgrowth of the small intestine can manifest itself through chronic diarrhea, malabsorption of nutrients, weight loss, and secondary malnutrition (see Dumic et al. 2019). Mitsui mentions that physical inactivity, in addition to age and the geographical location of the place of residence, is another risk factor for the development of bacterial overgrowth of the small intestine (see Mitsui et al. 2003). Altered motility of the small intestine also appears to be another risk factor for bacterial overgrowth. However, the motility of the small intestine is not restricted by the aging process itself, but primarily by medications and comorbidities (see Dumic et al. 2019).

In the area of the large intestine, there are diametric findings as to whether age can influence motility. While Madsen and Graff (2004) consider an age dependency of the motility of the large intestine to be given, the research results of Metcalf et al. (1987) contradict this. The suspected causes of slowed motility also include a decline in neurons and an increasing absence of neurotransmitters in the area of the large intestine (see Hanani et al. 2004; Takahashi et al. 2000). A much more clearly emerging age-dependent characteristic of the large intestine, however, is the change in the microbiota (see Magrone and Jirillo 2013). In old age, the composition of the individual strains of the microbiota changes away from the optimum. This results in the release of pro-inflammatory cytokines, which maintain a low-grade inflammation of the large intestine (see Larbi et al. 2008). This condition is supported by the fact that short-chain fatty acids, which are produced by the microbiota and have an anti-inflammatory and antineoplastic effect, are produced to a lesser extent by older people (see De Vuyst and Leroy 2011).

3.7.2 Effects of Medical Exercise Therapy on the Digestive System

Depending on the type, intensity, and training condition, medical exercise therapy can produce both negative and positive effects on the digestive system (see Bi and Triadafilopoulos. 2003).

Clark et al. (1989) found that physical stress is associated with an increase in gastroesophageal reflux. It should be noted that gastroesophageal reflux is mainly stimulated by stresses that involve a high degree of physical movement, such as running. Compared to running, the stimulation of gastroesophageal reflux during training on a bicycle ergometer is less. If food is consumed immediately before training, the occurrence of gastroesophageal reflux significantly increases. Therefore, it is advised against eating directly before physical stress (see Yazaki et al. 1996). The cause of gastroesophageal reflux is suspected to be a training-induced pressure reduction of the lower esophageal sphincter (see Peters et al. 1988).

Another factor that can be influenced by physical activity is the speed of gastric emptying. Studies show that endurance stresses below 70% of maximum oxygen uptake have no or only a slight stimulating effect on the speed of gastric emptying. Stresses above 70% of maximum oxygen uptake, on the other hand, slow down gastric emptying. Similarly, only very high endurance stresses inhibit the production of stomach acid (see Bi and Triadafilopoulos. 2003).

Cheng et al. (2003) found that regular moderate endurance training can reduce the risk of peptic duodenal ulcers in men. However, severe physical stresses during training or at work do not seem to contribute to prevention (see Shephard 2017).

In the area of the small intestine, high-intensity endurance stress can increase the risk of impaired nutrient absorption. In addition, strong endurance stress increases the risk of bleeding in the area of the small and large intestine (see Bi and Triadafilopoulos. 2003). However, the colon can also benefit from moderate physical activity in terms of reducing the risk of colon cancer (see Giovannucci et al. 1995). In addition, medical exercise therapy has a preventive character on diverticulitis (see Aldoori et al. 1995).

In summary, it can be concluded that intestinal ischemia during high-intensity endurance stress, together with possible dehydration, increases the risk of nausea, vomiting, abdominal pain, and bloody diarrhea. These symptoms occur 1.5 to 3 times more frequently in very well-trained athletes than in less well-trained individuals (see de Oliveira and Burini 2009).

3.8 Urinary System

3.8.1 Age-Dependent or Disease-Associated Changes in the Urinary System

From the age of 20, aging processes can be observed in the urinary system (see Chmielewski et al. 2016). From the age of 40, renal blood flow decreases by about 10% per decade. While the blood flow at the age of 40 is 600 ml/min/1.73 m^2, it decreases to 300 ml/min/1.73 m^2 at the age of 80 (see Macías-Núñez et al. 2008; Halter et al. 2009). Due to the large reserve capacity of the kidneys, these age-related changes do not negatively affect homeostasis or electrolyte concentration in healthy individuals (see Chmielewski et al. 2016).

However, in old age, it can happen that the functional reserve of the kidneys is exhausted. At this age, only about half of the glomeruli are still functioning. This is also reflected in the glomerular filtration rate, which decreases from 120 ml/min to 65 ml/min between the ages of 40 and 85 (see Weinstein and Anderson 2010). This is due to increasing glomerulosclerosis, tubulointerstitial fibrosis, and atrophy of the renal blood vessels. These structural changes also bring functional consequences. Processes of secretion and reabsorption can no longer proceed as required. This manifests itself in a deteriorated excretion of the urinary substances uric acid, urea, and creatinine. The ability to concentrate urine also decreases. These factors increase the risk of dehydration in older people (see Seeley and Stephens 2008).

Important for understanding the described changes in the kidneys is that comorbidities occurring in parallel with the aging process make a significant contribution to the reduction of kidney function. Known comorbidities include atherosclerosis, left ventricular dysfunction, heart failure, glucose intolerance, diabetes mellitus, and obesity. Smokers also carry an increased risk of accelerating renal degeneration (see Fliser 2008).

In addition to the changes in the kidneys, the issue of stress incontinence should also be addressed here. Urinary incontinence specifically affects women over the age of 65. About 1.5 million women over the age of 65 suffer from urinary incontinence. This corresponds to a percentage of about 14%. Risk factors for stress incontinence include obesity, changes in hormonal situation, previous births, and surgical interventions in the pelvic area (see Loertzer and Schneider 2013). On a structural level, a loosening of the ligament apparatus and insufficient neural control or reduced recruitment of the pelvic floor muscles can be mentioned pathophysiologically (see Loertzer and Schneider 2013).

The problem of stress incontinence, however, does not only occur in the third life tertile, but is also a noteworthy subject in female elite athletes. The prevalence of urinary incontinence in elite female athletes varies depending on the sport. Sports with a higher prevalence include compositional sports as well as ball and racket games. In both categories, prevalence values of up to 70% can be observed (see Schulte-Frei and Jäger 2018). Influencing factors include structural dysfunctions, training content, hormonal situation, and psychological influences.

3.8.2 Effects of Medical Exercise Therapy on the Urinary System

Physical activity in the form of combined endurance and strength training is capable of preventing or significantly slowing down comorbidities that negatively affect kidney function (see Schmitt et al. 2019).

For example, if it is possible to positively influence or prevent hyperglycemia and a diabetic metabolism through regular endurance training, this has immediate protective effects on kidney function. Training-induced reduced blood sugar levels can prevent pro-inflammatory and fibrotic signaling pathways. This reduces the risk of nephropathy (see Garud and Kulkarni 2014). Furthermore, by lowering blood pressure, oxidative stress can be reduced and endothelial function can be improved at the same time (see Mennuni et al. 2014).

Meredith et al. (1991) investigated the influence of endurance training on renal-sympathetic nerve activity. For this purpose, the participants practiced a training session on the bicycle ergometer three times a week over a one-month period at 60%–70% of their VO2max. In addition to a highly significant decrease in resting blood pressure, a significant improvement in VO2max was demonstrated. In addition, a reduction of total peripheral nerve activity by 24% was demonstrated. Specifically, renal-sympathetic nerve activity decreased by 41%. These 41% accounted for 66% of the effect on the entire organism. The reduction in renal-sympathetic nerve activity leads to a reduced reabsorption of sodium and can therefore influence blood pressure in a lowering manner (see Schmitt et al. 2019). In addition, the risk of kidney failure during training is minimized, as the vasoconstriction of the renal vessels is weakened (see Farrell et al. 2011).

In summary, a combination of endurance and strength training can be recommended for positively influencing kidney function (see Johansen 2005).

Specifically, medical training interventions that emphasize the pelvic floor muscles can have a direct influence on the urinary system. Training the targeted recruitment of the pelvic floor muscles can counteract stress incontinence (see Soave et al. 2019). It should be noted that targeted instruction is necessary for successful strengthening of the pelvic floor muscles. During training, visualization of the contraction through electromyography is recommended. The goals of medical exercise therapy include targeted recruitment of the pelvic floor muscles, extension of contraction times, and increased muscle strength (see Loertzer and Schneider 2013). Radzimińska et al. (2018) state in a systematic review, which includes information from 24 studies with a total of 2394 women, that training the pelvic floor muscles has a positive effect on urinary incontinence. In addition, the quality of life in people with urinary incontinence is increased. Jacomo et al. (2020) add that local and specific training of the pelvic floor muscles is the gold standard and no other forms of training lead to improved strength of the pelvic floor muscles.

3.9 Sexual System

3.9.1 Age-Dependent or Disease-Associated Changes in the Reproductive System

3.9.1.1 Age-Dependent or Disease-Associated Changes in the Male Reproductive System

After the testes gain volume between the ages of 11–30 years and subsequently maintain this volume between the ages of 30–60, the testicular volume consistently decreases from around the age of 60 (see Yang et al. 2011). While the average serum levels of gonadotropins are significantly increased with age, free testosterone in the serum is reduced (see Mahmoud et al. 2003). The increase in gonadotropins is largely due to a gradual loss of testicular function and can also be associated with an age-related reduction in Leydig cells (see Gunes et al. 2016). From the age of 40, a steady decrease in testicular metabolism can be observed (see Well et al. 2007).

Another widespread age-dependent change in the male reproductive system is benign prostatic hyperplasia. Approximately 80% of men over the age of 80 have benign prostatic hyperplasia (see Gunes et al. 2016).

Various semen parameters also undergo age-dependent changes. There is a negative correlation between daily sperm production, the total number of sperm, their lifespan, and increasing age. By the age of 50, daily sperm production is already reduced by about 30% (see Neaves et al. 1984).

3.9.1.2 Age-Dependent or Disease-Associated Changes in the Female Reproductive System

Perhaps the most significant age-dependent change in the female reproductive system is the process of menopause. Most women go through this process around the age of 51 (see Treloar 1981). Menopause begins at a time when the ovarian follicle reserve is almost depleted and initially manifests in increasingly irregular menstrual cycles. Once the follicle reserve is depleted, this also has immediate effects on the hormone system, as the follicles also produce a large proportion of the ovarian hormones and peptide hormones. Through the process of menopause, the plasma levels of these hormones drop rapidly and remain at a low level for the remaining lifetime (see Wise 2005).

The great loss of estrogens, progestogens, and peptide hormones not only has consequences for the female reproductive system but also affects other body structures and functions. In addition to bone and mineral metabolism, memory function and cognition are also negatively affected. Furthermore, there are negative consequences for the cardiovascular system as well as the immune system (see Wise 2005).

3.9.2 Effects of Medical Exercise Therapy on the Sexual System

3.9.2.1 Effects of Medical Exercise Therapy on the Male Sexual System

The evidence on the effect of medical exercise therapy on various semen parameters is predominantly heterogeneous. When reviewing existing literature on the topic, the type and intensity of training, in addition to diet, determine the effect. For example, if high-intensity training or specific activities are practiced, this leads to an increase in reactive oxygen species in the testes. This increases oxidative stress and leads to impaired semen parameters and fertility. Male libido can also be negatively affected by high-intensity endurance training (see Hackney et al. 2017). On the other hand, if training of low or moderate intensity is practiced, this leads to a reduction in the testicular reactive oxygen species and thus to a positive influence on semen parameters and fertility (see Belladelli et al. 2023).

To reduce the risk of suffering from benign prostatic hyperplasia, Williams (2008) recommends a weekly running distance of 16 to over 48 kilometers as a preventive measure. The research group around Nagakura (2022) also advocates daily physical activity as a component of prevention against benign prostatic hyperplasia.

Moderate to intense endurance training can be used as an effective means for erectile dysfunction. This information was calculated from a meta-analysis, which includes a population of a total of 478 participants (see Silva et al. 2017).

3.9.2.2 Effects of Medical Exercise Therapy on the Female Sexual System

A meta-analysis published by Mena et al. in 2019 concludes that physical activity is an affordable and practical way to supplement female fertility treatments (see Mena et al. 2019).

Even when early postmenopausal symptoms occur, dietary counseling and physical activity can improve quality of life (see Asghari et al. 2017). Within the climacteric, Hao et al. (2022) advocate regular intensive strength training. Women in the postmenopausal stage also benefit from physical training in terms of their bone density (see Kemmler et al. 2020). In terms of the form of training, proprioceptive training should also be implemented in addition to strength training (see Moreira et al. 2014). It has been shown that a twelve-week intervention program, which includes strength training, proprioceptive training, and endurance loads, has a function-promoting effect in postmenopausal women suffering from osteoporosis (see FilipoviĆ et al. 2021). Menopausal metabolic disorders can also be largely curbed with physical activity (see Marsh et al. 2023). For example, if postmenopausal hypertension occurs, aerobic endurance training is a suitable therapeutic measure (see Lin and Lee 2018).

3.10 Skin System

3.10.1 Age-Dependent or Disease-Associated Changes in the Skin System

The aging process of the skin is a multifactorial process. In addition to genetics and age, exposure to sunlight and its intensity also play a significant role in skin aging. Clinically, fine lines, altered pigmentation, and a loss of elasticity can be observed in aged skin. A significant reason for the thinning of the epidermis is the reduced proliferation of keratinocyte stem cells and their dwindling number (see Ho and Dreesen 2021). This aging phenomenon can be accelerated in women in the postmenopausal stage of life due to reduced estrogen levels (see Farage et al. 2013). The proliferation of keratinocytes is further negatively affected by the flattening of the transition zone between the epidermis and dermis, as the nutrient supply to the epidermis is worsened. At the same time, shear forces can be less well compensated (see Lavker et al. 1989).

The number or activity of melanocytes also changes with age. This can result in areas of the outer skin appearing hypopigmented or hyperpigmented (see Ortonne 1990).

The dermis also loses volume and thickness with increasing age. This is due to a reduced production of collagenous tissue. In addition, the construction of the elastic fibers also changes. This results in an increasing loss of elasticity and the appearance of wrinkles is favored (see Farage et al. 2013; Lavker et al. 1989). With increasing age, the oxidative stress of the skin increases and a pro-inflammatory milieu intensifies (see Ho and Dreesen 2021).

The aging process not only changes the epidermis and the dermis in isolation, but there is also an impairment of the cooperation between both skin layers. Specifically, the paracrine signal transmission between the dermal fibroblasts and the epidermal keratinocytes is slowed down (see Russo et al. 2020). Another age-related change in the skin system is the gradual degeneration of mitochondria. This process can be further driven by excessive exposure to UV radiation (see Krutmann and Schroeder 2009). It can be concluded that both increased oxidative stress during the aging process and mitochondrial aging are important influencing factors for potential diseases of the skin system (see Babbar et al. 2020).

3.10.2 Effects of Medical Training Therapy on the Skin System

Medical training therapy is capable of making a positive contribution to venous leg ulcers, psoriasis, and the process of skin aging (see Yeh et al. 2022).

By performing high-intensity aerobic endurance training, which exceeds a weekly training time of 4 hours, it becomes possible for the trainee to significantly slow down the thinning of the stratum corneum. An increased mitochondrial biogenesis, which can be detected after the aforementioned form of training, is another indicator for the slowing down of skin aging through targeted training intervention (see Crane et al. 2015).

A review by Yeroushalmi et al. (2022) deals with the influence of physical training on the disease pattern of psoriasis. The authors conclude that regular moderate to intensive physical activity can make a positive contribution to psoriasis. From a physiological point of view, it is suspected that the main effect results from the training-induced reduction of low-grade inflammation. Particularly overweight people suffering from psoriasis benefit from a diet and training-induced weight loss (see Naldi et al. 2014).

People suffering from venous leg ulcers can, if they have the ability to move, be recommended a combination of progressive strengthening exercises for the calf muscles and a walking activity of at least 30 minutes at least three times a week (see Jull et al. 2018).

Untrained people are not advised to do irregular high-intensity or very long anaerobic training. Tendentially, diseases such as androgenetic alopecia or skin cancer can even be favored by the training-induced oxidative stress (see Yeh et al. 2022).

3.11 Hormone System

3.11.1 Age-Dependent or Disease-Associated Changes in the Hormone System

In men, the gradual decline in serum testosterone levels begins between the ages of 30 and 40. From that starting point, serum testosterone levels decrease by about one percent per year (see Feldman et al. 2002). In females, the testosterone circulating in the blood system decreases vehemently between the ages of 20 and 45 (see Morley and Perry 2003). Testosterone plays an important role in the regeneration of skeletal muscle, particularly in protein synthesis. The age-related decline in testosterone levels leads to a reduction in muscle mass and muscle strength. This primarily affects the male sex (see Baumgartner et al. 1999).

Menopause is characterized by a significant drop in estrogen levels. From a physiological perspective, estrogens are characterized by positive effects on muscle strength and regeneration through the activation of satellite cells and their proliferation. These functions weaken postmenopausally (see Horstman et al. 2012).

Also age-related, the levels of dehydroepiandrosterone decrease. This is a natural steroid and precursor hormone, which is produced by the adrenal glands. The skeletal muscle is capable of converting dehydroepiandrosterone into active androgens or estrogens. At the same time, muscle growth and muscular regeneration are stimulated (see Maggio et al. 2013).

The aging process also brings about negative changes in the hypothalamic-pituitary-adrenal axis. Specifically, there is an increasing release of glucocorticoids from the adrenal cortex (see Vitale et al. 2013). Elevated levels of glucocorticoids inhibit protein synthesis within the skeletal muscle and stimulate proteolysis. These effects lead to a catabolic metabolic state (see Bodine and Furlow 2015).

These negative effects are supported by gradually declining levels of growth hormone (GH) and insulin-like growth factor 1 (IGF-1). This is due to a changed physiology of the hypothalamic-pituitary axis (see Vitale et al. 2016). The decline in GH and IGF-1 levels starts around the age of 30 and leads to a reduction of about 14% per additional decade in terms of GH (see Veldhuis et al. 1995).

A deficiency in vitamin D has negative consequences on muscle metabolism (see Halfon et al. 2015). If there is a vitamin D deficiency, there is an excessive release of parathyroid hormone. Animal experiments have shown that an elevated level of parathyroid hormone has a negative effect on energy and protein metabolism (see Baczynski et al. 1985). Research findings suggest a correlation between low vitamin D serum levels and reduced muscle strength or physical performance (see Janssen et al. 2002). In summary, it can be mentioned that people over 65 years of age with reduced 25-hydroxyvitamin-D levels or elevated levels of parathyroid hormone have a higher risk of sarcopenia (see Visser et al. 2003).

The amount of ghrelin produced in the stomach decreases with age. This leads to a suppression of appetite. This could result in a reduced protein intake and thus a promotion of sarcopenia (see Ueno et al. 2010).

As in other tissues, the insulin sensitivity of skeletal muscle decreases with increasing age (see Churchward-Venne et al. 2014). This can negatively affect the protein synthesis of skeletal muscle. At the same time, the risk of a diabetic metabolism increases (see Umegaki 2016).

Another risk factor for the development of sarcopenia is the age-related decline in oxytocin levels. In animal experiments, these can have a performance-reducing effect on muscle stem cells and the regeneration of skeletal muscle (see Elabd et al. 2014).

In summary, it can be concluded that various age-related hormonal influences affect the onset and speed of sarcopenia (see Vitale et al. 2016).

3.11.2 Effects of Medical Training Therapy on the Hormonal System

Janssen (2016) extensively studied the effects of various training interventions on the hormonal system. It is noted that physical training is capable of positively influencing the aging hormonal system. This fact becomes evident in various parts of the hormonal system. There is evidence that intense anaerobic training of short duration can temporarily significantly increase the levels of GH and IGF-1 (see Cappon et al. 1994; Amir et al. 2007). This stimulates the anabolic metabolism of skeletal muscle. This effect seems to benefit especially people with an already very good fitness level (see Amir et al. 2007). The levels of circulating GH can also be achieved gender-unspecifically through maximum or hypertrophy strength training (see Kraemer et al. 1991).

Physical activity is also capable of inducing changes in the male sexual hormones. Ten repeated intense sprints of 30 seconds each resulted in increased levels of circulating total testosterone, free testosterone, and dihydrotestosterone in young healthy men (see Smith et al. 2013). Elias et al. (1993) also found an increase in circulating testosterone in young active men through progressive high-intensity stress. In 102 predominantly sedentary men aged between 40 and 75 years, the effect of six times weekly aerobic endurance training on the hormonal system was examined. After a twelve-month intervention period, an increase in dihydrotestosterone value of 8.6% was observed. The values of free testosterone and testosterone did not change noticeably (Hawkins et al. 2008). In amateur athletes who ran the marathon distance, the testosterone value, serum levels of luteinizing hormone, and sex hormone-binding globulin decreased shortly after the stress (see Kuusi et al. 1984).

In the female reproductive system, physical activity can also have effects on the hormonal system. If high-intensity and high-volume training is regularly performed, this can negatively affect the menstrual cycle and reduce the release of sexual hormones. Regarding cancer diseases, it should be noted that low levels of sexual hormones are not necessarily to be considered negative (see McTiernan 2008). Women who consider themselves physically inactive and are above the median of the body mass index (BMI) have higher estrogen levels than active normal-weight individuals (McTiernan et al. 2006). In postmenopausal physically inactive and overweight women aged between 50 and 75 years, a twelve-month aerobic endurance training of moderate intensity significantly reduced estrogen levels. The training included five weekly training sessions of 45 minutes each (see McTiernan et al. 2004).

During physical training, the levels of circulating cortisol increase due to a response of the hypothalamic-pituitary-adrenal axis. The higher the stress, the more cortisol is released by the adrenal glands. The increased release of cortisol during physical activity has been researched as gender-independent in resistance training. Endurance-trained people show a reduced cortisol release during resistance training (see Kraemer and Ratamess 2005). A good fitness condition can prevent a slowing down of the reduction of cortisol levels after stress (see Traustadóttir et al. 2004).

A meta-analysis published in 2019 discusses the influence of training on the process of insulin resistance. It can be noted that regular aerobic endurance training is capable of therapeutically or preventively counteracting the process of insulin resistance (see Kumar et al. 2019). A key factor here is the improvement or maintenance of insulin sensitivity (see Conn et al. 2014).

In addition, reference should be made at this point in the book to Sect. 1.3.7. There you will find information on the topic of myokines.

References

Aldoori W, Giovannucci E, Rimm E, Ascherio A, Stampfer M, Colditz G, Willett W (February 1995) Prospective study of physical activity and the risk of symptomatic diverticular disease in men. Gut 36(2):276–282. https://doi.org/10.1136/gut.36.2.276

Amir R, Ben-Sira D, Sagiv M (1. June 2007) Igf-I and fgf-2 responses to wingate anaerobic test in older men. J Sports Sci Med 6(2):227–232

Anderson L, Oldridge N, Thompson D, Zwisler A-D, Rees K, Martin N, Taylor R (5. January 2016) Exercise-based cardiac rehabilitation for coronary heart disease: cochrane systematic review and meta-analysis. J Am Coll Cardiol 67(1):1–12. https://doi.org/10.1016/j.jacc.2015.10.044

Asghari M, Mirghafourvand M, Mohammad-Alizadeh-Charandabi S, Malakouti J, Nedjat S (February 2017) Effect of aerobic exercise and nutrition educationon quality of life and early menopause symptoms: a randomized controlled trial. Women Health 57(2):173–188. https://doi.org/10.1080/03630242.2016.1157128

Babbar M, Basu S, Yang B, Croteau D, Bohr V (2020) Mitophagy and DNA damage signaling in human aging. Mech Ageing Dev 186:111207

Baczynski R, Massry S, Magott M, el-Belbessi S, Kohan R, Brautbar N (November 1985) Effect of parathyroid hormone on energy metabolism of skeletal muscle. Kidney Int 28(5):722–727. https://doi.org/10.1038/ki.1985.190

Baumgartner R, Waters D, Gallagher D, Morley J, Garry P (1. March 1999) Predictors of skeletal muscle mass in elderly men and women. Mech Ageing

Dev 107(2):123–136. https://doi.org/10.1016/s0047-6374(98)00130-4

Bean J, Leveille S, Kiely D, Bandinelli S, Guralnik J, Ferrucci L (August 2003) A comparison of leg power and leg strength within the InCHIANTI study: which influences mobility more? J Gerontol A Biol Sci Med Sci 58(8):728–733. https://doi.org/10.1093/gerona/58.8.m728

Beckwée D, Delaere A, Aelbrecht S, Baert V, Beaudart C, Bruyere O, Sarcopenia Guidelines Development Group of the Bel (25. Apriel (2019) Exercise interventions for the prevention and treatment of sarcopenia. A systematic umbrella review. J Nutr Health Aging 23:494–502. https://doi.org/10.1007/s12603-019-1196-8

Beere P, Russell S, Morey M, Kitzman D, Higginbotham M (7. September 1999) Aerobic exercise training can reverse age-related peripheral circulatory changes in healthy older men. Circulation 10:1085–1094. https://doi.org/10.1161/01.cir.100.10.1085

Belladelli F, Basran S, Eisenberg M (July 2023) Male fertility and physical exercise. World J Mens Health 41(3):482–488. https://doi.org/10.5534/wjmh.220199

Berchtold N, Castello N, Cotman C (19. May 2010) Exercise and time-dependent benefits to learning and memory. Neuroscience 167(3):588–597. https://doi.org/10.1016/j.neuroscience.2010.02.050

Berry D, Phillips B, Cook Y, Schmitt F, Gilmore R, Patel R, Tyre E (November 1987) Sleep-disordered breathing in healthy aged persons: possible daytime sequelae. J Gerontol 42(6):620–626. https://doi.org/10.1093/geronj/42.6.620

Bi L, Triadafilopoulos G (September 2003) Exercise and gastrointestinal function and disease: an evidence-based review of risks and benefits. Clin Gastroenterol Hepatol 1(5):345–355. https://doi.org/10.1053/S1542-3565(03)00178-2

Biazus-Sehn L, Schuch F, Firth J, Stigger F (July-August 2020) Effects of physical exercise on cognitive function of older adults with mild cognitive impairment: a systematic review and meta-analysis. Arch Gerontol Geriatr 89:104048. https://doi.org/10.1016/j.archger.2020.104048

Bloch W (October 2019) Immunsystem und Sport – eine wechselhafte Beziehung. Dtsch Z Sportmed 70:217–218. https://doi.org/10.5960/dzsm.2019.399

Bodine S, Furlow J (2015) Glucocorticoids and skeletal muscle. Adv Exp Med Biol 872:145–176. https://doi.org/10.1007/978-1-4939-2895-8_7

Braskie M, Boyle C, Rajagopalan P, Gutman B, Toga A, Raji C, Thompson P (25. July 2014) Physical activity, inflammation, and volume of the aging brain. Neuroscience 273:199–209. https://doi.org/10.1016/j.neuroscience.2014.05.005

Cappon J, Brasel J, Mohan S, Cooper D (June 1994) Effect of brief exercise on circulating insulin-like growth factor I. J Appl Physiol (1985) 76(6):2490–6. https://doi.org/10.1152/jappl.1994.76.6.2490

Chakraborty A, Barajas S, Lammoglia G, Reyna A, Morley T, Johnson J, Rutkowski J (April 2019) Vascular endothelial growth factor-D (VEGF-D) overexpression and lymphatic expansion in murine adipose tissue improves metabolism in obesity. Am J Pathol 189(4):924–939. https://doi.org/10.1016/j.ajpath.2018.12.008

Cheng Y, Macera C, Davis D, Blair S (August 2000) Physical activity and peptic ulcers. Does physical activity reduce the risk of developing peptic ulcers? West J Med 173(2):101–7. https://doi.org/10.1136/ewjm.173.2.101

Chmielewski P, Strzelec B, Borysławski K, Chmielowiec K, Chmielowiec J, Dąbrowski P (2016) Effects of aging on the function of the urinary system: longitudinal changes with age in selected urine parameters in a hospitalized population of older adults. Anthropol Rev 79(3):331–345. https://doi.org/10.1515/anre-2016-0024

Churchward-Venne T, Breen L, Phillips S (March-April 2014) Alterations in human muscle protein metabolism with aging: protein and exercise as countermeasures to offset sarcopenia. BioFactors 40(2):199–205. https://doi.org/10.1002/biof.1138

Ciccocioppo R, Sabatino A, Luinetti O, Rossi M, Cifone M, Corazza G (July-August 2002) Small bowel enterocyte apoptosis and proliferation are increased in the elderly. Gerontology 48(4):204–208. https://doi.org/10.1159/000058351

Clark C, Kraus B, Sinclair J, Castell D (June 1989) Gastroesophageal reflux induced by exercise in healthy volunteers. JAMA 261(84):3599–3601

Colcombe S, Erickson K, Scalf P, Kim J, Prakash R, McAuley E, Kramer A (November 2006) Aerobic exercise training increases brain volume in aging humans. J Gerontol 61(11):1166–1170. https://doi.org/10.1093/gerona/61.11.1166

Conn V, Koopman R, Ruppar T, Phillips L, Mehr D, Hafdahl A (July 2014) Insulin sensitivity following exercise interventions: systematic review and meta-analysis of outcomes among healthy adults. J Prim Care Community Health 5(3):211–222. https://doi.org/10.1177/2150131913520328

Cotman C, Berchtold N, Christie L-A (September 2007) Exercise builds brain health: key roles of growth factor cascades and inflammation. Trends Neurosci 30(9):464–472. https://doi.org/10.1016/j.tins.2007.06.011

Cowansage K, LeDoux J, Monfils M-H (January 2010) Brain-derived neurotrophic factor: a dynamic gatekeeper of neural plasticity. Curr Mol Pharmacol 3(1):12–29. https://doi.org/10.2174/1874467211003010012

Crane J, MacNeil L, Lally J, Ford R, Bujak A, Brar I, Tarnopolsky M (August 2015) Exercise-stimulated interleukin-15 is controlled by AMPK and regulates skin metabolism and aging. Aging Cell 14(4):625–634. https://doi.org/10.1111/acel.12341

Cueni L, Detmar M (2008) Kein Datum. Lymphat Res Biol 6(3–4):109–122. https://doi.org/10.1089/lrb.2008.1008
Curlik D 2nd, Shors T (January 2013) Training your brain: Do mental and physical (MAP) training enhance cognition through the process of neurogenesis in the hippocampus? Neuropharmacology 64:506–514. https://doi.org/10.1016/j.neuropharm.2012.07.027
Davidson W Jr, Fee E (June 1990) Influence of aging on pulmonary hemodynamics in a population free of coronary artery disease. Am J Cardiol 65(22):1454–1458. https://doi.org/10.1016/0002-9149(90)91354-9
de Oliveira E, Burini R (September 2009) The impact of physical exercise on the gastrointestinal tract. Curr Opin Clin Nutr Metab Care 12(5):533–538. https://doi.org/10.1097/MCO.0b013e32832e6776
De Vuyst L, Leroy F (1. September 2011) Cross-feeding between bifidobacteria and butyrate-producing colon bacteria explains bifdobacterial competitiveness, butyrate production, and gas production. Int J Food Microbiol 149(1):73–80. https://doi.org/10.1016/j.ijfoodmicro.2011.03.003
Ding Q, Vaynman S, Akhavan M, Ying Z, Gomez-Pinilla F (7. July 2006) Insulin-like growth factor I interfaces with brain-derived neurotrophic factor-mediated synaptic plasticity to modulate aspects of exercise-induced cognitive function. Neuroscience 140(3):823–833. https://doi.org/10.1016/j.neuroscience.2006.02.084
Djukic M, Nau R, Sieber C (2014) Das alternde Immunsystem. Dtsch Med Wochenschr 139(40):1987–1990. https://doi.org/10.1055/s-0034-1370283
Drey M (01. September 2011) Sarcopenia – pathophysiology and clinical relevance. Wien Med Wochenschr 161:402–408. https://doi.org/10.1007/s10354-011-0002-y
D'Souza A (January 2007) Ageing and the gut. Postgrad Med J 83(975):44–53. https://doi.org/10.1136/pgmj.2006.049361
Dukowicz A, Lacy B, Levine G (February 2007) Small intestinal bacterial overgrowth: a comprehensive review. Gastroenterol Hepatol (N Y) 3(2):112–122
Dumic I, Nordin T, Jecmenica M, Lalosevic M, Milosavljevic T, Milovanovic T (17. January 2019) Gastrointestinal tract disorders in older age. Can J Gastroenterol Hepatol 2019:6757524. https://doi.org/10.1155/2019/6757524
Durazzo M, Campion D, Fagoonee S, Pellicano R (December 2017) Gastrointestinal tract disorders in the elderly. Minerva Med 108(6):575–591. https://doi.org/10.23736/S0026-4806.17.05417-9
Ebenbichler G, Kerschan-Schindl K (2009) Sicher Bewegen im Alter: Veränderungen der sensomotorischen Fähigkeiten. Physikalische Medizin, Rehabilitationsmedizin, Kurortmedizin 19(1):44–58. https://doi.org/10.1055/s-0028-1090078
Elabd C, Cousin W, Upadhyayula P, Chen R, Chooljian M, Li J, Conboy I (10. June 2014) Oxytocin is an age-specific circulating hormone that is necessary for muscle maintenance and regeneration. Nat Commun 5:4082. https://doi.org/10.1038/ncomms5082
Elias A, Wilson A, Pandian M, Rojas F, Kayaleh R, Stone S, James N (1993) Melatonin and gonadotropin secretion after acute exercise in physically active males. Eur J Appl Physiol Occup Physiol 66(4):357–361. https://doi.org/10.1007/BF00237782
Enright S, Unnithan V, Heward C, Withnall L, Davies D (1. March 2006) Effect of high-intensity inspiratory muscle training on lung volumes, diaphragm thickness, and exercise capacity in subjects who are healthy. Phys Ther 86(3):345–354. https://doi.org/10.1093/ptj/86.3.345
Erlich A, Tryon L, Crilly M, Memme J, Moosavi Z, Oliveira A, Hood D (September 2016) Function of specialized regulatory proteins and signaling pathways in exercise-induced muscle mitochondrial biogenesis. Integr Med Res 5(3):187–197. https://doi.org/10.1016/j.imr.2016.05.003
Fairey A, Courneya K, Field C, Bell G, Jones L, Mackey J (April 2005) Randomized controlled trial of exercise and blood immune function in postmenopausal breast cancer survivors. J Appl Physiol (1985) 98(4):1534–40. https://doi.org/10.1152/japplphysiol.00566.2004
Farage M, Miller K, Elsner P (2013) Characteristics of the aging skin. Adv. Wound Care (New Rochelle) 2:5–10
Farrell P, Joyner M, Caiozzo V (2011) ACSM's advanced exercise physiology, 2nd edn. Wolters Kluwer Health Adis (ESP)
Feldman H, Longcope C, Derby C, Johannes C, Araujo A, Coviello A, McKinlay J (February 2002) Age trends in the level of serum testosterone and other hormones in middle-aged men: longitudinal results from the Massachusetts male aging study. J Clin Endocrinol Metab 87(2):589–598. https://doi.org/10.1210/jcem.87.2.8201
Ferrari U, Drey M (2020) Sarkopenie: eine Herausforderung im Alter. Osteologie 29(02):143–149. https://doi.org/10.1055/a-1155-1461
Ferriolli E, Dantas R, Oliveira R, Braga F (August 1996) The influence of ageing on oesophageal motility after ingestion of liquids with different viscosities. Eur J Gastroenterol Hepatol 8(8):793–798
FilipoviĆ T, LazoviĆ M, BackoviĆ A, FilipoviĆ A, IgnjatoviĆ A, DimitrijeviĆ S, GopČeviĆ K (February 2021) A 12-week exercise program improves functional status in postmenopausal osteoporotic women: randomized controlled study. Eur J Phys Rehabil Med 57(1):120–130. https://doi.org/10.23736/S1973-9087.20.06149-3
Firth J, Stubbs B, Vancampfort D, Schuch F, Lagopoulos J, Rosenbaum S, Ward P (1. February 2018) Effect of aerobic exercise on hippocampal volume in humans: a systematic review and meta-analysis. Neuroimage 166:230–238. https://doi.org/10.1016/j.neuroimage.2017.11.007

Fiuza-Luces C, Santos-Lozano A, Joyner M, Carrera-Bastos P, Picazo O, Zugaza J, Lucia A (December 2018) Exercise benefits in cardiovascular disease: beyond attenuation of traditional risk factors. Nat Rev Cardiol 15(12):731–743. https://doi.org/10.1038/s41569-018-0065-1

Fliser D (2008) Nieren und Alter. Dtsch Med Wochenschr 133(37):1835–1838. https://doi.org/10.1055/s-0028-1082805

Freese J, Proschinger S (12. August 2020) Stärkung des Immunsystems durch Sport – eine Frage der Intensität. Erfahrungsheilkunde 69(04):223–229. https://doi.org/10.1055/a-1205-8025

Günnewig T, Erbguth F, Boelmans K (2022) Praktische Neurogeriatrie. Kohlhammer

Gaballa M, Jacob C, Raya T, Liu J, Simon B, Goldman S (September 1998) Large artery remodeling during aging: biaxial passive and active stiffness. Hypertension 32(3):437–443. https://doi.org/10.1161/01.hyp.32.3.437

Garud M, Kulkarni Y (May 2014) Hyperglycemia to nephropathy via transforming growth factor beta. Curr Diabetes Rev 10(3):182–189. https://doi.org/10.2174/1573399810666140606103645

Gatterer H, Faulhaber M (2019) Höhentraining. In Berghold F, Brugger H, Burtscher M, Domej W, Durrer B, Fischer R, . . . Sumann G (eds) Alpin- und Höhenmedizin. Springer, Berlin, S 423–431

Giovannucci E, Ascherio A, Rimm E, Colditz G, Stampfer M, Willett W (1. March 1995) Physical activity, obesity, and risk for colon cancer and adenoma in men. Ann Intern Med 122(5):327–334. https://doi.org/10.7326/0003-4819-122-5-199503010-00002

Gogniat M, Robinson T, Miller L (May 2021) Exercise interventions do not impact brain volume change in older adults: a systematic review and meta-analysis. Neurobiol Aging 101:230–246. https://doi.org/10.1016/j.neurobiolaging.2021.01.025

Gomez-Pinilla F, Vaynman S, Ying Z (December 2008) Brain-derived neurotrophic factor functions as a metabotrophin to mediate the effects of exercise on cognition. Eur J Neurosci 28(11):2278–2287. https://doi.org/10.1111/j.1460-9568.2008.06524.x

Goodpaster B, Park S, Harris T, Kritchevsky S, Nevitt M, Schwartz A, Newman A (October 2006) The loss of skeletal muscle strength, mass, and quality in older adults: the health, aging and body composition study. J Gerontol A Biol Sci Med Sci 61(10):1059–1064. https://doi.org/10.1093/gerona/61.10.1059

Grinton S (May 1994) Respiratory limitations in the aging population. SaveEmailSend to 87(5):47–49

Großkopf A, Simm A (19. September 2022) Alterung des Immunsystems. Z Gerontol Geriatr 55:553–557. https://doi.org/10.1007/s00391-022-02107-6

Guadagni V, Drogos L, Tyndall A, Davenport M, Anderson T, Eskes G, Poulin M, (26. May 2020) Aerobic exercise improves cognition and cerebrovascular regulation in older adults. Neurology 94(21):e2245–e2257. https://doi.org/10.1212/WNL.0000000000009478

Gunes S, Hekim G, Arslan M, Asci R (2016) Effects of aging on the male reproductive system. J Assist Reprod Genet 33:441–454. https://doi.org/10.1007/s10815-016-0663-y

Hackney A, Lane A, Register-Mihalik J, O'leary, C. (July 2017) Endurance exercise training and male sexual libido. Med Sci Sports Exerc 49(7):1383–1388. https://doi.org/10.1249/MSS.0000000000001235

Haemmerle M, Keller T, Egger G, Schachner H, Steiner W, Stokic D, Hantusch B (July 2013) Enhanced lymph vessel density, remodeling, and inflammation are reflected by gene expression signatures in dermal lymphatic endothelial cells in type 2 diabetes. Diabetes 62(7):2509–2529. https://doi.org/10.2337/db12-0844

Halfon M, Phan O, Teta D (2015) Vitamin D: a review on its effects on muscle strength, the risk of fall, and frailty. Biomed Res Int 2015:953241. https://doi.org/10.1155/2015/953241

Halter J, Ouslander J, Tinetti M, Studenski S, High K, Asthana S, Woolard N (2009) Hazzard's geriatric medicine and gerontology, 6th edn. McGraw-Hill, New York

Hanani M, Fellig Y, Udassin R, Freund H (June 2004) Age-related changes in the morphology of the myenteric plexus of the human colon. Auton Neurosci 113(1–2):71–78. https://doi.org/10.1016/j.autneu.2004.05.007

Hao S, Tan S, Li J, Li W, Li J, Liu Y, Hong Z (2022) The effect of diet and exercise on climacteric symptomatology. Asia Pac J Clin Nutr 31(3):362–370. https://doi.org/10.6133/apjcn.202209_31(3).0004

Harris T, Kiel D, Roubenoff R, Langlois J, Hannan M, Havlik R, Wilson P (February 1997) Association of insulin-like growth factor-I with body composition, weight history, and past health behaviors in the very old: the framingham heart study. J Am Geriatr Soc 45(2):133–139. https://doi.org/10.1111/j.1532-5415.1997.tb04497.x

Hawkins V, Foster-Schubert K, Chubak J, Sorensen B, Ulrich C, Stancyzk F, McTiernan A (February 2008) Effect of exercise on serum sex hormones in men: a 12-month randomized clinical trial. Med Sci Sports Exerc 40(2):223–233. https://doi.org/10.1249/mss.0b013e31815bbba9

Ho C, Dreesen O (September 2021). Faces of cellular senescence in skin aging. Mech Ageing Dev 198:111525. https://doi.org/10.1016/j.mad.2021.111525

Horstman A, Dillon E, Urban R, Sheffield-Moore M (November 2012) The role of androgens and estrogens on healthy aging and longevity. J Gerontol A Biol Sci Med Sci 67(11):1140–1152. https://doi.org/10.1093/gerona/gls068

Hu M, Turner D, Generaal E, Bos D, Ikram M, Ikram M, . . . Penninx B (18. August 2020) Exercise interventions for the prevention of depression: a systematic review of meta-analyses. BMC Public Health 20:1255. https://doi.org/10.1186/s12889-020-09323-y

Huonker M, Schmidt-Trucksäß A, Heiss H, Keul J (15. April 2014) Trainingseinflüsse auf altersbedingte strukturelle und funktionelle Veränderungen am Herzkreislaufsystem und an der Skelettmuskulatur. Z Gerontol Geriatr 35:151–156. https://doi.org/10.1007/s003910200019

Jacomo R, Nascimento T, da Siva M, Salata M, Alves A, da Cruz P, de Sousa J (October 2020) Exercise regimens other than pelvic floor muscle training cannot increase pelvic muscle strength-a systematic review. J Bodyw Mov Ther 24(4):568–574. https://doi.org/10.1016/j.jbmt.2020.08.005

JAMES T (July 1964) Pathology of the cardiac conduction system in hemochromatosis. N Engl J Med 271:92–94. https://doi.org/10.1056/NEJM196407092710209

Janssen H, Samson M, Verhaar H (April 2002) Vitamin D deficiency, muscle function, and falls in elderly people. Am J Clin Nutr 75(4):611–615. https://doi.org/10.1093/ajcn/75.4.611

Janssen J (2016) Impact of physical exercise on endocrine aging. In: Lanfranco F, Strasburger C (eds) Sports endocrinology, 47th edn. S.Karger AG, S 68–81. https://doi.org/10.1159/000445158

Jiang X, Nicolls M, Tian W, Rockson S (10. February 2018) Lymphatic dysfunction, leukotrienes, and lymphedema. Annu Rev Physiol 80:49–70. https://doi.org/10.1146/annurev-physiol-022516-034008

Jiang X, Tian W, Nicolls M, Rockson S (14. November 2019) The lymphatic system in obesity, insulin resistance, and cardiovascular diseases. Front Physiol 10:1402. https://doi.org/10.3389/fphys.2019.01402

Johansen K (2005) Exercise and chronic kidney disease: current recommendations. Sports Med 35(6):485–499. https://doi.org/10.2165/00007256-200535060-00003

Johnston A (February 2008) Resistance training, sarcopenia, and the mitochondrial theory of aging. Appl Physiol Nutr Metab 33(1):191–199. https://doi.org/10.1139/H07-141

Jull A, Slark J, Parsons J (1. November 2018) Prescribed exercise with compression vs compression alone in treating patients with venous leg ulcers: a systematic review and meta-analysis. JAMA Dermatol 154(11):1304–1311. https://doi.org/10.1001/jamadermatol.2018.3281

Kemmler W, Jakob F, Sieber C (2018) Sarkopenie. Arthritis und Rheuma 38(02):87–92. https://doi.org/10.1055/s-0038-1649286

Kemmler W, Shojaa M, Kohl M, von Stengel S (November 2020) Effects of different types of exercise on bone mineral density in postmenopausal women: a systematic review and meta-analysis. Calcif Tissue Int 107(5):409–439. https://doi.org/10.1007/s00223-020-00744-w

Kenney R (1989) The respiratory and cardiovascular systems. In: Kenney RA (ed) Physiology of aging. Mosby, Chicago

Kitzman D, Edwards W (March 1990) Age-related changes in the anatomy of the normal human heart. J Gerontol 45(2):M33–M39. https://doi.org/10.1093/geronj/45.2.m33

Klimaschewski L (2021) Altern und neurodegenerative Erkrankungen – warum gehen Nervenzellen verloren? In: Klimaschewski L (ed) Parkinson und Alzheimer heute. Springer, Berlin, S 31–114

Ko I, Jeong J, Kim Y, Jee Y, Kim S, Kim S, Chung K (June 2014) Aerobic exercise affects myostatin expression in aged rat skeletal muscles: a possibility of antiaging effects of aerobic exercise related with pelvic floor muscle and urethral rhabdosphincter. Int Neurourol J 18(2):77–85. https://doi.org/10.5213/inj.2014.18.2.77

Koopman R, Verdijk L, van Loon L (2011) Exercise and nutritional interventions to combat age-related muscle loss. In: Lynch G (ed) Sarcopenia – age-related muscle wasting and weakness. Springer, Dordrecht, S 289–315

Kraemer W, Ratamess N (2005) Hormonal responses and adaptations to resistance exercise and training. Sports Med 35(4):339–361. https://doi.org/10.2165/00007256-200535040-00004

Kraemer W, Gordon S, Fleck S, Marchitelli L, Mello R, Dziados J, Fry A (April 1991) Endogenous anabolic hormonal and growth factor responses to heavy resistance exercise in males and females. Int J Sports Med 12(2):228–235. https://doi.org/10.1055/s-2007-1024673

Krutmann J, Schroeder P (2009) Role of mitochondria in photoaging of human skin: the defective powerhouse model. J Investig Dermatol Symp Proc 14:44–49

Kumar A, Maiya A, Shastry B, Vaishali K, Ravishankar N, Hazari A, Jadhav R (March 2019) Exercise and insulin resistance in type 2 diabetes mellitus: a systematic review and meta-analysis. Ann Phys Rehabil Med 62(2):98–103. https://doi.org/10.1016/j.rehab.2018.11.001

Kuusi T, Kostiainen E, Vartiainen E, Pitkänen L, Ehnholm C, Korhonen H, Puska P (June 1984) Acute effects of marathon running on levels of serum lipoproteins and androgenic hormones in healthy males. Metabolism 33(6):527–531. https://doi.org/10.1016/0026-0495(84)90007-6

Lakatta E (May 1986) Diminished beta-adrenergic modulation of cardiovascular function in advanced age. Cardiol Clin 4(2):185–200

Landrigan J-F, Bell T, Crowe M, Clay O, Mirman D (2020) Lifting cognition: a meta-analysis of effects of resistance exercise on cognition. Psychol Res 84:1167–1183. https://doi.org/10.1007/s00426-019-01145-x

Langer D, Ciavaglia C, Faisal A, Webb K, Neder J, Gosselink R, O'Donnell D (August 2018) Inspiratory muscle training reduces diaphragm activation and dyspnea during exercise in COPD. J Appl Physiol 125(2):243–685. https://doi.org/10.1152/japplphysiol.01078.2017

Larbi A, Franceschi C, Mazzatti D, Solana R, Wikby A, Pawelec G (April 2008) Aging of the immune system as a prognostic factor for human longevity. Physiology (Bethesda) 23:64–74. https://doi.org/10.1152/physiol.00040.2007

Lauretani F, Russo C, Bandinelli S, Bartali B, Cavazzini C, Di Iorio A, Ferrucci L (November 2003) Age-associated changes in skeletal muscles and their effect on mobility: an operational diagnosis of sarcopenia. J Appl Physiol (1985) 95(5):1851–60. https://doi.org/10.1152/japplphysiol.00246.2003

Lavker R, Zheng P, Dong G (1989) Morphology of aged skin. Clin Geriatr Med 5:53–67

LEV, M. (January 1954) Aging changes in the human sinoatrial node. J Gerontol 9(1):1–9. https://doi.org/10.1093/geronj/9.1.1

Levy W, Cerqueira M, Abrass I, Schwartz R, Stratton J (July 1993) Endurance exercise training augments diastolic filling at rest and during exercise in healthy young and older men. Circulation 88(1):116–126. https://doi.org/10.1161/01.cir.88.1.116

Lewis B (March 2000) Small intestinal bleeding. Gastroenterol Clin North Am 29(1):67–95

Lin Y-Y, Lee S-D (25. August 2018) Cardiovascular benefits of exercise training in postmenopausal hypertension. Int J Mol Sci 19(9):2523. https://doi.org/10.3390/ijms19092523

Ling S, Conwit R, Ferrucci L, Metter E (July 2009) Age-associated changes in motor unit physiology: observations from the baltimore longitudinal study of aging. Arch Phys Med Rehabil 90(7):1237–1240. https://doi.org/10.1016/j.apmr.2008.09.565

Loertzer H, Schneider P, (18. May 2013) Belastungsinkontinenz der Frau im Alter. Urologe 52:813–820. https://doi.org/10.1007/s00120-013-3167-8

Lopez-Lopez C, LeRoith D, Torres-Aleman I, (29. June 2004) Insulin-like growth factor i is required for vessel remodeling in the adult brain. Proc Natl Acad Sci U S A 101(26):9833–9838. https://doi.org/10.1073/pnas.0400337101

Macías-Núñez J, Cameron J, Oreopoulos D (2008) The aging kidney in health and disease, 1st edn. Springer, New York

Madsen J, Graff J (March 2004) Effects of ageing on gastrointestinal motor function. Age Ageing 33(2):154–159. https://doi.org/10.1093/ageing/afh040

Maggio M, Lauretani F, Ceda G (January 2013) Sex hormones and sarcopenia in older persons. Curr Opin Clin Nutr Metab Care 16(1):3–13. https://doi.org/10.1097/MCO.0b013e32835b6044

Magrone T, Jirillo E (5. August 2013) The interaction between gut microbiota and age-related changes in immune function and inflammation. Immun Ageing 10(1):31. https://doi.org/10.1186/1742-4933-10-31

Mahmoud A, Goemaere S, El-Garem Y, Pottelbergh I, Comhaire F, Kaufman J (January 2003) Testicular volume in relation to hormonal indices of gonadal function in community-dwelling elderly men. J Clin Endocrinol Metab 88(1):179–184. https://doi.org/10.1210/jc.2002-020408

Marcomichelakis J, Withers R, Newman G, O'Brien K, Emanuel R (November-December 1983) The relation of age to the thickness of the interventricular septum, the posterior left ventricular wall and their ratio. Int J Cardiol 4(4):405–419. https://doi.org/10.1016/0167-5273(83)90190-0

Marsh M, Novaes Oliveira M, Vieira-Potter V (14. January 2023) Adipocyte metabolism and health after the menopause: the role of exercise. Nutrients 15(2):444. https://doi.org/10.3390/nu15020444

McClaran S, Babcock M, Pegelow D, Reddan W, Dempsey J (May 1995) Longitudinal effects of aging on lung function at rest and exercise in healthy active fit elderly adults. J Appl Physiol 78(5):1957–68. https://doi.org/10.1152/jappl.1995.78.5.1957

McDermott M (March 2018) Exercise rehabilitation for peripheral artery disease: a review. J Cardiopulm Rehabil Prev 63–69. https://doi.org/10.1097/HCR.0000000000000343

McDonald D (10. August 2018) Tighter lymphatic junctions prevent obesity. Science 361(6402):551–552. https://doi.org/10.1126/science.aau5583

McKenzie D (May 2012) Respiratory physiology: adaptations to high-level exercise. Br J Sports Med 46(6):381–384. https://doi.org/10.1136/bjsports-2011-090824

McTiernan A (March 2008) Mechanisms linking physical activity with cancer. Nat Rev Cancer 8(3):205–211. https://doi.org/10.1038/nrc2325

McTiernan A, Tworoger S, Rajan K, Yasui Y, Sorenson B, Ulrich C, Schwartz R (July 2004) Effect of exercise on serum androgens in postmenopausal women: a 12-month randomized clinical trial. Cancer Epidemiol Biomarkers Prev 13(7):1099–1105

McTiernan A, Wu L, Chen C, Chlebowski R, Mossavar-Rahmani Y, Modugno F, Investigators WHI (September 2006) Relation of BMI and physical activity to sex hormones in postmenopausal women. Obesity (Silver Spring) 14(9):1662–1677. https://doi.org/10.1038/oby.2006.191

Mena G, Mielke G, Brown W (11. September 2019) The effect of physical activity on reproductive health outcomes in young women: a systematic review and meta-analysis. Hum Reprod Update 25(5):541–563. https://doi.org/10.1093/humupd/dmz013

Mennuni S, Rubattu S, Pierelli G, Tocci G, Fofi C, Volpe M (February 2014) Hypertension and kidneys: unraveling complex molecular mechanisms underlying hypertensive renal damage. J Hum Hypertens 28(2):74–79. https://doi.org/10.1038/jhh.2013.55

Meredith I, Friberg P, Jennings G, Dewar E, Fazio V, Lambert G, Esler M (November 1991) Exercise training lowers resting renal but not cardiac sympathetic activity in humans. Hypertension 18(5):575–582. https://doi.org/10.1161/01.hyp.18.5.575

Metcalf A, Phillips S, Zinsmeister A, MacCarty R, Beart R, Wolff B (January 1987) Simplified

assessment of segmental colonic transit. Gastroenterology 92(1):40–47. https://doi.org/10.1016/0016-5085(87)90837-7
Metter E, Conwit R, Tobin J, Fozard J (September 1997) Age-associated loss of power and strength in the upper extremities in women and men. J Gerontol A Biol Sci Med Sci 52(5):267–276. https://doi.org/10.1093/gerona/52a.5.b267
Mitsui T, Kagami H, Kinomoto H, Ito A, Kondo T, Shimaoka K (April 2003) Small bowel bacterial overgrowth and rice malabsorption in healthy and physically disabled older adults. J Hum Nutr Diet 16(2):119–122. https://doi.org/10.1046/j.1365-277x.2003.00424.x
Moreira L, de Oliveira M, Lirani-Galvão A, Marin-Mio R, dos Santos R, Lazaretti-Castro M (July 2014) Physical exercise and osteoporosis: effects of different types of exercises on bone and physical function of postmenopausal women. Arq Bras Endocrinol Metabol 58(5):514–522. https://doi.org/10.1590/0004-2730000003374
Moriondo A, Mukenge S, Negrini D (July 2005) Transmural pressure in rat initial subpleural lymphatics during spontaneous or mechanical ventilation. Am J Physiol Heart Circ Physiol 289(1):H263–H269. https://doi.org/10.1152/ajpheart.00060.2005
Morley J, Perry H 3rd (May 2003) Androgens and women at the menopause and beyond. J Gerontol A Biol Sci Med Sci 58(5):M409–M416. https://doi.org/10.1093/gerona/58.5.m409
Mottillo S, Filion K, Genest J, Joseph L, Pilote L, Poirier P, Eisenberg M, (28. September 2010) The metabolic syndrome and cardiovascular risk a systematic review and meta-analysis. J Am Coll Cardiol 56(14):1113–1132. https://doi.org/10.1016/j.jacc.2010.05.034
Musumeci, G. (2017). Sarcopenia and exercise "The state of the art". J Funct Morphol Kinesiol 2(4):40. https://doi.org/10.3390/jfmk2040040
Nagakura Y, Hayashi M, Kajioka S (December 2022) Lifestyle habits to prevent the development of benign prostatic hyperplasia: analysis of japanese nationwide datasets. Prostate Int 10(4):200–206. https://doi.org/10.1016/j.prnil.2022.06.004
Nagler R, Hershkovich O (January 2005) Relationships between age, drugs, oral sensorial complaints and salivary profile. Arch Oral Biol 50(1):7–16. https://doi.org/10.1016/j.archoralbio.2004.07.012
Naldi L, Conti A, Cazzaniga S, Patrizi A, Pazzaglia M, Lanzoni A, Psoriasis Emilia Romagna Study Group (March 2014) Diet and physical exercise in psoriasis: a randomized controlled trial. Br J Dermatol 170(3):634–642. https://doi.org/10.1111/bjd.12735
Neaves W, Johnson L, Porter J, Parker C Jr, Petty C (October 1984) Leydig cell numbers, daily sperm production, and serum gonadotropin levels in aging men. J Clin Endocrinol Metab 59(4):756–763. https://doi.org/10.1210/jcem-59-4-756
Nelson N (December 2016) Breast cancer-related lymphedema and resistance exercise: a systematic review. J Strength Cond Res 30(9):2656–2665. https://doi.org/10.1519/JSC.0000000000001355
Neudecker J, Baumann F (2016) Krafttraining bei sekundärem Lymphödem – kraftvoll gegen Ödeme. physiopraxis 14(09):44–47. https://doi.org/10.1055/s-0042-111600
Nicastro H, Zanchi N, da Luz C, Lancha A Jr (November 2011) Functional and morphological effects of resistance exercise on disuse-induced skeletal muscle atrophy. Braz J Med Biol Res 44(11):1070–1079. https://doi.org/10.1590/s0100-879x2011007500125
Niemann C, Godde B, Staudinger U, Voelcker-Rehage C (5. December 2014) Exercise-induced changes in basal ganglia volume and cognition in older adults. Neuroscience 281:147–163. https://doi.org/10.1016/j.neuroscience.2014.09.033
Ortonne J (1990) Pigmentary changes of the ageing skin. Br J Dermatol 122(35):21–28
Otto S, Ebner F (2016) Onkologie – „Bewege Dich und Dein Immunsystem – was bewirkt körperliche Aktivität?" Geburtshilfe Frauenheilkd 76(01):23–25. https://doi.org/10.1055/s-0035-1552484
Parlesak A, Klein B, Schecher K, Bode J, Bode C (June 2013) Prevalence of small bowel bacterial overgrowth and its association with nutrition intake in nonhospitalized older adults. J Am Geriatr Soc 51(6):768–773. https://doi.org/10.1046/j.1365-2389.2003.51259.x
Parsons B, Ijaz U, D'Amore R, Burkitt M, Eccles R, Lenzi L, Pritchard D (2. November 2017) Comparison of the human gastric microbiota in hypochlorhydric states arising as a result of Helicobacter pylori-induced atrophic gastritis, autoimmune atrophic gastritis and proton pump inhibitor use. PLoS Pathog 13(11):e1006653. https://doi.org/10.1371/journal.ppat.1006653
Payette H, Roubenoff R, Jacques P, Dinarello C, Wilson P, Abad L, Harris T (September 2003) Insulin-like growth factor-1 and interleukin 6 predict sarcopenia in very old community-living men and women: the Framingham Heart Study. J Am Geriatr Soc 51(9):1237–1243. https://doi.org/10.1046/j.1532-5415.2003.51407.x
Peters O, Peters P, Clarys J, DeMeirleir K, Devis G (May 1988) Esophageal motility and exercise. Gastroenterology 94(5):A351–A351
Philippot A, Dubois V, Lambrechts K, Grogna D, Robert A, Jonckheer U, De Volder A (15. March 2022) Impact of physical exercise on depression and anxiety in adolescent inpatients: a randomized controlled trial. J Affect Disord 301:145–153. https://doi.org/10.1016/j.jad.2022.01.011
Pontoppidan H, Beecher H (31. December 1960) Progressive loss of protective reflexes in the airway with the advance of age. JAMA 174:2209–2213. https://doi.org/10.1001/jama.1960.03030180029007
Radzimińska A, Strączyńska A, Weber-Rajek M, Styczyńska H, Strojek K, Piekorz Z (17 May 2018) The impact of pelvic floor muscle training on the quality of life of women with urinary incontinence:

a systematic literature review. Clin Interv Aging 13:957–965. https://doi.org/10.2147/CIA.S160057

Raine J, Bishop J (March 1963) A-a difference in O2 tension and physiological dead space in normal man. J Appl Physiol 18:284–288. https://doi.org/10.1152/jappl.1963.18.2.284

Robson K, Glick M (September 2003) Dysphagia and advancing age: are manometric abnormalities more common in older patients? Dig Dis Sci 48(9):1709–1712. https://doi.org/10.1023/a:1025430625252

Rogers, M., Hagberg, J., Martin 3rd, W., Ehsani, A., & Holloszy, J. (May 1990). Decline in VO2max with aging in master athletes and sedentary men. *J Appl Physiol (1985), 68*(5), S. 2195–9. https://doi.org/10.1152/jappl.1990.68.5.2195

Rolland Y, Czerwinski S, Van Kan G, Morley J, Cesari M, Onder G, Vellas B, (August-September 2008) Sarcopenia: its assessment, etiology, pathogenesis, consequences and future perspectives. J Nutr Health Aging 12(7):433–450. https://doi.org/10.1007/BF02982704

Rooyackers O, Adey D, Ades P, Nair K (December 1996) Effect of age on in vivo rates of mitochondrial protein synthesis in human skeletal muscle. Proc Natl Acad Sci U S A 93(26):15364–15369. https://doi.org/10.1073/pnas.93.26.15364

Rosano C, Guralnik J, Pahor M, Glynn N, Newman A, Ibrahim T, Aizenstein H (3. March 2017) Hippocampal response to a 24-month physical activity intervention in sedentary older adults. Am J Geriatr Psychiatry 25(3):209–217. https://doi.org/10.1016/j.jagp.2016.11.007

Roth S, Ferrell R, Hurley B (2000) Strength training for the prevention and treatment of sarcopenia. J Nutr Health Aging 4(3):143–155

Roubenoff R (February 2001) Origins and clinical relevance of sarcopenia. Can J Appl Physiol 26(1):78–89. https://doi.org/10.1139/h01-006

Roubenoff R, Harris T, Abad L, Wilson P, Dallal G, Dinarello C (January 1998) Monocyte cytokine production in an elderly population: effect of age and inflammation. J Gerontol A Biol Sci Med Sci 53(1):20–26. https://doi.org/10.1093/gerona/53a.1.m20

Roubenoff R, Parise H, Payette H, Abad L, Agostino R, Jacques P, Harris T (October 2003) Cytokines, insulin-like growth factor 1, sarcopenia, and mortality in very old community-dwelling men and women: the Framingham Heart Study. Am J Med 115(6):429–435. https://doi.org/10.1016/j.amjmed.2003.05.001

Russo B, Brembilla N, Chizzolini C (2020) Interplay between keratinocytes and fibroblasts: a systematic review providing a new angle for understanding skin fibrotic disorders. Front Immunol 11:648

Ryan S, Vincent T, Mitchell R, Filley G, Dart G (1965) Ductectasia; an asymptomatic pulmonary change related to age. Med Thorac 22:181–187

Rywik T, Blackman M, Yataco A, Vaitkevicius P, Zink R, Cottrell E, Fleg J (December 1999) Enhanced endothelial vasoreactivity in endurance-trained older men. J Appl Physiol (1985) 87(6):2136–42. https://doi.org/10.1152/jappl.1999.87.6.2136

Saffrey M, (1. Oktober, (2013) Cellular changes in the enteric nervous system during ageing. Dev Biol 382(1):344–355. https://doi.org/10.1016/j.ydbio.2013.03.015

Schmitt E, Johnson E, Yusifova M, Bruns D (1. November 2019) The renal molecular clock: broken by aging and restored by exercise. Am J Physiol Renal Physiol 317(5):F1087–F1093. https://doi.org/10.1152/ajprenal.00301.2019

Schmitz K, Ahmed R, Troxel A, Cheville A, Lewis-Grant L, Smith R, Chittams J (22. December 2010) Weight lifting for women at risk for breast cancer-related lymphedema: a randomized trial. JAMA 304(24):2699–2705. https://doi.org/10.1001/jama.2010.1837

Schmitz K, Ahmed R, Troxel A, Cheville A, Smith R, Lewis-Grant L, Greene Q (13. August 2009) Weight lifting in women with breast-cancer-related lymphedema. N Engl J Med 361(7):664–673. https://doi.org/10.1056/NEJMoa0810118

Schmitz K, Courneya K, Matthews C, Demark-Wahnefried W, Galvão D, Pinto B, College A, of Sports Medicine (July 2010) American college of sports medicine roundtable on exercise guidelines for cancer survivors. Med Sci Sports Exerc 42(7):1409–1426. https://doi.org/10.1249/MSS.0b013e3181e0c112

Schulte-Frei B, Jäger L (2018) Inkontinenz bei Leistungssportlerinnen. physioscience 14(03):105–111. https://doi.org/10.1055/a-0658-0190

Seefried L, Genest F (2017) Funktionsdiagnostik der Sarkopenie. Osteologie 26(01):13–17. https://doi.org/10.1055/s-0037-1622080

Seeley R, Stephens T, Tate P (2008) Anatomy & physiology, 8th edn. McGraw-Hill, New York

Sharma G, Goodwin J (2006) Effect of aging on respiratory system physiology and immunology. Clin Interv Aging 1(3):253–260. https://doi.org/10.2147/ciia.2006.1.3.253

Shephard R (January 2017) Peptic ulcer and exercise. Sports Med 47(1):33–40. https://doi.org/10.1007/s40279-016-0563-4

Shimamoto C, Hirata I, Hiraike Y, Takeuchi N, Nomura T, Katsu K-I (November–December 2002) Evaluation of gastric motor activity in the elderly by electrogastrography and the (13)C-acetate breath test. Gerontology 48(6):381–386. https://doi.org/10.1159/000065500

Short K, Bigelow M, Kahl J, Singh R, Coenen-Schimke J, Raghavakaimal S, Nair K (12. April 2005) Decline in skeletal muscle mitochondrial function with aging in humans. Proc Natl Acad Sci U S A 102(15):5618–5623. https://doi.org/10.1073/pnas.0501559102

Short K, Vittone J, Bigelow M, Proctor D, Nair K (January 2004) Age and aerobic exercise training effects on whole body and muscle protein metabolism. Am J Physiol Endocrinol Metab 286(1):E92–101. https://doi.org/10.1152/ajpendo.00366.2003

Silva A, Sousa N, Azevedo L, Martins C (October 2017) Physical activity and exercise for erectile dysfunction: systematic review and meta-analysis. Br J Sports Med 51(19):1419–1424. https://doi.org/10.1136/bjsports-2016-096418

Smith A, Toone R, Peacock O, Drawer S, Stokes K, Cook C (15. May 2013) Dihydrotestosterone is elevated following sprint exercise in healthy young men. J Appl Physiol 114(10):1435–40. https://doi.org/10.1152/japplphysiol.01419.2012

Smith K, Ainslie P (1. November 2017) Regulation of cerebral blood flow and metabolism during exercise. Exp Physiol 102(11):1356–1371. https://doi.org/10.1113/EP086249

Soave I, Scarani S, Mallozzi M, Nobili F, Marci R, Caserta D, (16. January 2019) Pelvic floor muscle training for prevention and treatment of urinary incontinence during pregnancy and after childbirth and its effect on urinary system and supportive structures assessed by objective measurement techniques. Arch Gynecol Obstet 299:609–623. https://doi.org/10.1007/s00404-018-5036-6

Sobin S, Fung Y, Tremer H (April 1985) Collagen and elastin fibers in human pulmonary alveolar walls. J Appl Physiol (1985) 64(4): 1659–75. https://doi.org/10.1152/jappl.1988.64.4.1659

Souza H, Rocha T, Pessoa M, Rattes C, Brandão D, Fregonezi G, Dornelas A (December 2014) Effects of Inspiratory muscle training in elderly women on respiratory muscle strength, diaphragm thickness and mobility. J Gerontol 69(12):1545–1553. https://doi.org/10.1093/gerona/glu182

Spiering B, Kraemer W, Anderson J, Armstrong L, Nindl B, Volek J, Maresh C (2008) Resistance exercise biology: manipulation of resistance exercise programme variables determines the responses of cellular and molecular signalling pathways. Sports Med 38(7):527–540. https://doi.org/10.2165/00007256-200838070-00001

Svennerholm L, Boström K, Jungbjer B (October 1997) Changes in weight and compositions of major membrane components of human brain during the span of adult human life of swedes. Acta Neuropathol 94(4):345–352. https://doi.org/10.1007/s004010050717

Takahashi T, Qoubaitary A, Owyang C, Wiley J (November 2000) Decreased expression of nitric oxide synthase in the colonic myenteric plexus of aged rats. Brain Res 883(1):15–21. https://doi.org/10.1016/s0006-8993(00)02867-5

Tolep K, Higgins N, Muza S, Criner G, Kelsen S (August 1995) Comparison of diaphragm strength between healthy adult elderly and young men. Am J Respir Crit Care Med 152(2):677–682. https://doi.org/10.1164/ajrccm.152.2.7633725

Traustadóttir T, Bosch P, Cantu T, Matt K (July 2004) Hypothalamic-pituitary-adrenal axis response and recovery from high-intensity exercise in women: effects of aging and fitness. J Clin Endocrinol Metab 89(7):3248–3254. https://doi.org/10.1210/jc.2003-031713

Treloar A (December 1981) Menstrual cyclicity and the pre-menopause. Maturitas 3(3–4):249–264. https://doi.org/10.1016/0378-5122(81)90032-3

Tsunoda K, Abe K, Goto T, Yasujima M, Sato M, Omata K, Yoshinaga K (February 1896) Effect of age on the renin-angiotensin-aldosterone system in normal subjects: simultaneous measurement of active and inactive renin, renin substrate, and aldosterone in plasma. J Clin Endocrinol Metab 62(2):384–389. https://doi.org/10.1210/jcem-62-2-384

Turner J, Mead J, Wohl M (December 1968) Elasticity of human lungs in relation to age. J Appl Physiol 25(6):664–671. https://doi.org/10.1152/jappl.1968.25.6.664

Ueno H, Shiiya T, Nakazato M (July 2010) Translational research of ghrelin. Ann N Y Acad Sci 1200:120–127. https://doi.org/10.1111/j.1749-6632.2010.05509.x

Umegaki H (March 2016) Sarcopenia and frailty in older patients with diabetes mellitus. Geriatr Gerontol Int 16(3):293–299. https://doi.org/10.1111/ggi.12688

Vaitkevicius P, Fleg J, Engel J, O'Connor F, Wright J, Lakatta L, Lakatta E (October 1993) Effects of age and aerobic capacity on arterial stiffness in healthy adults. Circulation 88(4 Pt 1):1456–1462. https://doi.org/10.1161/01.cir.88.4.1456

Valenzuela P, Ruilope L, Santos-Lozano A, Wilhelm M, Kränkel N, Fiuza-Luces C, Lucia A (1. June 2023) Exercise benefits in cardiovascular diseases: from mechanisms to clinical implementation. Eur Heart J 44(21):1874–1889. https://doi.org/10.1093/eurheartj/ehad170

Van der Borght K, Kóbor-Nyakas D, Klauke K, Eggen B, Nyakas C, Van der Zee E, Meerlo P (October 2009) Physical exercise leads to rapid adaptations in hippocampal vasculature: temporal dynamics and relationship to cell proliferation and neurogenesis. Hippocampus 19(10):928–936. https://doi.org/10.1002/hipo.20545

Veldhuis J, Liem A, South S, Weltman A, Weltman J, Clemmons D, Pincus S (November 1995) Differential impact of age, sex steroid hormones, and obesity on basal versus pulsatile growth hormone secretion in men as assessed in an ultrasensitive chemiluminescence assay. J Clin Endocrinol Metab 80(11):3209–3222. https://doi.org/10.1210/jcem.80.11.7593428

Verdú E, Ceballos D, Vilches J, Navarro X (December 2000) Influence of aging on peripheral nerve function and regeneration. J Peripher Nerv Syst 5(4):191–208. https://doi.org/10.1046/j.1529-8027.2000.00026.x

Verdijk L, Snijders T, Beelen M, Savelberg H, Meijer K, Kuipers H, Van Loon L (November 2010) Characteristics of muscle fiber type are predictive of skeletal muscle mass and strength in elderly men. J Am Geriatr Soc 58(11):2069–2075. https://doi.org/10.1111/j.1532-5415.2010.03150.x

Visser M, Deeg D, Lips P, Longitudinal Aging Study Amsterdam (December 2003) Low vitamin D and high parathyroid hormone levels as determinants of loss of muscle strength and muscle mass (sarcopenia): the longitudinal aging study Amsterdam. J Clin Endocrinol Metab 88(12):5766–5772. https://doi.org/10.1210/jc.2003-030604

Vitale G, Cesari M, Mari D (November 2016) Aging of the endocrine system and its potential impact on sarcopenia. Eur J Intern Med 35:10–15. https://doi.org/10.1016/j.ejim.2016.07.017

Vitale G, Salvioli S, Franceschi C (April 2013) Oxidative stress and the ageing endocrine system. Nat Rev Endocrinol 9(4):228–240. https://doi.org/10.1038/nrendo.2013.29

Wang C, Swerdloff R, Iranmanesh A, Dobs A, Snyder P, Cunningham G, Testosterone Gel Study Group (August 2000) Transdermal testosterone gel improves sexual function, mood, muscle strength, and body composition parameters in hypogonadal men. J Clin Endocrinol Metab 85(8):2839–2853. https://doi.org/10.1210/jcem.85.8.6747

Wei J (10. December 1992) Age and the cardiovascular system. N Engl J Med 327(24):1735–1739. https://doi.org/10.1056/NEJM199212103272408

Wei J, Spurgeon H, Lakatta E (June 1984) Excitation-contraction in rat myocardium: alterations with adult aging. Am J Physiol 246(6 Pt 2):H784–H791. https://doi.org/10.1152/ajpheart.1984.246.6.H784

Weinstein J, Anderson S (July 2010) The aging kidney: physiological changes. Adv Chronic Kidney Dis 17(4):302–307. https://doi.org/10.1053/j.ackd.2010.05.002

Well D, Yang H, Houseni M, Iruvuri S, Alzeair S, Sansovini M, Torigian D (May 2007) Age-related structural and metabolic changes in the pelvic reproductive end organs. Semin Nucl Med 37(3):173–184. https://doi.org/10.1053/j.semnuclmed.2007.01.004

Williams P (October 2008) Effects of running distance and performance on incident benign prostatic hyperplasia. Med Sci Sports Exerc 40(10):1733–1739. https://doi.org/10.1249/MSS.0b013e31817b8eba

Wise P (2005) Chapter 21 – aging of the female reproductive system. Handbook of the biology of aging, 6th edn. S 570–590. https://doi.org/10.1016/B978-012088387-5/50024-8

Wokke J, Jennekens F, van den Oord C, Veldman H, Smit L, Leppink G (March 1990) Morphological changes in the human end plate with age. J Neurol Sci 95(3):291–310. https://doi.org/10.1016/0022-510x(90)90076-y

Yan Z, Lira V, Greene N (July 2012) Exercise training-induced regulation of mitochondrial quality. Exerc Sport Sci Rev 40(3):159–164. https://doi.org/10.1097/JES.0b013e3182575599

Yang H, Chryssikos T, Houseni M, Alzeair S, Sansovini M, Iruvuri S, Alavi A (April 2011) The effects of aging on testicular volume and glucose metabolism: an investigation with ultrasonography and FDG-PET. Mol Imaging Biol 13(2):391–398. https://doi.org/10.1007/s11307-010-0341-x

Yazaki E, Shawdon A, Beasley I, Evans D (December 1996) The effect of different types of exercise on gastro-oesophageal reflux. Aust J Sci Med Sport 28(4):93–96

Yeh C, Flatley E, Elkattawy O, Berger L, Rao B (July 2022) Exercise in dermatology: exercise's influence on skin aging, skin cancer, psoriasis, venous ulcers, and androgenetic alopecia. J Am Acad Dermatol 87(1):183–184. https://doi.org/10.1016/j.jaad.2021.07.023

Yeroushalmi S, Hakimi M, Chung M, Bartholomew E, Bhutani T, Liao W (2. July 2022) Psoriasis and exercise: a review. Psoriasis (Auckl) 12:189–197. https://doi.org/10.2147/PTT.S349791

Yoo S-Z, No M-H, Heo J-W, Park D-H, Kang J-H, Kim S, Kwak H-B (24. August 2018) Role of exercise in age-related sarcopenia. J Exerc Rehabil 14(4):551–558. https://doi.org/10.12965/jer.1836268.134

Zaugg M, Lucchinetti E (1. March 2000) Respiratory function in the elderly. Anesthesiol Clin North America 18(1):47–58. https://doi.org/10.1016/S0889-8537(05)70148-6

Zhao J-L, Jiang W-T, Wang X, Cai Z-D, Liu Z-H, Liu G-R (September 2020) Exercise, brain plasticity, and depression. CNS Neurosci Ther 26(9):885–895. https://doi.org/10.1111/cns.13385

Zimmer P, Baumann F, Bloch W, Zopf E, Schulz S, Latsch J, Schenk A (February 2016) Impact of a half marathon on cellular immune system, pro-inflammatory cytokine levels, and recovery behavior of breast cancer patients in the aftercare compared to healthy controls. Eur J Haematol 96(2):152–159. https://doi.org/10.1111/ejh.12561

4 Process of Assessment

Contents

Trailer

The fourth chapter delves into the heart of medical training therapy: the process of assessment. This crucial chapter unfolds the methods and tools that professionals use to gain a comprehensive overview of their patients' physical condition, laying the foundation for tailored therapy plans.

S. Wolfram and R. Bauer, *Evidence-Based Medical Exercise Therapy*,
https://doi.org/10.1007/978-3-662-70774-6_4

At the beginning, the chapter focuses on the assessment of strength status, a key aspect for creating individual training programs. It guides through the various technical and formula-based methods for measuring strength, from device-based determinations to renowned formulas such as Epley, Brzycki, and Lombardi, which allow for precise estimation of maximum strength. This section not only provides a detailed insight into the theory behind each method, but also practical instructions for calculating the ideal training weight for various training goals.

The next section focuses on the assessment of endurance status, another critical area for planning effective training therapies. Both device-based and non-device-based tests are presented, including the Harvard Step Test and the Cooper Test, which provide professionals with valuable data on cardiorespiratory fitness. In addition, the role of effort and Borg scales in assessing perceived exertion and performance is discussed.

The assessment of the coordinative status is addressed next, highlighting both device-based and non-device-based methods for evaluating coordination. This section emphasizes the importance of coordination for overall physical performance and how it can be assessed in practice.

In conclusion, the chapter focuses on joint mobility, an often overlooked but essential factor for health and performance. It explains how mobility can be effectively measured and evaluated to identify limitations and plan targeted interventions.

This chapter is an indispensable guide for anyone involved in medical training therapy. It not only provides a solid foundation for assessing physical abilities, but also practical tools that therapists, trainers, and patients alike can use to maximize health and performance. Get ready to master the art and science of assessment and revolutionize the effectiveness of your training programs.

4.1 Assessment of Strength Status

The goal of determining strength status can be achieved through both device-based and non-device-based approaches. For the determination of maximum strength, the one-repetition-maximum (1RM) is a crucial parameter. The 1RM is the training weight that can be moved once at maximum effort. To determine this value, the initially estimated maximum training weight can be set and then tested whether the weight can be moved once. With this approach, untrained individuals have a higher risk of injury (see Shaw et al. 1995). From this perspective, it is helpful to calculate the value of the 1RM based on the training weight and the number of repetitions associated with it. Various formulas exist for this purpose, all of which have in common that the number of repetitions should not exceed 10 during testing, otherwise the calculated values are no longer meaningful (see Reynolds et al. 2006). It should also be considered that the formulas have a standard deviation of about 5 kg. The actual value of the 1RM could therefore be slightly above or below the calculated training weight (see Kravitz et al. 2003; Mann et al. 2012). Various formulas exist for calculating maximum strength, which differ only slightly from each other in the end result. The different formulas are presented in Sect. 4.1.2–4.1.8.

4.1.1 Device-Based Determination of Strength

The determination of strength status can be achieved through various device-based procedures. These include the dynamometer, isokinetic dynamometry, and force plates.

The hand dynamometer, for example, is a valid tool for assessing grip strength (see Lupton-Smith et al. 2022). Isokinetic dynamometry is often used to assess the lower extremity (see Brígido-Fernández et al. 2022). Vertical jumping on force plates also allows conclusions to be drawn about the development of force (see Bellicha et al. 2022).

4.1.2 The Epley Formula

The Epley formula is 1RM = Training weight x (1 + (Repetition number ÷ 30)). Minimal variations can also be found in the literature (see Martín-Hernández et al. 2013). So, for example, if a person were to manage 7 repetitions on the leg press at a training weight of 100 kg, the Epley formula could be adjusted as follows: 1RM = 100(1 + (7:30)). The 1RM is 123.33 kg after solving the equation.

4.1.3 The Brzycki Formula

The Brzycki formula is 1RM = Training weight × 36 ÷ (37-Repetition number). Nascimento et al. (2007) concluded that the Brzycki formula has good validity for a repetition number of 7–10. These findings were obtained from men who were minimally to moderately active in the bench press exercise. So, for example, if a person were to perform 7 repetitions on the leg press with a training weight of 100 kg, the Brzycki formula could be adjusted as follows: 1RM = 100 × 36 ÷ (37−7). The 1RM is 120 kg after solving the equation.

4.1.4 The Lander Formula

The Lander formula is 1RM = 100 × Training weight ÷ (101.3 − 2.67123 × Repetition number) (see Wood et al. 2009). So, for example, if a person were to perform 7 repetitions on the leg press with a training weight of 100 kg, the Lander formula could be adjusted as follows: 1RM = 100 × 100 ÷ (101.3−2.67123 × 7). The 1RM is 121.06 kg after solving the equation.

Additional formulas were established by Lombardi, Mayhew/Ball/Arnold et al., O'Connor et al., and Wathen (see Wood et al. 2009).

The 1RM corresponds to a performance capacity of 100%. Determining this value is of enormous importance in maximal strength training but can also be used as a calculation basis for the load control of other types of strength, such as endurance strength.

Practical Tip

Regardless of the formula used, when determining the 1RM, care should be taken to ensure that complete fatigue is reached by the tenth repetition at the latest during the exercise. An eleventh repetition should therefore no longer be possible. This approach can minimize inaccuracies.

4.1.5 Lombardi Formula

The Lombardi formula can be used to calculate the 1RM. It is as follows: 1RM = Lifted weight (W) × Repetitions $(R)^{0.10}$. So, for example, if a total of 7 repetitions are possible with a weight of 100 kg, the Lombardi formula can be adjusted as follows: 1RM = 100 kg × $7^{0.10}$. After solving the formula, the following result can be noted: 1RM = 121.48 kg (see Lombardi 1989).

Using the „Prone-Bench-Pull-Exercise", García-Ramos et al. (2019) examined, among other things, the reliability and validity of the Lombardi formula. The measured coefficient of variation of 3.44% and the intraclass correlation coefficient of 0.94 suggest a high value of the Lombardi formula and thus support its use.

4.1.6 Mayhew Formula

The Mayhew formula can be used to calculate the 1RM. It is as follows: 1RM = (100 × Training weight) ÷ ((52.2 + (41.9 × $e^{-0.055 \times \text{Repetition number}}$)). The letter e stands for the natural logarithm and is approximately 2.71828. So, for example, if a total of 7 repetitions are possible with a weight of 100 kg, the Mayhew formula can be adjusted as follows:

$(100 \times 100\ \text{kg}) \div ((52.2 + (41.9 \times e^{-0.055 \times 7}))$. After solving the formula, the following result can be noted: 1RM = 123.89 kg. Mayhew et al. (1992) found in a study, which included cross-validations, that the Mayhew formula has good predictive power for different populations in relation to bench pressing. A standard error of ±3.1 to ±5.6 kg was found.

4.1.7 Wathen Formula

The Wathen formula can be used to calculate the 1RM. It is as follows: 1RM = (100 × Training weight) ÷ ((48.8 + (53.8 × e–$^{0.075 \text{ x repetition number}}$)). The letter e stands for the natural logarithm and is to be given as approximately 2.71828. So, for example, if a total of 7 repetitions are possible with a weight of 100 kg, the Wathen formula can be adjusted as follows: $(100 \times 100\ \text{kg}) \div ((48.8 + (53.8 \times e^{-0.075 \times 7}))$. After resolving the formula, the following result can be noted: 1RM = 124.03 kg (cf. Wathen 1994).

4.1.8 O'Connor Formula

The O'Connor formula can be used to calculate the 1RM. It is as follows: 1RM = Training weight x (1 + 0.025 × repetition number). So, for example, if a total of 7 repetitions are possible with a weight of 100 kg, the O'Connor formula can be adjusted as follows: 1RM = 100 x (1 + 0.025 × 7). After resolving the formula, the following result can be noted: 1RM = 117.5 kg (cf. O'Connor 1989).

The use of the O'Connor formula is particularly suitable for young adults with prior experience in the field of strength training (cf. Neto et al. 2017).

4.1.9 The OMNIBUS Resistance Exercise Scale

Another way to objectively validate the subjective effort during strength training is the OMNIBUS Resistance Exercise Scale (OMNI-Res). On an 11-point scale, the subjectively perceived effort is indicated from 0 „easy“ to 10 „extremely hard“. If the points from 1–10 are multiplied by 10, this corresponds, with a standard deviation of ± 0.2 to ± 0.4, to the percentage of the 1RM (cf. Robertson et al. 2003). Fig. 4.1 provides an overview of the OMNIBUS Resistance Exercise Scale.

4.1.10 The Perceived Velocity Scale

In addition to subjective effort, subjective movement speed can also be measured. The perceived movement speed (English: perceived velocity) during strength training can be assessed with a scale from 0.1–1.6 using the Perceived Velocity Scale. In wording, it can be differentiated with intermediate stages from „very slow“ to „maximum fast“ (cf. Bautista et al. 2014).

Effort level in figures	Verbal description
0	Extremely light
1	
2	light
3	
4	reasonably light
5	
6	reasonably heavy
7	
8	heavy
9	
10	Extremely heavy

Fig. 4.1 OMNIBUS Resistance Exercise Scale. (Own illustration 2023)

Perceived speed of exercise execution in figures	Verbal description of the perceived speed
0.1	
0.2	Very slow
0.3	
0.4	slowly
0.5	
0.6	
0.7	
0.8	Power zone
0.9	
1	
1.1	fast
1.2	
1.3	very fast
1.4	
1.5	
1.6	Maximum speed

Fig. 4.2 Perceived Velocity Scale. (Own illustration 2023)

Fig. 4.2 provides an overview of the Perceived Velocity Scale.

4.1.11 Calculation of Training Weight for Endurance Strength Training, Maximum Strength Training, Speed Strength Training, Reactive Strength Training

The basis for calculating the training weight suitable for the chosen type of strength is the 1RM. The process of determining the 1RM is explained in Sect. 4.1. The different types of strength differ not only in the way they are performed, but also in the number of repetitions and the percentage intensity chosen based on the 1RM. Precise information about these variables and the effects of the different types of strength is provided in the entire Chap. 2. At this point, the focus should be on calculating the training weight of the different types of strength. The intensity values of the different types of strength play a crucial role in this.

The stimulus intensity in aerobic endurance strength training can be declared at 30–50%. Submaximal endurance strength training uses an approximate intensity range of 50–75%. Maximum strength endurance goes beyond the 75% mark of the 1RM (see Ehlenz et al. 1998). For example, if a 1RM of about 100 kg is calculated for an exercise and a strength endurance training of 60% is chosen, the training weight would be set at 60 kg. The training weight can be fine-tuned to the training goal in interaction with the subjective effort and the number of repetitions that can be performed.

Regarding maximum strength training, a distinction can be made between hypertrophy training and intramuscular coordination training. In hypertrophy training, an intensity between 60%–90% can be called up (see Fry et al. 2004). This intensity range can also be transferred to reactive strength training. In intramuscular coordination training, the intensity increases to 90–100% of the 1RM. The intensity indication of 90–100% can be transferred to speed strength (see Haas and Fox 2005).

4.2 Assessment of Endurance Status

To determine the endurance status, the bicycle ergometer or the treadmill is usually used as training equipment. The determination of lactate values, spirometry with respiratory gas analysis, and the electrocardiogram (EKG) offer possibilities to measure the strain on the cardiovascular system, the respiratory system via ventilation, and the energy metabolism. Lactate measurements and the determination of VO2max are available as the most accurate measurement methods of cardiorespiratory endurance ability.

4.2.1 Apparatus Determination of Endurance

The apparatus determination of endurance can be carried out both by means of lactate measurement and through spirometric respiratory gas analysis. Sect. 4.2.1.1 and 4.2.1.2 provide a more detailed insight into the topic.

4.2.1.1 Lactate Measurement

When measuring lactate levels, it is important to document the training device used, as the training device influences the results. For athletes, the training device can be adapted to the sport. For example, cyclists can use the bicycle ergometer, while marathon runners choose the treadmill.

During the test, the performance to be achieved is gradually increased. Various procedures are available for the process of increase. The load can be increased continuously in stages, there can be interval-like increasing loads with a load-break ratio, or a constant duration load with increasing performance on several test days. The first method, the so-called step test, is the most common. The heart rate gradually increases with the increased performance. The EKG can take over the measurement of the heart currents. At the same time, the measurement of the performance-dependent lactate value is possible through blood drops from the earlobe. Various thresholds can be derived through recurring lactate measurements during the performance increase while simultaneously measuring the heart rate. When the lactate value reaches 2 mmol/l, the heart rate measured at this point represents the aerobic threshold. If the value of 4 mmol/l is reached with further increasing performance, this marks the anaerobic threshold. These threshold values originate from empirical data and provide a rough insight into the performance capacity of the person to be tested (see Laube 2011). For an even more precise determination of the anaerobic threshold, the maximum lactate steady state can be determined (see Wackerhage et al. 2022).

> **Practical Tip**
> Performance checks using lactate measurements allow conclusions to be drawn about targeted individual training control. More information on this topic is provided by Sect. 2.5.3.1 and 2.5.3.2. One advantage of this approach is that it does not lead to exhaustion.

4.2.1.2 Spirometric Respiratory Gas Analysis

Another way to measure endurance is to determine the maximum oxygen uptake in milliliters per kilogram per minute (relative VO2max). The VO2max value is composed of the cardiac output and the difference in oxygen partial pressure between arterial and venous blood (see Levine 2008). Under exhaustion and taking into account body weight, the relative VO2max value can be determined using spirometric respiratory gas analysis (see Jouannot 2008). The relative VO2max value makes it possible to make comparisons between people of different body weights. Depending on age, there are different norm values for the relative VO2max (see Shvartz and Reibold 1990; Silva et al. 2016).

Laube (2011) refers to the lactate thresholds in the performance diagnostics of endurance as net criteria, while the VO2max value can be considered as a gross criterion. The values are therefore related to each other but are to be interpreted as individual sizes.

4.2.2 Harvard Step Test

If neither a lactate test nor a spirometric respiratory gas analysis can be performed to assess endurance, non-apparatus tests must be used. These include, for example, the Harvard Step Test, the Walk Test, the Cooper Test, the Conconi Test, the PWC Test, and the IPN Test. The following presents some of these tests in their theoretical test execution.

The Harvard Step Test offers a way to roughly predict the relative VO2max. To do this, the standing test person practices steps on a step for a maximum period of 5 minutes. The step should be adjusted to the body size to lead to a knee flexion angle of 90° during ascent. 30 steps must be performed in one minute. The execution time is measured in seconds. An early termination is given by leaving the rhythm of the specification of 30 steps per minute in a period of 15 seconds. Subsequently, the heartbeats between 60–90 seconds after the load are counted. In addition, the heartbeats between 120–150 seconds after the load and between 180–210 seconds after the load are counted. The obtained values can then be inserted into the short or long version of the Physical Fitness Index formula.

The short Physical Fitness Index formula is (100 × test time in seconds) ÷ (5.5 × heartbeats between 60–90 s). So if the test person were to run the full 5 minutes of the test and have a total of 90 heartbeats between seconds 60–90 after the test, the formula could be filled in as follows: (100 × 300) ÷ (5.5 × 90). After resolving the formula, an approximate relative VO2max value of 60.60 ml/min/kg would result.

The long Physical Fitness Index formula is (100 × test time in seconds) ÷ (2 × the sum of all heartbeats between 60–90 s/120–150 s/180–210 s). If a person were to stop the test after 240 seconds and had 90 heartbeats between seconds 60–90, 80 heartbeats between seconds 120–150, and 70 heartbeats between seconds 180–210, the formula could be filled in as follows (100 × 240) ÷ (2 x (90 + 80 + 70)). After resolving the formula, an approximate relative VO2max value of 50 ml/min/kg would result.

In a study comparing the above-mentioned Harvard Step Test with a spirometric respiratory gas analysis in determining the relative VO2max, a positive correlation coefficient of r = 0.905 was found. The standard deviation of the Harvard Step Test was ± 4.07 ml/kg1/min-1. These results speak for a good validity of the Harvard Step Test when the step height is adjusted to the body size of the person to be tested (see Ismail 2011).

4.2.3 2 km Walk Test

Another test that can also be used for an approximate calculation of cardiorespiratory fitness is the 2 km walk test. In this test, the test subject is asked to walk a distance of 2 km as quickly as possible. It is important that the test subject does not run at any point, but only walks as quickly as possible. Therefore, there is ground contact at all times during the walk. Immediately after completing the 2 km distance, the heart rate is measured. In addition, both the BMI and the age of the test subject are required. Once all the information is available after the test, the values can be implemented into different formulas depending on the gender.

The following index formula applies to the male gender: 420 – ((test time in minutes x 11.6) + (test time in seconds x 0.2) + (heart rate after completion x 0.56) + (BMI value x 2.6)) – (age in years x 0.2). If a 30-year-old man with a BMI of 32 took 14 minutes and 10 seconds to cover the 2 km distance and had a stress heart rate of 166 at the end of the distance, the formula could be filled in as follows: 420 – ((14 x 11.6) + (10 x 0.2) + (166 x 0.56) + (32 x 2.6)) – (30 x 0.2). After solving the formula, an index value of 88.64 is calculated. The index classification of the UKK Institute states that a value below 70 is below average, a value between 70 and 89 is slightly below average, a value between 90-110 is average, a value between 111–130 is slightly above average, and a value above 130 is above average.

Furthermore, the following formula from the UKK Institute can be used to determine the relative VO2max value in men: 184.9 – (4.65 x time in minutes) – (0.22 x stress heart rate) – (0.26 x age in years) – (1.05 x Body Mass Index). If the data described above is inserted into the formula, the following result is obtained: 184.9 – (4.65 x 14) – (0.22 x 166) – (0.26 x 30) – (1.05 x 32).

When the formula is solved, a relative VO2max of 41.88 ml/min/kg is calculated.

The following index formula applies to the female gender: 350 – ((test time in minutes x 8.1) + (test time in seconds x 0.14) + (heart rate after completion x 0.36) + (BMI value x 1.0)) – (age in years x 0.3). If a 30-year-old woman with a BMI of 32 took 14 minutes and 10 seconds to cover the 2 km distance and had a stress heart rate of 166 at the end of the distance, the formula could be filled in as follows: 350 – ((14 x 8.1) + (10 x 0.14) + (166 x 0.36) + (32 x 1.0)) – (30 x 0.3). After solving the formula, an index value of 153.44 is calculated. The index classification of the UKK Institute states that a value below 70 is below average, a value between 70 and 89 is slightly below average, a value between 90–110 is average, a value between 111–130 is slightly above average, and a value above 130 is above average.

Furthermore, the following formula from the UKK Institute can be used to determine the relative VO2max value in women: 116.2 – (2.98 x time in minutes) – (0.11 x stress heart rate) – (0.14 x age in years) – (0.39 x body mass index). If the data described above is inserted into the formula, the following result is obtained: 116.2 – (2.98 x 14) – (0.11 x 166) – (0.14 x 30) – (0.39 x 32). When the formula is solved, a relative VO2max of 39.54 ml/min/kg is calculated (see UKK-Institute 2023).

In a validity study of the 2 km walking test, it was shown that the 2 km distance performs better compared to shorter distances. In addition, absolute correlation coefficients of 0.77 for the female gender and 0.69 for the male gender were found compared to spirometric respiratory gas analysis. The 2 km walk test shows good validity especially in untrained and overweight people without additional diseases (see Laukkanen et al. 1992).

4.2.4 Cooper Test

The implementation of the Cooper Test determines a value that allows statements about general endurance. The duration of the test is a total of 12 minutes. During this time, the participants must cover the greatest possible distance for them, either walking or running. Subsequently, the distance covered, taking into account the gender and age, is compared with corresponding standard values. The test can determine a starting value in meters. In addition, the value can be interpreted based on the existing standard values. The test shows a test-retest reliability correlation coefficient of 0.92 (see Maksud and Coutts 1971). This indicates good repeatability of the Cooper Test. It is important to have as similar conditions as possible for the test implementation in terms of surface, gradient, and temperature. For untrained or inexperienced runners and adolescents, conclusions from the Cooper Test results on aerobic capacity should be made with caution (see Maksud and Coutts 1971). The publication by Carl Magnus Swahn (no date) served as the basis for the standard values presented in Figs. 4.3a and 4.3b.

4.2.5 Conconi Test

The Conconi Test can be practiced using activities such as running or training on a bicycle ergometer. When running, a distance of 200 m is run at a constant speed. On the bicycle ergometer, a certain wattage would be maintained for two minutes each. At the end of this first stage, the heart rate is measured. After the first stage, the intensity is increased. When running, by about 1 km/h, on the ergometer by 20 watts. This procedure is repeated in 12–16 stages, each building on the previous one. The heart rate is measured at the end of each stage. As soon as the intensity can no longer be maintained for 2 minutes, the test is finished. The data are then plotted in a coordinate system. The X-axis represents the heart rate, while the Y-axis represents the intensity (km/h or watts). The measured heart rate values at the corresponding intensity are plotted in the coordinate system and then connected linearly. The point at which the heart rate values no longer increase linearly is referred to as the deflection point (see Conconi et al. 1996). The deflection point can be used as a rough indicator of the anaerobic threshold (see Pereira et al. 2016).

4.2.6 Physical-Working-Capacity-Test

The Physical-Working-Capacity-Test (PWC) is a submaximal test, usually performed on a bicycle ergometer. The aim of the test procedure is to reach a predetermined target heart rate during the test. The level of the target heart rate varies depending on the fitness level of the person being tested. For people with a low fitness level, the target heart rate of 130 (PWC130) is chosen. For amateur athletes, the target heart rate of 150 (PWC150) is preferred. For professional athletes, the target heart rate of 170 (PWC170) is used. The test begins with a starting power of 50 watts. Subsequently, the wattage is increased by 25 watts every three minutes. At the end of each

Cooper test (amateur athletes and young people)						
Age	Gender	Very good	Good	Average	Bad	Very bad
13-14 years	Male	> 2700 m	2400–2700 m	2200–2399 m	2100–2199 m	< 2100 m
	Female	> 2000 m	1900–2000 m	1600–1899 m	1500–1599 m	< 1500 m
15-16 years	Male	> 2800 m	2500–2800 m	2300–2499 m	2200–2299 m	< 2200 m
	Female	> 2100 m	2000–2100 m	1700–1999 m	1600–1699 m	< 1600 m
17-19 years	Male	> 3000 m	2700–3000 m	2500–2699 m	2300–2499 m	< 2300 m
	Female	> 2300 m	2100–2300 m	1800–2099 m	1700–1799 m	< 1700 m

Fig. 4.3a Cooper Test standard values Part 1. (Own illustration 2023)

Cooper test (amateur athletes and young people)						
Age	Gender	Very good	Good	Average	Bad	Very bad
20–29 years	Male	> 2800 m	2400–2800 m	2200–2399 m	1600–2199 m	< 1600 m
	Female	> 2700 m	2200–2700 m	1800–2199 m	1500–1799 m	< 1500 m
30–39 years	Male	> 2700 m	2300–2700 m	1900–2299 m	1500–1899 m	< 1500 m
	Female	> 2500 m	2000–2500 m	1700–1999 m	1400–1699 m	< 1400 m
40–49 years	Male	> 2500 m	2100–2500 m	1700–2099 m	1400–1699 m	< 1400 m
	Female	> 2300 m	1900–2300 m	1500–1899 m	1200–1499 m	< 1200 m
50+ years	Male	> 2400 m	2000–2400 m	1600–1999 m	1300–1599 m	< 1300 m
	Female	> 2200 m	1700–2200 m	1400–1699 m	1100–1399 m	< 1100 m

Fig. 4.3b Cooper Test standard values Part 2. (Own illustration 2023)

load stage, the heart rate is measured and documented. The test ends when the target heart rate is reached at the end of a stage. The values are then inserted into the following formula:

Performance (target heart rate) = wattage of the penultimate stage + (wattage of the last stage – wattage of the penultimate stage) x ((target heart rate – heart rate at the end of the penultimate load stage) ÷ (heart rate at the end of the last load stage – heart rate at the end of the penultimate load stage)). The following formula will be filled with values using an example. The PWC170 is tested. The penultimate wattage is 225 watts, the last wattage is 250 watts. The heart rate at the end of the penultimate load stage is 155. The heart rate at the end of the last load stage is 176. If the presented values are inserted into the formula, the following equation is created: Performance (target heart rate) = 225 + (250–225) x ((170–155) ÷ (176–155)). After solving the formula, the following result is obtained: Performance (target heart rate) = 242.85 watts. If the calculated performance is divided by the body weight of the person being tested, a value that takes into account body weight is obtained (242.85 watts ÷ 80 kg = 3.04 watts/kg. Fig. 4.4shows an overview of these standard values. The standard values were taken from the Academy of Sports (2023).

Heid and Zipf (1984) were able to demonstrate a highly significant linear correlation between the PWC170 and the anaerobic threshold.

4.2.7 Borg Scales

Another way to infer the strain on the cardiorespiratory system during endurance activity is through the Borg scales (see Borg 1970). On a scale of 6–20, the degree of perceived exertion (English: rating of perceived exertion – Borg-RPE) can be categorized from „very, very light" to „very, very hard". With a consistent standard deviation of ± 0.2 to ± 0.4, the aerobic and anaerobic threshold can be inferred from the given value. A value of 10.1 corresponds to the aerobic threshold in patients with metabolic syndrome, while a value of 15.6 corresponds to the anaerobic threshold (see Irving et al. 2006).

Useful visualizations can be found in Fig. 4.5.

Another Borg scale is the Category Ratio Scale (Borg-CR). Here, the degree of fatigue due to cardiorespiratory strain can be objectified. On a scale of 0–10, a classification from 0 „nothing" to 10 „very, very strong/intense" can be made (see Borg 1982).

Useful visualizations can be found in Fig. 4.6.

PWC test start	PWC with Target heart rate 130	PWC with Target heart rate 150	PWC with Target heart rate 170
Very good	> 2.0	> 2.5	> 3.0
Above average	1.5–2.0	2.0–2.5	2.5–3.0
Average	1.0–1.5	1.5– 2.0	2.0–2.5
Below average	0.5–1.0	1.0–1.5	1.5–2.0
Weak	< 0.5	< 1.0	< 1.5

Fig. 4.4 PWC-Test standard values. (Own illustration 2023)

Perception of exertion in figures	Verbal description of the feeling of exertion
6	
7	very, very light
8	
9	very light
10	
11	fairly light
12	
13	somewhat heavy
14	
15	heavy
16	
17	Very heavy
18	
19	very, very heavy
20	

Fig. 4.5 Borg-RPE scale. (Own illustration 2023)

Perception of fatigue in figures	Verbal description of the feeling of fatigue
0	nothing
0.5	just noticeable
1	very weak
2	weak
3	moderate
4	little strong
5	strong
6	
7	very strong
8	
9	
10	Very, very strong

Fig. 4.6 Borg-CR scale. (Own illustration 2023)

4.2.8 Effort Scale-Sport

The Effort Scale-Sport is a further development of the Borg-RPE scale. The adjective „effortful" provides an accurate description for the purpose of measuring the degree of effort. In addition to the accurate verbal description, the Effort Scale-Sport has the advantage that each effort level from 1–10 is assigned a verbal description. For successful use, the trainee must be asked after the training how strenuous the previous training session was. In addition to documenting the values, a coordination or practice phase with the Effort Scale-Sport is recommended (see Büsch et al. 2021).

Useful visualizations can be found in Fig. 4.7.

4.3 Assessment of Coordination Status

In the assessment of coordination status, the instrumental evaluation of coordination can be distinguished from the non-instrumental evaluation. Sect. 4.3.1 and 4.3.2 provide a deeper insight into the topic.

Effort level in figures	Verbal description
1	Not exhausting at all
2	Extremely little effort
3	Very little effort
4	not very strenuous
5	moderately strenuous
6	exhausting
7	very strenuous
8	Extremely exhausting
9	Maximum effort
10	so exhausting that I have to stop

Fig. 4.7 Effort Scale-Sport. (Own illustration 2023)

4.3.1 Instrumental Determination of Coordination

The function of the sensorimotor system depends on its structures. If structures degenerate or are injured, this can lead to a functional scar of the sensorimotor system (cf. Laube 2011). In view of medical training therapy, the ability of the motor system's coordination is of central importance. It is therefore a matter of whether or to what intensity motor units can be activated.

For diagnostics, the combination of electromyography (EMG) and dynamography as well as kinesiological electromyography can be used (cf. Medved and Cifrek 2011; Soderberg and Knutson 2000). For example, it has been shown that patients after reconstruction of the anterior cruciate ligament have a lower EMG amplitude of the quadriceps femoris muscle (cf. Pamukoff et al. 2017).

4.3.2 Non-Instrumental Assessment of Coordination

For the most objective data collection in the absence of instrumental examination methods in relation to coordination, a variety of tests are available.

To assess the risk of falling or balance, for example, the Berg Balance Test (cf. Downs et al. 2013), the Romberg Test (cf. Halmágyi and Curthoys 2021), the Star Excursion Balance Test (cf. Powden et al. 2019) as well as the tandem stand (cf. Joo et al. 2019) and tandem walk (cf. Santo et al. 2023) can be used.

If the goal is to gain information about walking ability and mobility, the implementation of the Timed-Up-and-Go Test (cf. Rodrigues et al. 2023), the Dynamic Gait Index (cf. Mehta et al. 2019), the 6-minute walk test (cf. Hamilton and Haennel 2000) as well as the Figure-8 Walk Test (cf. Lowry et al. 2022) is recommended.

For the assessment of body control and reach, the Interactive Functional Reach Test is suitable (cf. Galen et al. 2015).

Short explanations of the tests can be taken from the assessment list in this book.

4.4 Assessment of Joint Mobility

Various instruments such as the goniometer, the inclinometer or even the smartphone are available for assessing joint mobility. Hanks and Myers (2023) compared a goniometer with a medical inclinometer and a construction inclinometer in a study. It was found that both inclinometers are significantly faster at measuring joint mobility than the goniometer. The inclinometers also have better reliability. The correlation of the measured values between the goniometer and the inclinometers is to be classified as poor to moderate. The measured degree numbers differed between the inclinometers and the goniometer by an average of 4 degrees. Therefore, it is recommended to use the instrument of the initial test for retests. Due to the higher reliability and speed of measuring the range of motion, the measurement by inclinometer is described as the new gold standard (cf. Hanks and Myers 2023).

In a publication from 2019, joint mobility measurement by a goniometer was compared with a smartphone goniometer software. It was found from measurements on the upper ankle joint that the smartphone goniometer software has a higher inter- and intra-tester reliability compared to the traditional goniometer (cf. Alawna et al. 2019). A photography-based goniometry software for the smartphone was also able to generate high inter- and intra-tester reliability for joint mobility measurements at the knee joint (cf. Ferriero et al. 2013).

▶ **Practical Tip**
Goniometers provide usable results when measuring joint mobility. However, smartphone software and inclinometers offer better reliability values at an increased execution speed.

References

Academy of Sports (27 November 2023) https://www.academyofsports.de/de/. Von https://www.academyofsports.de/de/lexikon/pwc-test/. Accessed 27 Nov 2023

Alawna M, Unver B, Yuksel E (January 2019) The Reliability of a Smartphone Goniometer Application Compared With a Traditional Goniometer for Measuring Ankle Joint Range of Motion. J Am Podiatr Med Assoc 109(1):22–29. https://doi.org/10.7547/16-128

Bautista I, Chirosa I, Chirosa L, Martín I, González A, Robertson R (September 2014) Development and validity of a scale of perception of velocity in resistance exercise. J Sports Sci Med 13(3):542–549

Bellicha A, Giroux C, Ciangura C, Menoux D, Thoumie P, Oppert J-M, Portero P (January 2022) Vertical Jump on a Force Plate for Assessing Muscle Strength and Power in Women With Severe Obesity: Reliability, Validity, and Relations With Body Composition. J Strength Cond Res 36(1):75–81. https://doi.org/10.1519/JSC.0000000000003432

Borg G (1970) Perceived exertion as an indicator of somatic stress. Scand J Rehabil Med 2(2):92–98

Borg G (1982) Psychophysical bases of perceived exertion. Med Sci Sports Exerc 14(5):377–381

Brígido-Fernández I, San José F-M, Charneco-Salguero G, Cárdenas-Rebollo J, Ortega-Latorre Y, Carrión-Otero O, Fernández-Rosa L (December 2022) Knee Isokinetic Profiles and Reference Values of Professional Female Soccer Players. Sports (Basel) 10(12):204. https://doi.org/10.3390/sports10120204

Büsch D, Utesch T, Marschall F (4 October 2021) Development and evaluation of the “Anstrengungsskala Sport” (Effort Scale Sport). Ger J Exerc Sport Res 52:173–178. https://doi.org/10.1007/s12662-021-00757-z

Conconi F, Grazzi G, Casoni I, Guglielmini C, Borsetto C, Ballarin E, Manfredini F (October 1996) The Conconi test: methodology after 12 years of application. Int J Sports Med 17(7):509–519. https://doi.org/10.1055/s-2007-972887

Downs S, Marquez J, Chiarelli P (June 2013) The Berg Balance Scale has high intra- and inter-rater reliability but absolute reliability varies across the scale: a systematic review. J Physiother 59(2):93–99. https://doi.org/10.1016/S1836-9553(13)70161-9

Ehlenz H, Grosser M, Zimmermann E (1998) Krafttraining. Grundlagen, Methoden, Übungen, Leistungssteuerung, Trainingsprogramme, BLV Verlagsgesellschaft München

Ferriero G, Vercelli S, Sartorio F, Lasa S, Ilieva E, Brigatti E, Foti C (June 2013) Reliability of a smartphone-based goniometer for knee joint goniometry. Int J Rehabil Res 36(2):146–151. https://doi.org/10.1097/MRR.0b013e32835b8269

Fry A (2004) The role of resistance exercise intensity on muscle fibre adaptations. Sports Med 34(10):663–679. https://doi.org/10.2165/00007256-200434100-00004

Galen S, Pardo V, Wyatt D, Diamond A, Brodith V, Pavlov A (August 2015) Validity of an Interactive Functional Reach Test. Games Health J 4(4):278–284. https://doi.org/10.1089/g4h.2015.0002

García-Ramos A, Barboza-González P, Ulloa-Díaz D, Rodriguez-Perea A, Martinez-Garcia D, Guede-Rojas F, Weakley J (October 2019) Reliability and validity of different methods of estimating the one-repetition maximum during the free-weight prone bench pull exercise. J Sports Sci 37(19):2205–2212. https://doi.org/10.1080/02640414.2019.1626071

Haas H-J, Fox T (2005) Muskelaufbau Schritt für Schritt. Physiopraxis 3(1):26–28. https://doi.org/10.1055/s-0032-1307863

Halmágyi G, Curthoys I (September 2021) Vestibular contributions to the Romberg test: Testing semicircular canal and otolith function. Eur J Neurol 28(9):3211–3219. https://doi.org/10.1111/ene.14942

Hamilton D, Haennel R (May–June 2000) Validity and reliability of the 6-minute walk test in a cardiac rehabilitation population. J Cardiopulm Rehabil

20(3):156–164. https://doi.org/10.1097/00008483-200005000-00003

Hanks J, Myers B (1 August 2023) Validity, Reliability, and Efficiency of a Standard Goniometer, Medical Inclinometer, and Builder's Inclinometer. Int J Sports Phys Ther 18(4):989–996. https://doi.org/10.26603/001c.83944

Heid J, Zipf K (1984) Die Beziehung zwischen der aerob-anaeroben Schwelle und der PWC 170 im Vitamaxima-Test auf dem Fahrradergometer. Franz I-W, Mellerowicz H, Noack W(Hrsg) Training und Sport zur Prävention und Rehabilitation in der technisierten Umwelt. Springer, Berlin, Heidelberg, S 649–654

Irving B, Rutkowski J, Brock D, Davis C, Barrett E, Gaesser G, Weltman A (July 2006) Comparison of Borg- and OMNI-RPE as markers of the blood lactate response to exercise. Med Sci Sports Exerc 38(7):1348–1352. https://doi.org/10.1249/01.mss.0000227322.61964.d2

Ismail W (July 2011) Evaluating the Validity and Reliability of Harvard Step Test to Predict VO2max in Terms of the Step Height According to the Knee Joint Angle. J Appl Sports Sci 1(2):126–132. https://doi.org/10.21608/jass.2011.84908

Joo B, Marquez J, Osmotherly P (6 December 2021) Ten-Second Tandem Stance Test: A Potential Tool to Assist Walking Aid Prescription and Falls Risk in Balance Impaired Individuals. Arch Rehabil Res Clin Transl 4(1):100173. https://doi.org/10.1016/j.arrct.2021.100173

Jouannot P (May 2001) VO2 max: technique and practical importance. Presse Med 30(17):835–840

Kravitz L, Akalan C, Nowicki K, Kinzey S (February 2003) Prediction of 1 repetition maximum in high-school power lifters. J Strength Cond Res 17(1):167–172. https://doi.org/10.1519/1533-4287(2003)017<0167:pormih>2.0.co;2

Laube W (2011) Physiologie, Leistungsphysiologie, Pathophysiologie. In: Hütter-Becker A, Dölken M (Hrsg) Biomechanik. Thieme, Bewegungslehre, Leistungsphysiologie, Trainingslehre, Stuttgart, S 129–332

Laukkanen R, Oja P, Pasanen M, Vuori I (April 1992) Validity of a two kilometre walking test for estimating maximal aerobic power in overweight adults. Int J Obes Relat Metab Disord 16(4):263–268

Levine B (1 January 2008) VO2max: what do we know, and what do we still need to know? J Physiol 586(1):25–34. https://doi.org/10.1113/jphysiol.2007.147629

Lombardi V (1989) Beginning weight training. W.C. Brown, Dubuque, IA

Lowry K, Woods T, Malone A, Krajek A, Smiley A, Van Swearingen J (April 2022) The Figure-of-8 Walk Test used to detect the loss of motor skill in walking among persons with Parkinson's disease. Physiother Theory Pract 38(4):552–560. https://doi.org/10.1080/09593985.2020.1774948

Lupton-Smith A, Fourie K, Mazinyo A, Mokone M, Nxaba S, Morrow B (26 September 2022) Measurement of hand grip strength: A cross-sectional study of two dynamometry devices. S Afr J Physiother 78(1):1768. https://doi.org/10.4102/sajp.v78i1.1768

Maksud M, Coutts K (1971) Application of the Cooper Twelve-Minute Run-Walk Test to Young Males. Res Q Am Asso. Health Phys Educ Rec 42(1):54–59 https://doi.org/10.1080/10671188.1971.10615035

Mann J, Stoner J, Mayhew J (October 2012) NFL-225 test to predict 1RM bench press in NCAA Division I football players. J Strength Cond Res 26(10):2623–2631. https://doi.org/10.1519/JSC.0b013e31826791ef

Martín-Hernández J, Marín P, Menéndez H, Ferrero C, Loenneke J, Herrero A (March 2013) Muscular adaptations after two different volumes of blood flow-restricted training. Scand J Med Sci Sports 23(2):e114-120. https://doi.org/10.1111/sms.12036

Mayhew J, Ball T, Arnold M, Bowen J (November 1992) Relative Muscular Endurance Performance as a Predictor of Bench Press Strength in College Men and Women. J Strength Cond Res 6(4):200–206

Medved V, Cifrek M (09 September 2011) Kinesiological Electromyography, IntechOpen Verlag, London 349-366. Biomech App. https://doi.org/10.5772/21282

Mehta T, Young H-J, Lai B, Wang F, Kim Y, Thirumalai M, Rimmer J (15 February 2019) Comparing the Convergent and Concurrent Validity of the Dynamic Gait Index with the Berg Balance Scale in People with Multiple Sclerosis. Healthcare (Basel) 7(1):27. https://doi.org/10.3390/healthcare7010027

Nascimento M, Cyrino E, Romanzini M, Nakamura F (January 2007) Validation of the Brzycki equation for the estimation of 1-RM in the bench press. Revista Brasileira de Medicina do Esporte 13(1):40e–42e

Neto F, Guanais P, Dornelas E, Coutinho A, Costa R (09 May 2017) Validity of one-repetition maximum predictive equations in men with spinal cord injury. Spinal Cord 55:950–956

O'Connor B, Simmons J, O'Shea P (1989) Weight training today. West, St. Paul, MN

Pamukoff D, Pietrosimone B, Ryan E, Lee D, Blackburn J (May 2017) Quadriceps Function and Hamstrings Co-Activation After Anterior Cruciate Ligament Reconstruction. J Athl Train 52(5):422–428. https://doi.org/10.4085/1062-6050-52.3.05

Pereira P, Carrara V, Rissato G, Duarte J, Guerra R, Azevedo P (May 2016) The relationship between the heart rate deflection point test and maximal lactate steady state. J Sports Med Phys Fitness 56(5):497–502

Powden C, Dodds T, Gabriel E (September 2019) THE RELIABILITY OF THE STAR EXCURSION BALANCE TEST AND LOWER QUARTER Y-BALANCE TEST IN HEALTHY ADULTS: A SYSTEMATIC REVIEW. Int J Sports Phys Ther 14(5):683–694

Reynolds J, Gordon T, Robergs R (August 2006) Prediction of one repetition maximum strength from multiple repetition maximum testing and anthropometry. J Strength Cond Res 20(3):584–592. https://doi.org/10.1519/R-15304.1

Robertson R, Goss F, Rutkowski J, Lenz B, Dixon C, Timmer J, Andreacci J (February 2003) Concurrent validation of the OMNI perceived exertion scale for resistance exercise. Med Sci Sports Exerc 35(2):333–341. https://doi.org/10.1249/01.MSS.0000048831.15016.2A

Rodrigues F, Teixeira J, Forte P (March 2023) The Reliability of the Timed Up and Go Test among Portuguese Elderly. Healthcare (Basel) 11(7):928. https://doi.org/10.3390/healthcare11070928

Santo A, Joyce M, Lynall R (September 2023) Tandem gait test-retest reliability among healthy physically active young adults. PM R 15(9):1098–1105. https://doi.org/10.1002/pmrj.12909

Shaw C, McCully K, Posner J (July–August 1995) Injuries during the one repetition maximum assessment in the elderly. J Cardiopulm Rehabil 15(4):283–287. https://doi.org/10.1097/00008483-199507000-00005

Shvartz E, Reibold R (January 1990) Aerobic fitness norms for males and females aged 6 to 75 years: a review. Aviat Space Environ Med 61(1):3–11

Silva C, Franklin B, Forman D, Araújo C (January 2016) Influence of age in estimating maximal oxygen uptake. J Geriatr Cardiol 13(2):126–131

Soderberg G, Knutson L (1 May 2000) A Guide for Use and Interpretation of Kinesiologic Electromyographic Data. Phys Ther 80(5):485–498. https://doi.org/10.1093/ptj/80.5.485

Swahn C (kein Datum) https://web.archive.org/. von https://web.archive.org/web/20171026004646/. http://www.coopertestchart.com/wp-content/uploads/2017/04/cooper-test.pdf. Accessed 27 Nov 2023

UKK Institute (24 November 2023) UKK Institute. Von https://ukkinstituutti.fi/en/products-services/fitness-tests/ukk-2-km-walk-test/ Accessed 24 Nov 2023

Wackerhage H, Gehlert S, Schulz H, Weber S, Ring-Dimitriou S, Heine O (22 July 2022) Lactate Thresholds and the Simulation of Human Energy Metabolism: Contributions by the Cologne Sports Medicine Group in the 1970s and 1980s. Front Physiol 13:899670. https://doi.org/10.3389/fphys.2022.899670

Wathen D (1994) Load assignment. In: Baechle T (Hrsg) Essential. Human Kinetics, Champaign, IL, S 435–446

Wood T, Maddalozzo G, Harter R (18 November 2009) Accuracy of Seven Equations for Predicting 1-RM Performance of Apparently Healthy, Sedentary Older Adults. Meas Phys Educ Exerc Sci 6(2):67–94. https://doi.org/10.1207/S15327841MPEE0602_1

Orthopedic-Surgical Body Area-Related or Disease-Associated Test Procedures and Medical Exercise Therapy

5

Contents

Supplementary Information The electronic version of this chapter contains additional material, which can be accessed via the following link https://doi.org/10.1007/978-3-662-70774-6_5. The videos can be played by clicking on the DOI link in the legend of a corresponding figure, or by scanning this link with the SN More Media App.

S. Wolfram and R. Bauer, *Evidence-Based Medical Exercise Therapy*,
https://doi.org/10.1007/978-3-662-70774-6_5

Trailer

The fifth chapter guides you through the specialized world of disease-associated medical training therapy, a central area that bridges the gap between medical treatment and physical rehabilitation. It provides detailed insights into the application of targeted exercises for the treatment and relief of complaints associated with a variety of musculoskeletal diseases.

From the pelvis to the wrist, each region of the body is carefully examined, with specific diseases and the most effective training approaches for improving functionality and reducing pain being presented. This chapter illustrates how individually tailored training therapies can significantly improve the quality of life for those affected.

The section on the pelvic/hip joint area covers common diseases such as coxarthrosis, femoroacetabular impingement, and hip dysplasia, demonstrating how targeted movements and strengthening exercises can lead to better mobility and fewer complaints.

In the area of the knee joint, readers are familiarized with the challenges of gonarthrosis, patellofemoral pain syndrome, and cruciate ligament ruptures. Each condition is addressed with an individual exercise program aimed at restoring the stability and function of the knee.

The chapter continues to examine the lower leg and foot, including the treatment of ankle instability, Achilles tendonitis, and foot deformities. It shows how adapted therapies can not only alleviate symptoms but also address the causes of the problems.

Another focus is on the lumbar spine area, where conditions such as lumbar radiculopathy, low back pain, and spondylolisthesis are treated. The importance of exercises to strengthen the core muscles and improve posture is emphasized to effectively combat back pain.

The sections on the thoracic and cervical spine as well as the shoulder girdle and elbow joint provide valuable insights into dealing with specific diseases such as ankylosing spondylitis, scoliosis, glenohumeral instability, and impingement syndrome.

Finally, the wrist area is addressed, with carpal tunnel syndrome being the focus. Practical exercises are presented that can help alleviate symptoms and improve hand function.

This comprehensive chapter is an indispensable guide for anyone involved in medical training therapy or interested in physical rehabilitation for specific diseases. It underscores the power of movement as medicine and offers practical, evidence-based strategies for promoting healing and well-being.

5.1 Pelvic/Hip Joint Area

5.1.1 Coxarthrosis

A meta-analysis comparing the sole medical training intervention with normal care showed that people with cox- and gonarthrosis benefit primarily from training therapy in the first two months. It was shown that medical training therapy leads to a significant decrease in pain as well as an improvement in function and quality of life (see Goh et al. September 2019). For the most positive therapy effect, an individually adapted training plan is essential. In addition, the first twelve therapy sessions, which include at least two training units per week, should be conducted under supervision. In addition to correct training execution, patient education is also an important factor. This increases the chance of long-term integration of medical training therapy into the daily lives of those affected (see Skou and Roos 2019). Individually adapted medical training therapy is recommended in the course of hip arthrosis as preparation for a possible operation as well as a measure of postoperative care (see van Doormaal et al. 2020).

The question of which training intervention is the most promising option depends on the desired outcome. A 2019 published meta-analysis concluded that aerobic training as well as coordination exercises are capable of best alleviating pain and simultaneously improving function. Pure strength and flexibility training, on the other hand, influences various outcomes such as pain, function, performance, and quality of life at a moderate intensity (see Hansen et al. 2020; see Goh et al. May 2019). If the training interventions of aerobic endurance training, coordination training, strength and flexibility training are mixed, this has a lower therapeutic value than the respective single intervention with regard to the mentioned outcomes. However, if the implementation of the single intervention is not possible, the mixture of training forms still offers a better effect than no training intervention (see Goh et al. May 2019). Over a period of three months with weekly 150 minutes of aerobic endurance training, its function-improving and pain-relieving effect in people with coxarthrosis was confirmed (see Hall et al. 2022).

Individuals with hip osteoarthritis typically exhibit a reduced function of the Musculus gluteus medius et minimus (see Zacharias et al. 2020). It has been shown that a progressive training program can increase the activity of these two muscles during walking. Specific command giving during gait training can be supplemented by backward walking training. This can then be followed by targeted strength training through controlled lunges and bridging exercises. For global and local strengthening, bilateral squats, deadlifts, and the so-called "Hip-Hitching" can contribute. In Hip-Hitching, the training person stands on a step with, for example, the right leg and lets the left half of the pelvis drop. The pelvis is then moved back into a horizontal position by muscle work of the Musculus gluteus medius et minimus on the right side (see Rostron et al. 2023).

Other research findings suggest that a rapid concentric execution of the training exercises is superior to a slower execution. Training with the Theraband in hip extension, hip abduction, hip flexion, and knee extension, a rapid execution of the concentric exercise component resulted in a reduction of the time of the Timed-up-and-go test and a reduced echo intensity of the Musculus gluteus maximus (see Fukumoto et al. 2014). In another research work on the speed of exercise execution, it was shown that rapid exercise execution increases muscle strength and walking speed and increases stride cadence. In contrast, slow exercise execution could increase stride length, enhance hip extension, alleviate pain, and significantly reduce the dorsal extension moment in the upper ankle joint (see Fukumoto et al. 2017). If the goal in medical training therapy is to increase walking speed, this should ideally be achieved by increasing stride cadence. Compared to increasing individual steps, the hip joint load and pain perception are reduced (see Tateuchi et al. 2021).

In rehabilitation after the insertion of a total hip endoprosthesis, maximal strength training of the lower extremity shows very good results in terms of muscle strength increase with good tolerance. Three training sessions per week over a total period of three months on the leg press and the abductor machine led to a significant increase in maximal strength in postoperative patients. This was done with 4–5 repetitions at a weight of 85%–90% of the 1RM (see Winther et al. 2018). Husby et al. (2010) recommend continuous maximal strength training after the implantation of a total hip endoprosthesis, complemented by regular endurance training.

Self-stretches of the hip flexors, hip extensors, and hip abductors can also have a positive effect on pain, mobility, and muscle tone in coxarthrosis (see Ceballos-Laita et al. 2022).

Depending on the desired outcome, assessments can include the Harris-Hip-Score (see Fukumoto et al. 2017), the Timed-up-and-go test (see Fukumoto et al. 2014), the 6-Point-Likert-Scale, and the visual analogue scale (see Hoeksma et al. 2004). More detailed information on the individual assessments can be taken from the assessment list in the appendix of this book.

Useful visualizations can be taken from Fig. 5.2, 5.3, 5.4, 5.5, 5.6, 5.7, 5.8, 5.9 and 5.10.

Summary for Practice

Medical training therapy alleviates pain in coxarthrosis and leads to an improvement in functions and thus quality of life.

This requires an individual training plan with at least two training sessions per week. The focus should be on aerobic training and coordination exercises. Pure strength and flexibility training should only be performed at a moderate intensity. The training sessions should always pursue only one goal and should not be mixed in their approaches.

The focus is on strengthening the M. gluteus medius and minimus. Specific exercises in the context of coxarthrosis are lunges, bridging, squats, deadlifts, and hip hitching.

During execution, quick concentric exercise runs should be performed now and then. This can be done, for example, with a theraband in all directions of movement. A slow execution increases the stride length and can alleviate pain.

After surgery and the use of a hip TEP, the focus should be on maximal strength training with supplementary endurance training.

Fig. 5.1 provides an overview of the information mentioned.

5.1.2 Femoroacetabular Impingement

The approach of medical training therapy for femoroacetabular impingement pursues a mix of strength and stretching interventions. It is important not to provoke pain during training (see Wall et al. 2013). Specifically, postural alignment should be improved, the strength and endurance of the trunk increased, the strength and motor control of the hip surrounding musculature optimized, and the flexibility of the lower extremity musculature increased. In the latter point, the muscles that have anatomical connections to the pelvis have the highest priority (see Terrell and Lynn 2019; Kemp et al. 2018; Aoyama et al. 2019; Pennock et al. 2018; Hoit et al. 2020; Mansell et al. 2018). Initial successes can be expected within a period of 6–12 weeks.

To improve coordination, balance exercises such as single-leg stance training can be used (see Kemp et al. 2019).

To improve posture and body awareness, pelvic tilts to the ventral or dorsal can be used. The starting position can be progressively adjusted. After initial training in supine position, the transition can be made to quadruped position and later to sitting or standing (see Terrell and Lynn 2019; Aoyama et al. 2019). The pelvic tilts can

Categories	Evidence-based training recommendation
Units	3 training sessions per week á 45-60 minutes per session
Exercises	Aerobic + coordination training / Strength and flexibility exercises (gluteus medius and minimus muscles) / lunges / Bridging / Squat / Deadlift / Hip- Hitching / Leg Press and Abductor machine as an instrument following the use of a hip TEP
Exercise parameters	Pure strength training after hip TEP insertion 4-5 repetitions with 85-90% of 1RM / regular endurance training approx. 150 minutes per week
Elongation	Self-stretching of the hip flexors, hip extensors, hip abductors

Fig. 5.1 Summary of MTT in Coxarthrosis or Hip Arthroplasty

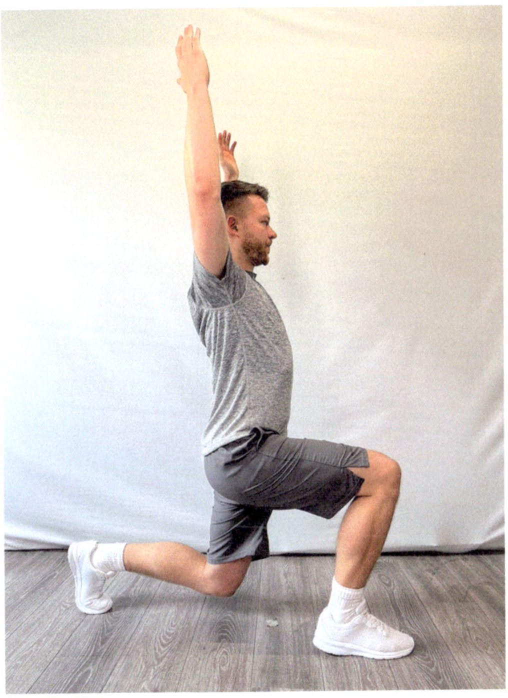

Fig. 5.2 MTT in Coxarthrosis—Lunges

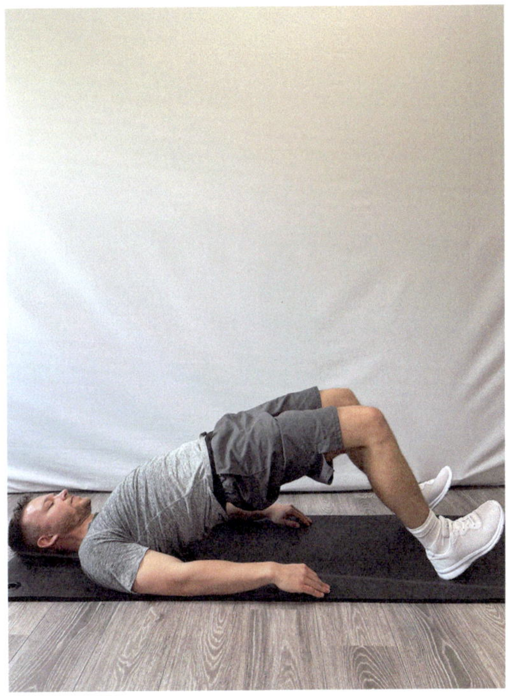

Fig. 5.3 MTT in Coxarthrosis—Bridging Exercises

be combined with inhalation and exhalation (see Terrell et al. 2021). The goal is a neutral pelvic position.

Another important component in the non-surgical management of femoroacetabular impingement is trunk stability training. The central point here is the establishment of a recruitment ability of the transversus abdominis muscle, the multifidus muscles, the respiratory diaphragm, and the pelvic floor musculature (see

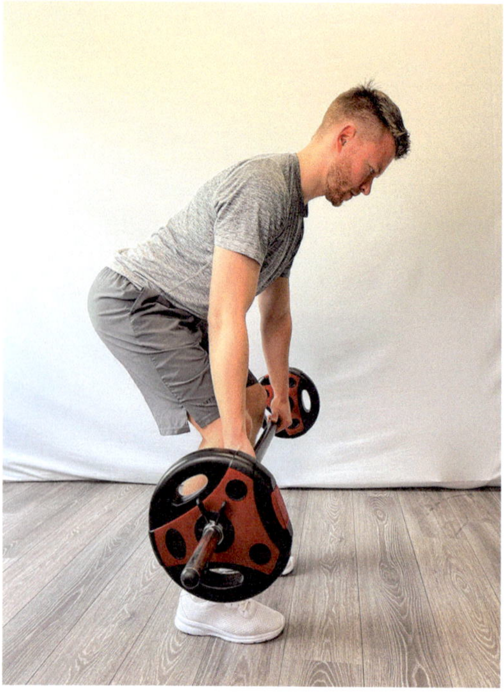

Fig. 5.4 MTT in Coxarthrosis—Deadlifts

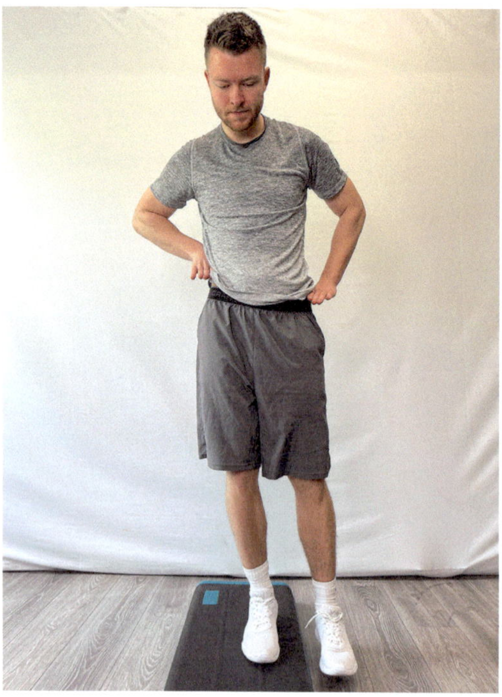

Fig. 5.5 MTT in Coxarthrosis—Hip Hitching

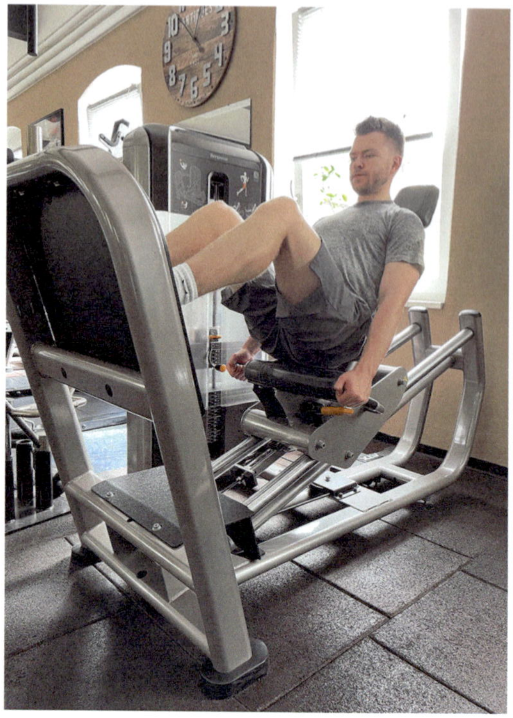

Fig. 5.6 MTT in Coxarthrosis—Leg Press

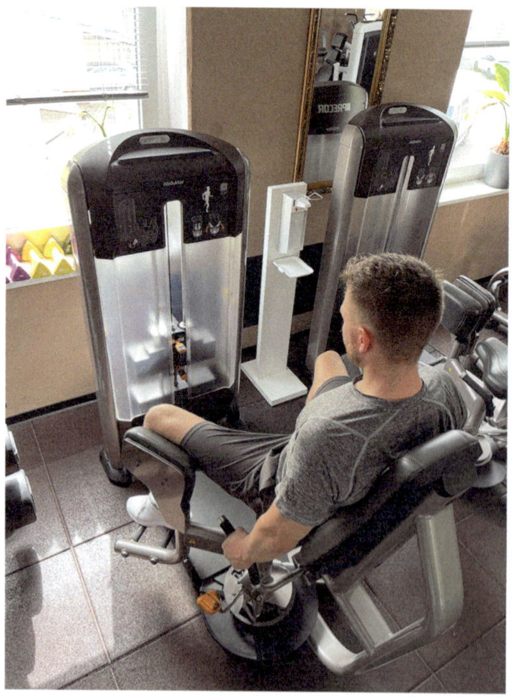

Fig. 5.7 MTT in Coxarthrosis—Abductor Machine

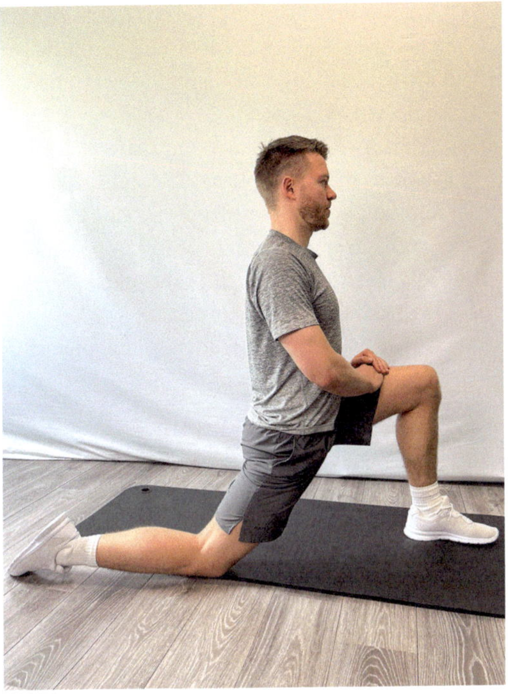

Fig. 5.8 MTT in Coxarthrosis—Self-Stretching Hip Flexors

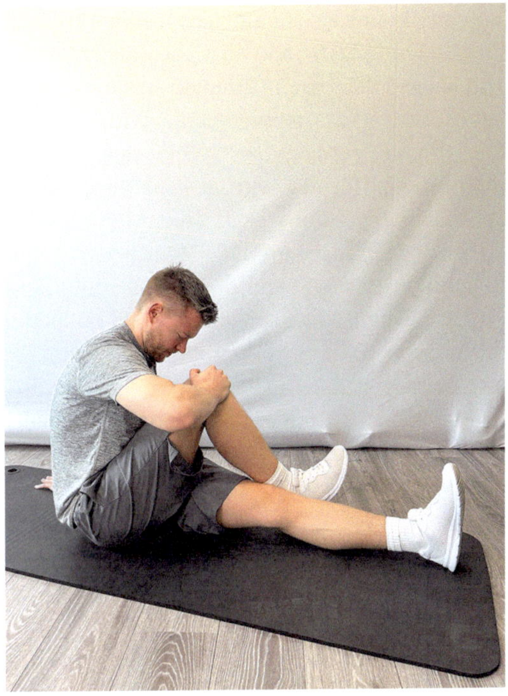

Fig. 5.10 MTT in Coxarthrosis—Self-Stretching Hip Abductors

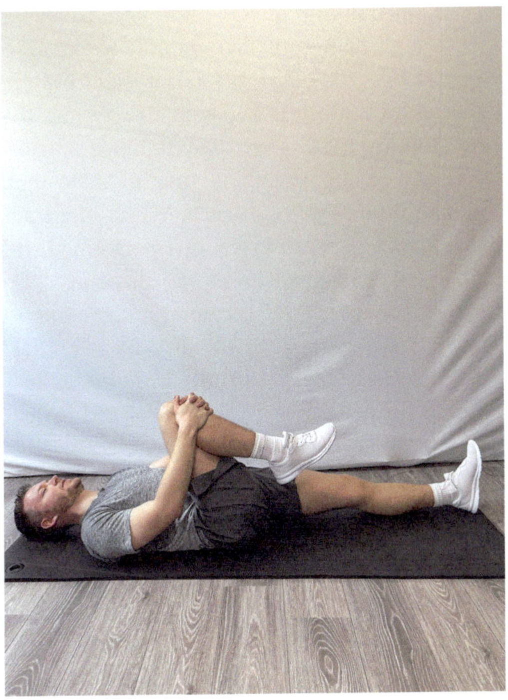

Fig. 5.9 MTT in Coxarthrosis—Self-Stretching Hip Extensors

Terrell and Lynn 2019). The first step should be the targeted activation of the mentioned musculature. Specifically for the transversus abdominis muscle, the use of a biofeedback system is recommended. Pressure biofeedback devices or musculoskeletal ultrasound can be used for this purpose (see Raj 5th and Thomas 2023; la Fuente et al. 2020). Once targeted recruitment of the deep stabilizing musculature is possible, strengthening exercises of the trunk can be performed with the maintained tension of those muscles. Examples would be opposing extension and retraction of the limbs in quadruped position, forearm support, side support, alternating opposing extension and retraction of the limbs in supine position, trunk rotation exercises in lunge position with a held medicine ball, and tension exercises of the limbs in supine position with a Pezziball in various variations (see Terrell et al. 2021).

In terms of strengthening the hip surrounding musculature, in addition to the thigh muscles, the hip abductors, hip external rotators, and hip extensors should also be emphasized. Freke et al. (2016) add that the hip abductors also show a decrease in strength in symptomatic femoroacetabular impingement. With three to four training sessions per week, each exercise should be performed with at least three sets of up to ten repetitions each (see Mansell et al. 2018). If working with one's own body weight, in addition to single and double leg bridging in supine position, external rotation and abduction movements of the upper leg in side position can also be practiced. In addition to side steps with a resistance band, exercises that target the quadriceps femoris muscle or the ischiocrural muscles can also be integrated (see Terrell et al. 2021).

To increase flexibility and mobility, self-stretches and auto-mobilizations can be used. Self-stretches should reach the iliopsoas muscle, the ischiocrural muscle group, and the piriformis muscle. Due to the pathophysiology of femoroacetabular impingement, a stretch of the piriformis muscle in over 90° hip flexion and external rotation is favored. Auto-mobilizations can be performed in hip abduction, hip adduction, and hip flexion with extended knee joint (see Terrell et al. 2021).

Useful visualizations can be taken from Fig. 5.12, 5.13, 5.14, 5.15, 5.16, 5.17, 5.18, 5.19, 5.20, 5.21, 5.22 and Fig. 5.23.

Summary for Practice

Medical training therapy for femoroacetabular impingement should be a mix of strength and stretching exercises. The goal is to improve the postural alignment of the pelvis. This is achieved through strength and endurance training of the trunk, as well as strengthening exercises for the muscles surrounding the hip. Furthermore, the flexibility of the muscles in the lower extremity should be increased.

It is important to note that no pain should occur during the execution and the focus should be placed on the correct pelvic position.

Exercises such as active pelvic tilting, balance exercises, and single-leg stance can support this.

Trunk stability can be optimally trained through a biofeedback system. The focus should be on the m. transversus abdominis, the mm. multifidii, the respiratory diaphragm, and the pelvic floor muscles.

In addition to strengthening the thigh muscles, emphasis should also be placed on strengthening the hip abductors, external rotators, and extensors.

Fig. 5.11 provides an overview of the mentioned information.

5.1.3 Hip Dysplasia

Jacobsen et al. (2022) discuss in their publication the acceptance and effectiveness of medical training therapy in people diagnosed with hip dysplasia. It was recognized that the subjects responded very positively to the combination of training intervention and education with a high degree of therapy adherence. Over a period of six months, a total of eight training sessions took place under guidance. In the first two months, there were two training sessions each, and in the following four months, there was one training session each. Within the training sessions, four exercises were performed with individually adapted levels of difficulty. The four exercises include bridging, side support, squats, and a one-legged stability exercise. Each exercise should be performed at home at least three times a week with three sets and at least five repetitions each. The implementation of the described training program led to clinically relevant improvements in terms of pain, strength, and function (see Jacobsen et al. 2022).

Mortensen et al. (2018) explored the effects of progressive strength training in people with hip dysplasia. The training period lasted a total of eight weeks and included a total of 20 training sessions with five sessions within two

Categories	Evidence-based training recommendation
Units	3-4 training sessions per week á 45-60 minutes per session
Exercises	One- and two-legged bridging in supine position / exercises in external rotation and abduction movements in lateral position / side steps against resistance / leg extension / leg flexors
Exercise parameters	Each exercise at least 3 sets with a maximum of 10 repetitions
Elongation	Self-stretching iliopsoas muscle, ischiocrural muscles, piriformis muscle (in over 90° hip flexion and external rotation)

Fig. 5.11 Summary of MTT for femoroacetabular impingement

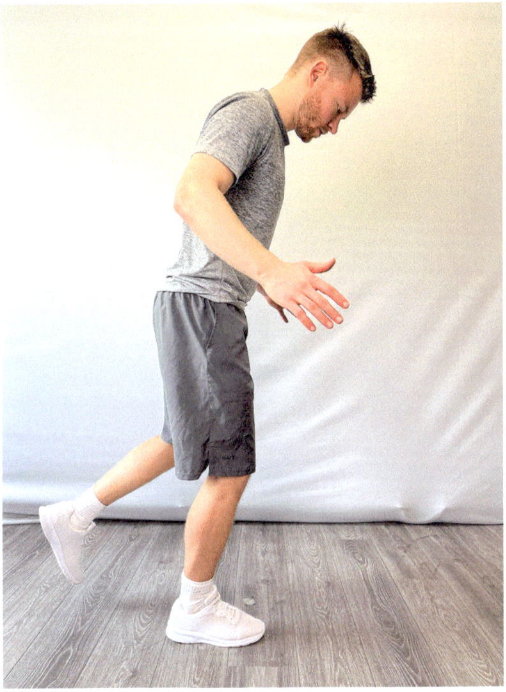

Fig. 5.12 MTT for femoroacetabular impingement—Single-leg stance

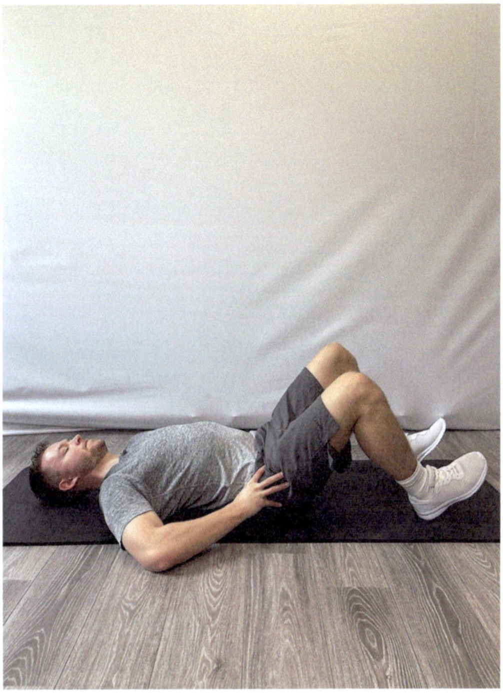

Fig. 5.13 MTT for femoroacetabular impingement—Ventral pelvic tilt

weeks. A training session lasted between 45 and 60 minutes. After a warm-up of 5–10 minutes on the bicycle ergometer, the strength training followed. This consisted of the leg press bilaterally, leg curl bilaterally, leg extension bilaterally, and a one-legged training of the hip flexors and lunges. Training was carried out with 3–4 sets at 8–21 repetitions. The training weight was progressively adjusted during the course of the study. This type of training led to an improving pain situation, better function, and an increase in strength of the hip flexors over time.

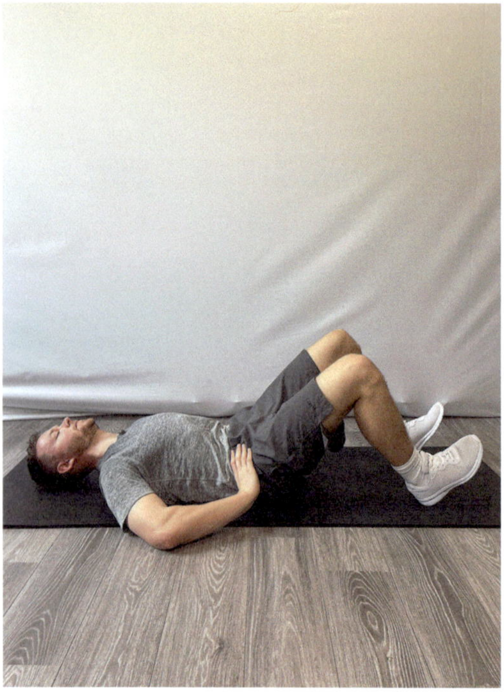

Fig. 5.14 MTT for femoroacetabular impingement—Dorsal pelvic tilt

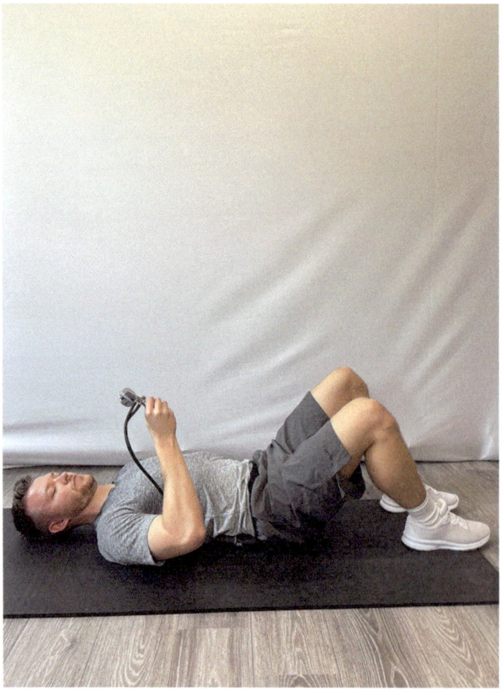

Fig. 5.15 MTT for femoroacetabular impingement—Trunk stability training with biofeedback

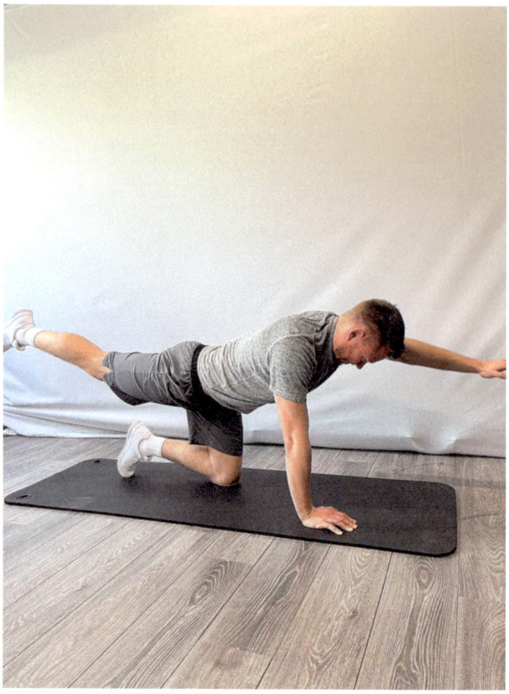

Fig. 5.16 MTT for femoroacetabular impingement—Opposite extension of the extremities in quadruped position

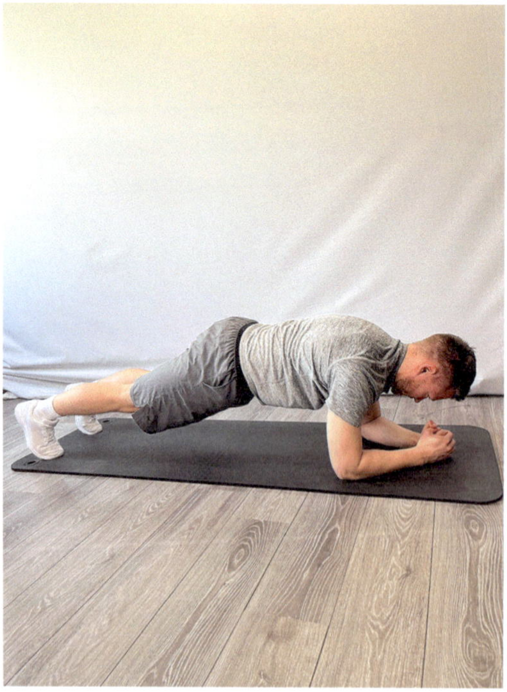

Fig. 5.17 MTT for femoroacetabular impingement—Forearm support

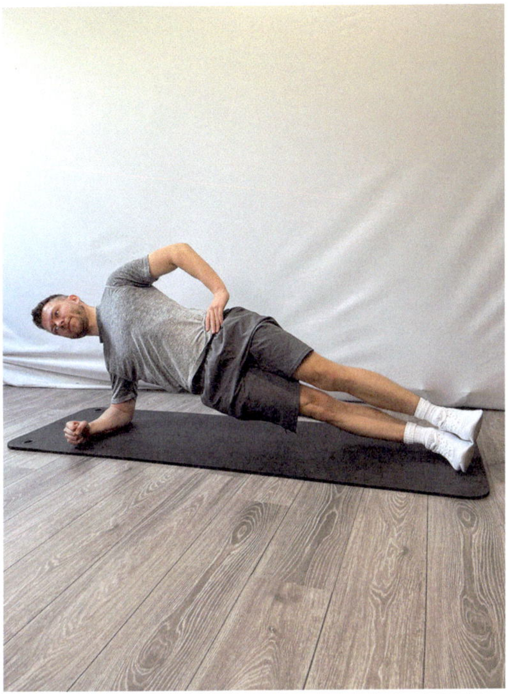

Fig. 5.18 MTT for femoroacetabular impingement—Side support

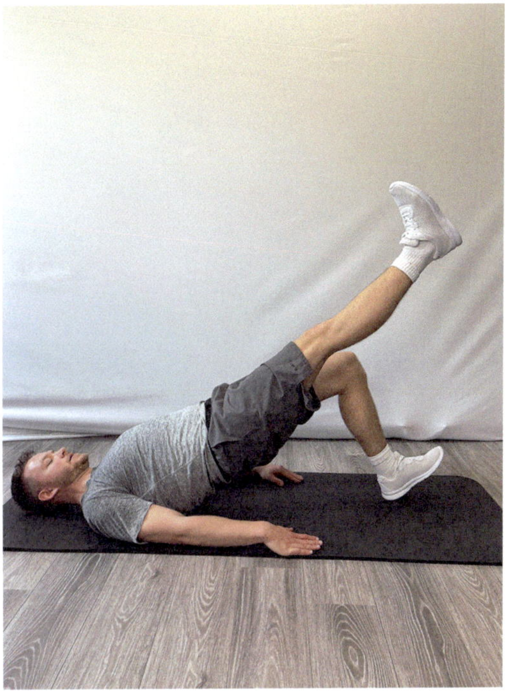

Fig. 5.20 MTT for femoroacetabular impingement—Single-leg bridging

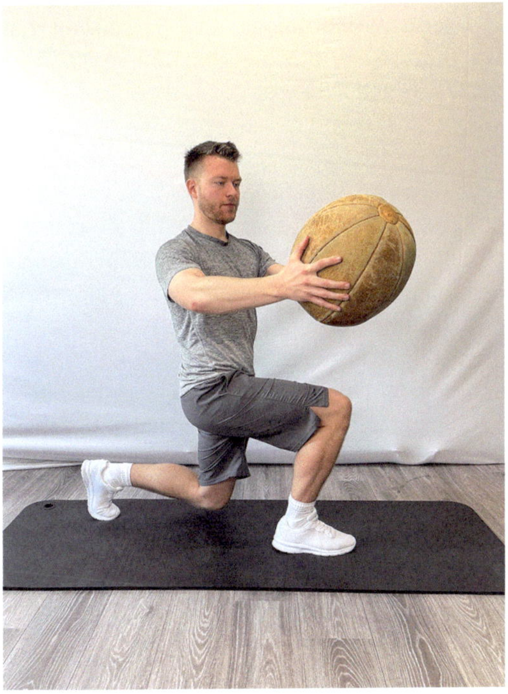

Fig. 5.19 MTT for femoroacetabular impingement—trunk rotation exercise in lunge with medicine ball

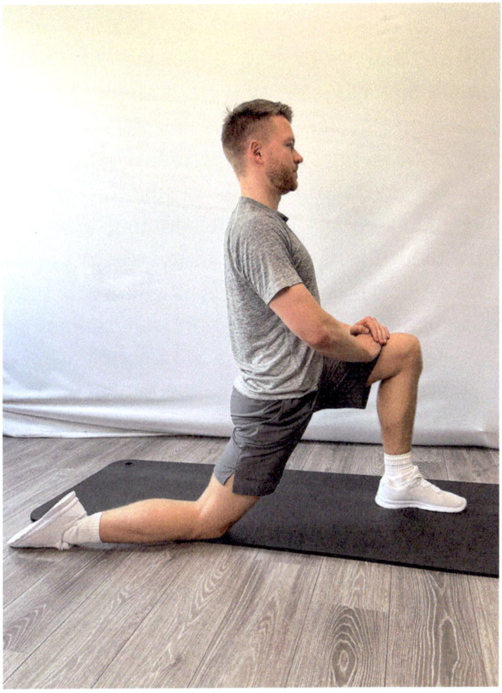

Fig. 5.21 MTT for femoroacetabular impingement—Self-stretching M. iliopsoas

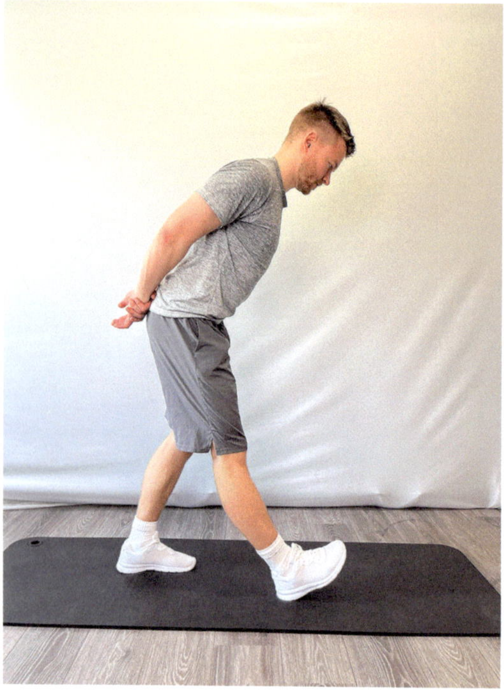

Fig. 5.22 MTT for femoroacetabular impingement—Self-stretching Mm. ischiocrurales

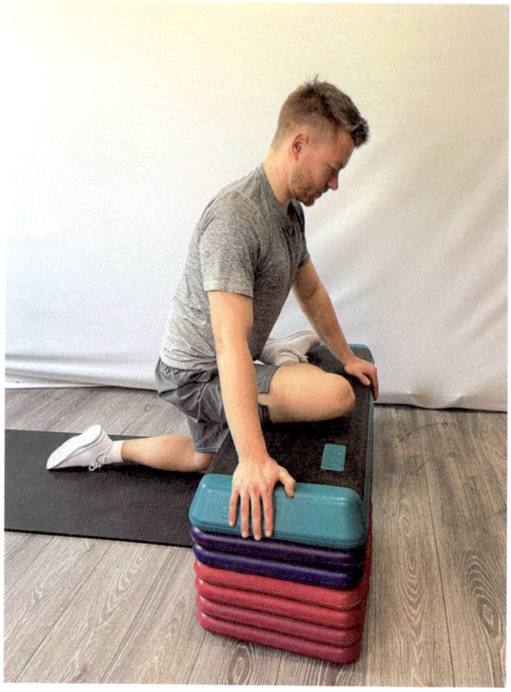

Fig. 5.23 MTT for femoroacetabular impingement—Self-stretching M. piriformis

In a clinical examination, Diasuke et al. (2013) deal with the influence of three-month hip abductor strength training in people with acetabular dysplasia. After the twelve-week intervention period, it was shown that the average strength of the hip abductors increased by 16%. In addition, a significant reduction in pain intensity was achieved, measured on the visual analogue scale. The researchers conclude that targeted training of the abductor muscles of the hip joint can lead to improved stability of the pelvis during walking (see Diasuke et al. 2013).

Assessments that can be used include the Hip-and-Groin-Outcome-Score, the Y-Balance-Test, and the Hop-for-Distance-Test (see Jacobsen et al. 2022). Other hop tests can also be used (see Mortensen et al. 2018). More detailed information on the individual assessments can be found in the assessment list in the appendix of this book.

Useful visualizations can be taken from Fig. 5.25, 5.26, 5.27, 5.28, 5.29, 5.30, 5.31, 5.32, 5.33 and 5.34.

Summary for Practice

Medical training therapy for hip dysplasia can relieve pain and improve strength and functions. Regular training under guidance and independently should be emphasized. The training therapy should start with aerobic warm-up training and then transition into strength training. The weight should be progressively adjusted. The focus is on the hip and knee joint extensors as well as the hip flexors and hip abductors. An improved gait pattern and the mentioned assessments can provide insights into the targeted training.

Fig. 5.24 provides an overview of the mentioned information.

Categories	Evidence-based training recommendation
Units	At least 3 training sessions per week á 45-60 minutes per session
Exercises	Bridging / side support / squat / one-legged stability exercises / Leg press / leg curl double leg / Leg extension, both legs / Hip flexor training unilateral / Lunges / abductor machine
Exercise parameters	10 minutes warm-up / strength training 3-4 sets of 8-21 repetitions each / adjust training weight progressively

Fig. 5.24 Summary of MTT in Hip Dysplasia

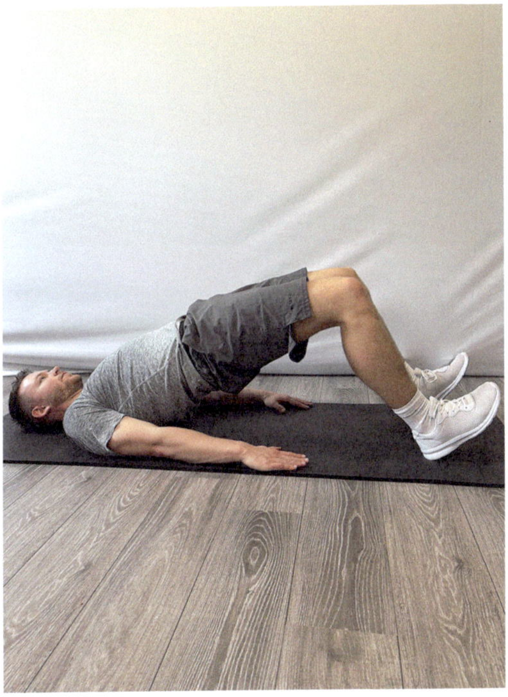

Fig. 5.25 MTT in Hip Dysplasia—Bridging

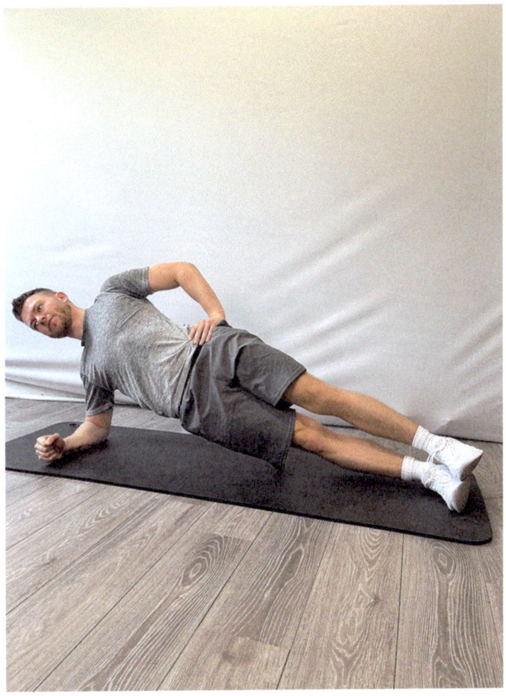

Fig. 5.26 MTT in Hip Dysplasia—Side Support

5.1.4 Perthes Disease

A central goal in the conservative or postoperative care of Perthes disease is the improvement or preservation of the mobility of the affected hip joint. Restrictions in movement affect the extension, abduction, and internal rotation of the hip joint, as well as the lumbar spine (see Hefti 2015). In addition to restrictive mobility, a weakness of the lower extremity and the trunk is often noticeable. The coordinative performance, especially the balance ability, is also reduced in most cases (see Krieg et al. 2018). Due to the young age of the patients, limited compliance with medical exercise therapy can be expected.

Various balance exercises, which address the lower extremity and the trunk, are recommended. Active stretching of the hip flexors, hip

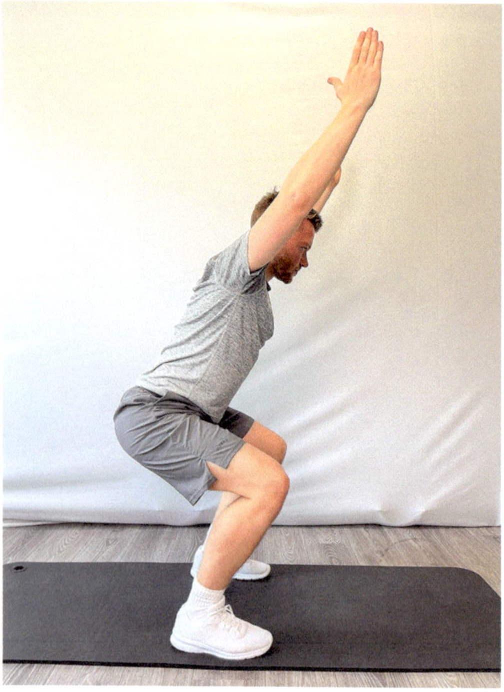

Fig. 5.27 MTT in Hip Dysplasia—Squatting

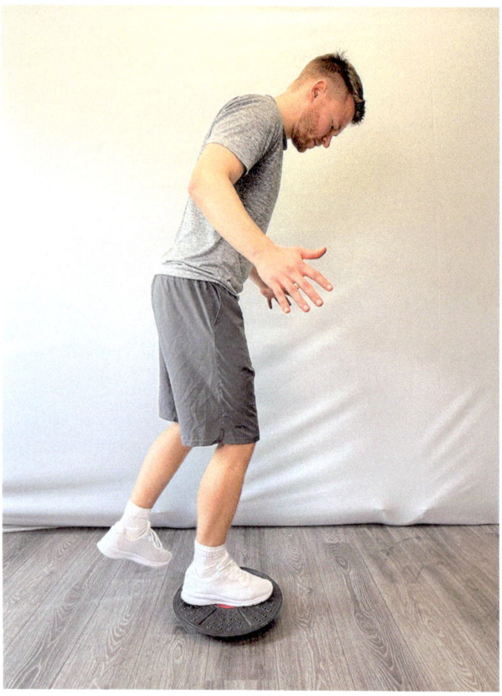

Fig. 5.28 MTT in Hip Dysplasia—Single Leg Stability Exercise

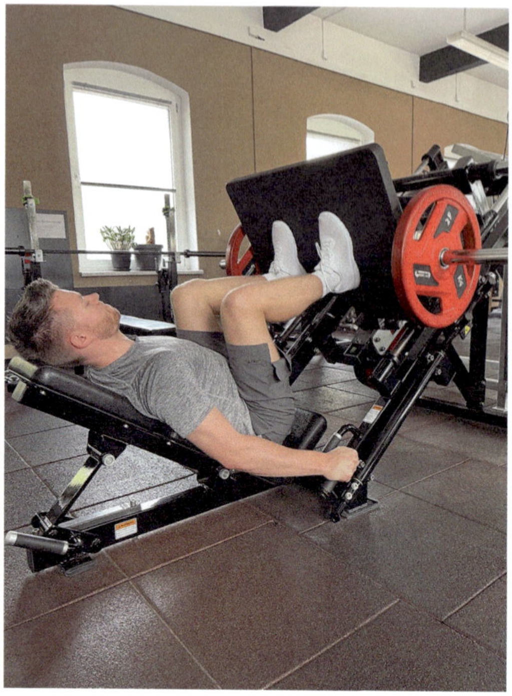

Fig. 5.29 MTT in Hip Dysplasia—Bilateral Leg Press

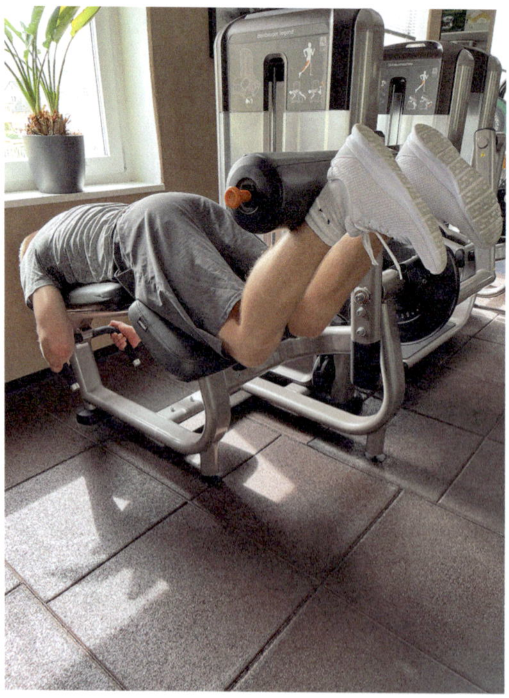

Fig. 5.30 MTT in Hip Dysplasia—Bilateral Hamstring Curl

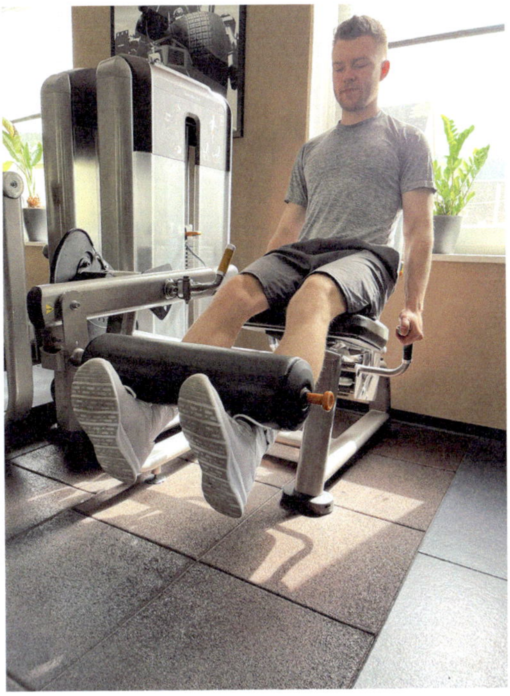

Fig. 5.31 MTT in Hip Dysplasia—Bilateral Leg Extension

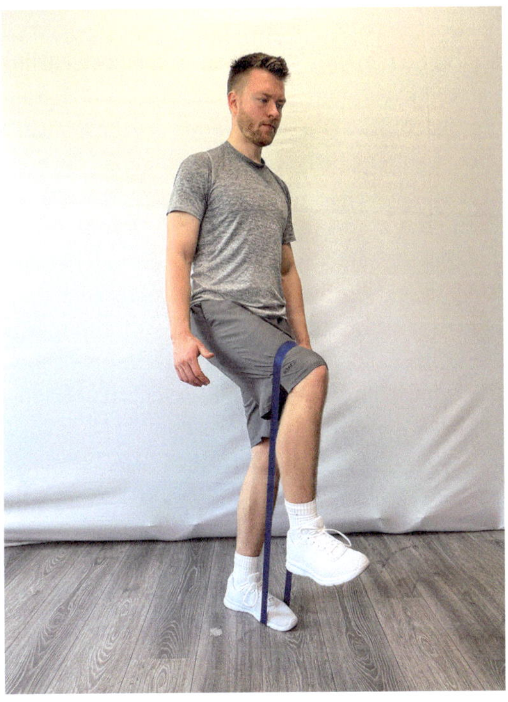

Fig. 5.32 MTT in Hip Dysplasia—Single Leg Hip Flexor Strengthening

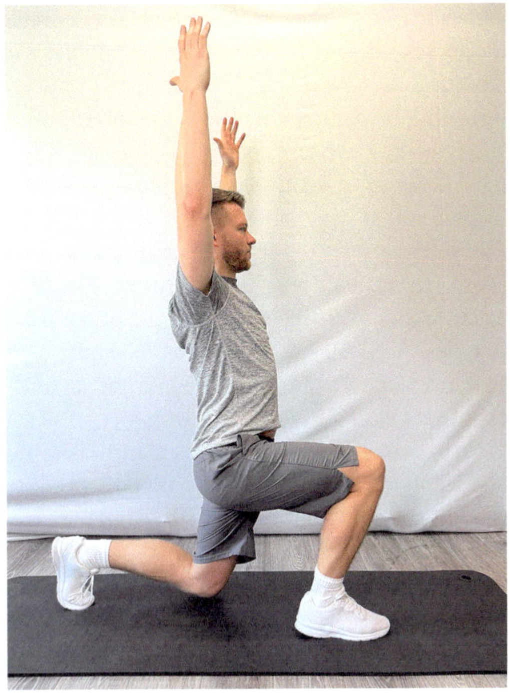

Fig. 5.33 MTT in Hip Dysplasia—Lunges

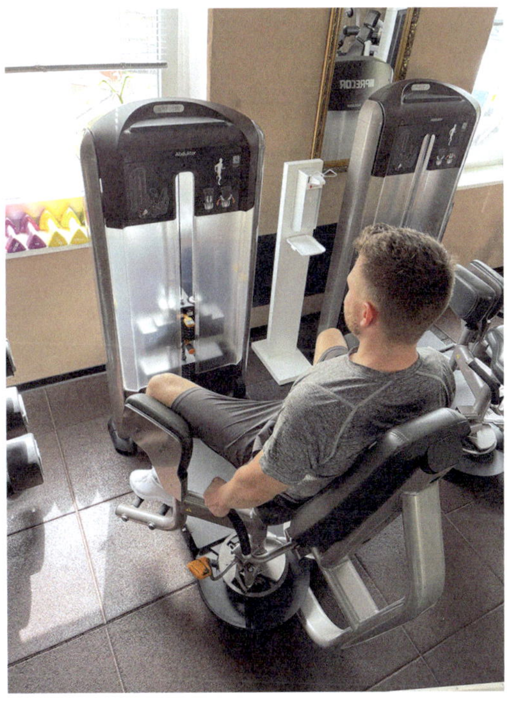

Fig. 5.34 MTT in Hip Dysplasia—Abductor Machine

adductors, and hip external rotators are suitable means for influencing the restrictive mobility of the hip joint. Once mobility has been improved through active stretching, auto-mobilizations or strengthening exercises can be used in the newly gained range of motion. In addition to squats, lunges are also suitable. Light dumbbells can increase the intensity of the training over time (see Krieg et al. 2018). Another focus of medical exercise therapy is the strengthening of the trunk muscles. This can be done, for example, with forearm support. Jumping should be avoided (see Krieg et al. 2018).

In a comparative study, medical exercise therapy led to a significant improvement in mobility, muscle strength, and articular dysfunction (see Brech and Guarnieiro 2006).

Melin et al. (2023) recommend stretching exercises in all stages of the disease, while there are divergent statements regarding the implementation of strengthening exercises in the initial phase or in the fragmentation stages. A complete weight relief of the affected hip joint is uniformly not recommended (see Melin et al. 2023).

Useful visualizations can be found in Fig. 5.36, 5.37, 5.38, 5.39, 5.40 and 5.41.

Summary for Practice

The goal of medical exercise therapy in Perthes disease is primarily to improve or maintain the mobility of the affected hip joint. From a scientific point of view, balance exercises that address the lower extremity and the trunk are recommended. Furthermore, stretching of the hip flexors, adductors, and external rotators supports the process. These can be performed at any stage. In the newly gained range of motion, auto-mobilizations and strengthening exercises can subsequently be performed. Squats and lunges are suitable for this. During the initial and fragmentation stages of Perthes disease, strength training should be carried out with caution as it could potentially worsen the condition in the short term. A slow and careful increase is therefore important. For training the trunk, science recommends forearm support. Jumping should be avoided.

Fig. 5.35 provides an overview of the mentioned information.

5.2 Knee Joint Area

5.2.1 Gonarthrosis

In a systematic review, the effect of medical training therapy on people with knee osteoarthritis was examined. It was recognized that training programs are a suitable means for analgesia and simultaneously increase strength. In addition to Pilates, aerobic endurance training and strength training are advocated. Initial effects can be expected in a training period between 8–12 weeks, provided that three to five training sessions of at least one hour of training time are carried out weekly. Training sessions can be practiced both in water and on land (cf. Raposo

Categories	Evidence-based training recommendation
Exercises	Balance exercises / Automobilizations / Squats / Lunges / Forearm support
Exercise parameters	No jumps / stretching before mobilization before strengthening
Elongation	Hip joint flexors, adductors, external rotators

Fig. 5.35 Summary of MTT in Perthes Disease

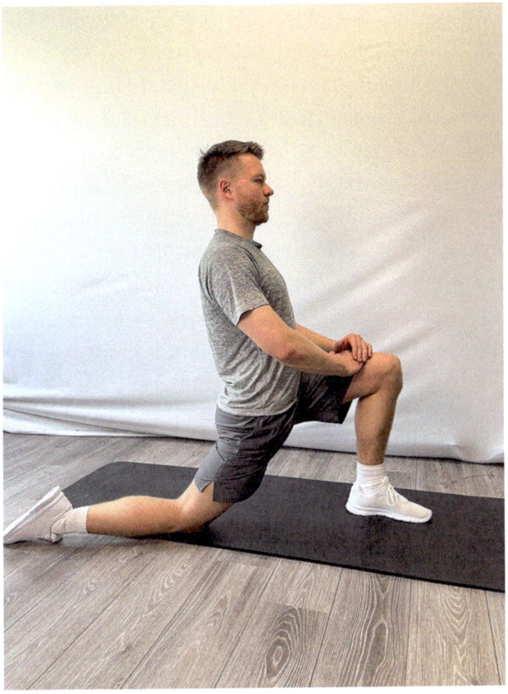

Fig. 5.36 MTT in Perthes Disease—Stretching Hip Flexors

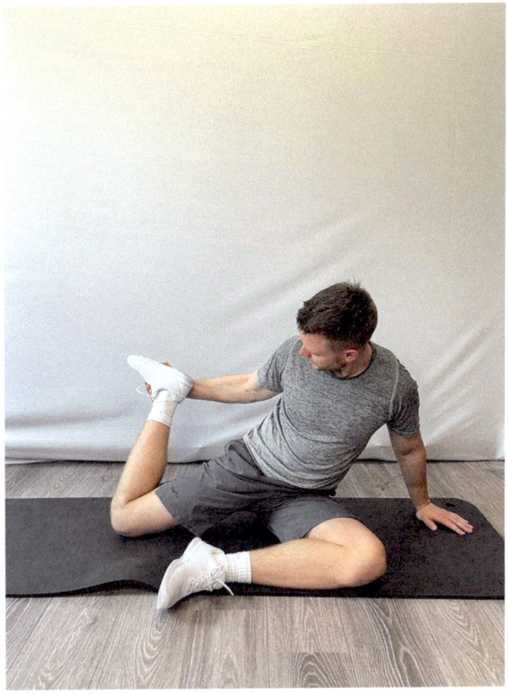

Fig. 5.38 MTT in Perthes Disease—Stretching Hip External Rotators

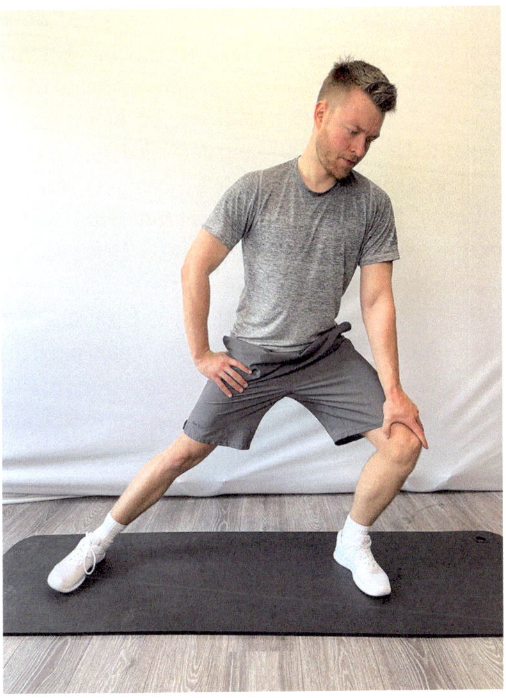

Fig. 5.37 MTT in Perthes Disease—Stretching Hip Adductors

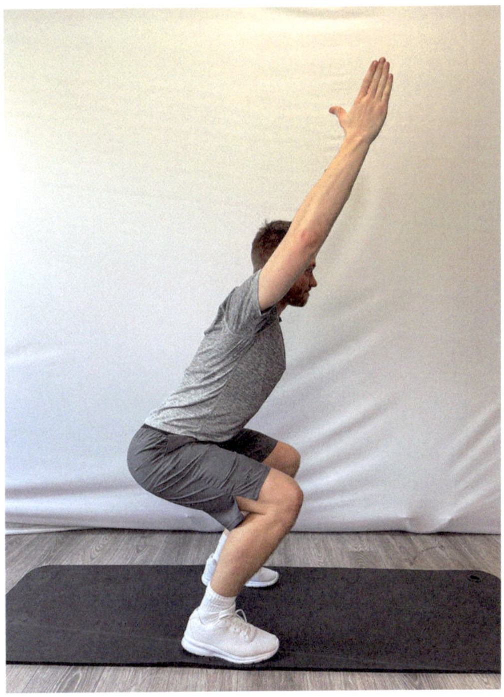

Fig. 5.39 MTT in Perthes Disease—Knee Bend

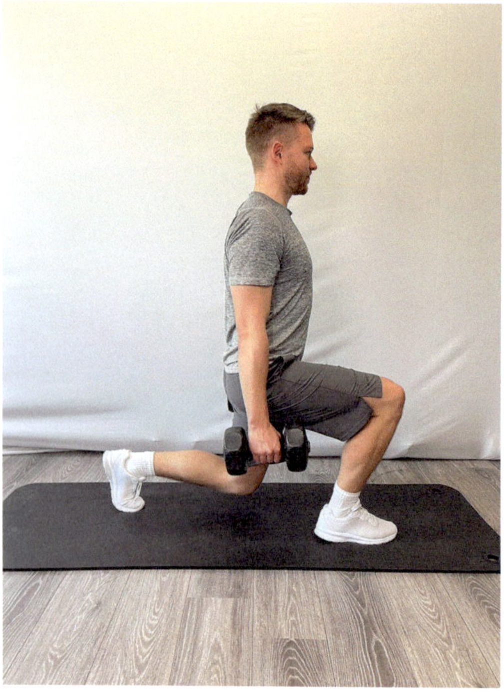

Fig. 5.40 MTT in Perthes Disease—Lunges with Dumbbells

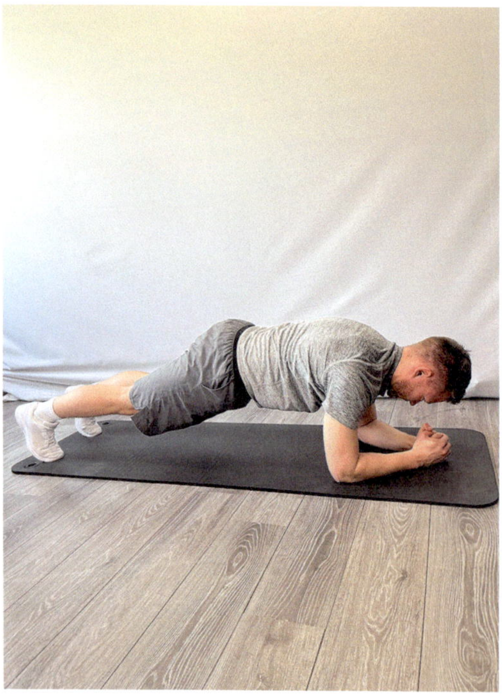

Fig. 5.41 MTT in Perthes Disease—Forearm Support

et al. 2021; Bartels et al. 2016; Rewald et al. 2020). Aerobic endurance training on the bicycle ergometer can be used specifically against pain and for sports-related functional improvement (cf. Luan et al. 2021). Ferreira et al. (2019) describe medical training therapy, especially strength training, as the most efficient non-pharmacological and non-surgical therapy strategy for gonarthrosis. Training in combination with education was able to improve symptoms and the function of the affected knee joints equivalently in an eight-week intervention period compared to four saline injections (cf. Bandak et al. 2022). Even compared to anti-inflammatory drugs and the intake of opioids, medical training therapy can assert itself as the best conservative therapy measure (cf. Thorlund et al. 2022). Due to the high safety and the absence of side effects, medical training therapy should be the conservative therapy of choice (cf. Weng et al. 2023).

Proprioceptive training can be used to alleviate pain in knee osteoarthritis. Three to four training sessions of 30–40 minutes each are recommended per week. Exercise selection can include, among others, single-leg stance, walking on heels, walking on tiptoes, and balance exercises on different surfaces, such as a trampoline. The difficulty level can be increased by closing the eyes (see Jeong et al. 2019).

There is evidence that strength training relieves pain and improves function over a period of eight to twelve weeks. However, no statements can be made about the optimal number of repetitions, set number, and training frequency (see Turner et al. 2020). High-intensity training does not appear to be superior to low-intensity training in terms of pain, function, and quality of life (see Hua et al. 2023).

Over a period of four months, the effectiveness of concentric muscular training was compared to the eccentric approach in a randomized controlled study with a sample of 54 individuals. The participants were between 60–85 years old and 61% were female.

The concentric group trained twice a week at an intensity of 60% of the 1RM. For each exercise, one set of 12 repetitions was performed per training session. The exercises included leg press, knee extension, knee flexion, calf press, chest press, shoulder press, and rowing.

The eccentric group differed from the concentric group only in the number of repetitions, which was eight. It was found that both forms of training are capable of relieving pain and positively influencing the function of arthritic knees. In addition to the tolerability of the training form, the load patterns of activities to be trained and the available equipment depend on the choice between a concentric or eccentric focus (see Vincent et al. 2019). In another randomized controlled study, the effects described above were confirmed. Additionally, it was recognized that concentric training more effectively relieves pain during and after walking than eccentric training (see Vincent and Vincent 2020).

Muscular stretching exercises of the lower extremity can be used as a measure to alleviate pain in knee osteoarthritis. To achieve the maximum analgesic effect, it is recommended to perform stretching exercises alone within a training session rather than a combination of strength training and stretching exercises (see Luan et al. 2022).

Torstensen et al. (2023) examined the influence of training duration on the results in knee osteoarthritis. The training program consisted of global (aerobic), semi-global, and joint-specific exercises, which were performed by both groups three times a week for twelve weeks. Group A performed eleven exercises with a training duration of 70 to 90 minutes. Group B, on the other hand, performed five exercises per training session with a training duration of 20–30 minutes. Both forms of training led to improvements in the Knee Injury and Osteoarthritis Outcome Score (KOOS) and quality of life. The longer training form was superior in improving function in sports and leisure activities, as well as in the outcome of quality of life after six and twelve months (see Torstensen et al. 2023). It can therefore be concluded that a training duration of 20–30 minutes is also effective.

In overweight individuals with arthritic knees, a twelve-week training of the quadriceps femoris muscle contributed to an improvement in pain and function. Training with one's own body weight is considered equivalent to training with external training weights (see Bennell et al. 2020).

The KOOS and the quality of life (QoL) can be used as assessments, among others (see Bandak et al. 2022; Torstensen et al. 2023). More detailed information on the individual assessments can be found in the assessment list in the appendix of this book.

Useful visualizations can be found in Fig. 5.43, 5.44, 5.45, 5.46, 5.47, 5.48, 5.49, 5.50 and 5.51.

Summary for Practice

Medical training therapy is the conservative treatment of choice for gonarthrosis. In particular, strength training in combination with aerobic endurance training, stretching, and proprioceptive training, lead to pain relief and functional improvement. Compared to saline injections or the intake of anti-inflammatory drugs or opioids, medical training therapy offers a method with fewer side effects and more effectiveness. The focus of the training is on strength training, which is equipped with exercises such as the leg press, the knee extender and flexor, the calf press, and the chest press, shoulder press, and rowing. Training of the M. quadriceps femoris is particularly recommended for overweight individuals. In this context, it is also important to know that even a short training session of 20–30 minutes can already achieve positive effects.

Fig. 5.42 provides an overview of the mentioned information.

5.2.2 Patellofemoral Pain Syndrome/Runner's Knee

Medical training therapy for people with patellofemoral pain syndrome/Runner's knee aims to reduce or better control the valgus position of the femorotibial joint. In addition to targeted

Categories	Evidence-based training recommendation
Units	3-5 training sessions per week á 45-60 minutes per session
Exercises	Aerobic endurance training with the bicycle ergometer / one-legged stand / walking on heels / walking on tiptoes / balance exercises on the trampoline / leg press / knee extensions / knee flexors / calf press / chest press / shoulder press / rowing
Exercise parameters	20 to 90 minutes per session / concentric training is more effective than eccentric strength training / focus on the quadriceps femoris muscle in overweight patients
Elongation	Stretching the muscles of the lower extremities

Fig. 5.42 Summary of MTT in Gonarthrosis

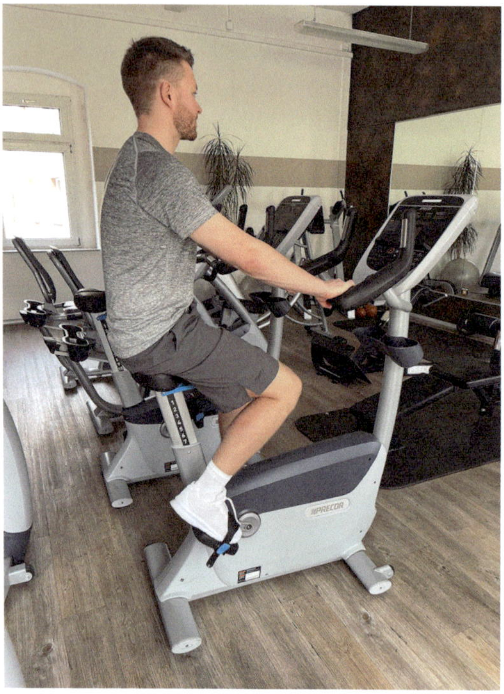

Fig. 5.43 MTT in Gonarthrosis—Exercise Bike

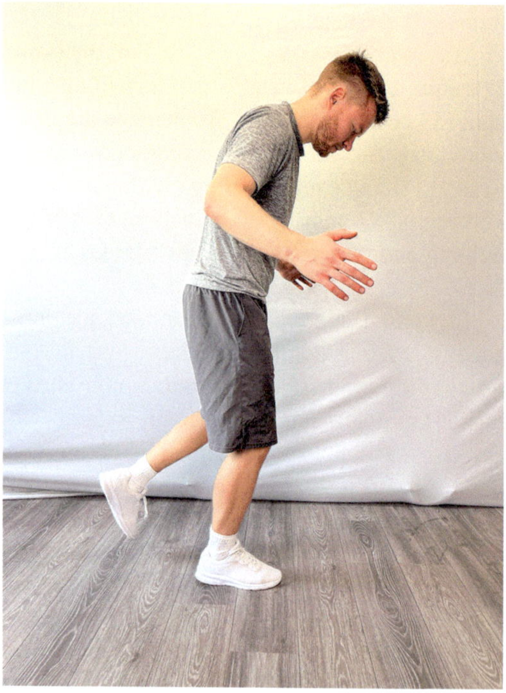

Fig. 5.44 MTT in Gonarthrosis—One-Leg Stand

training of the thigh muscles, the hip abductors and hip external rotators should be addressed (see Rogan et al. 2019). In addition to strength training, proprioceptive content should also be incorporated into the therapy (see Alammari et al. 2023).

Emamvirdi et al. (2019) examined the influence of valgus control training on patellofemoral pain syndrome in 64 active women aged between 18 and 25 years. During the intervention period of six weeks, the training intensity was progressively increased. The number of

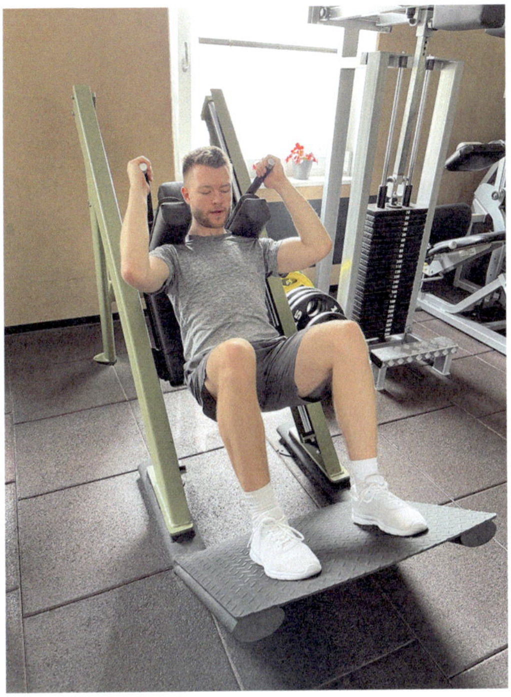

Fig. 5.45 MTT in Gonarthrosis—Leg Press

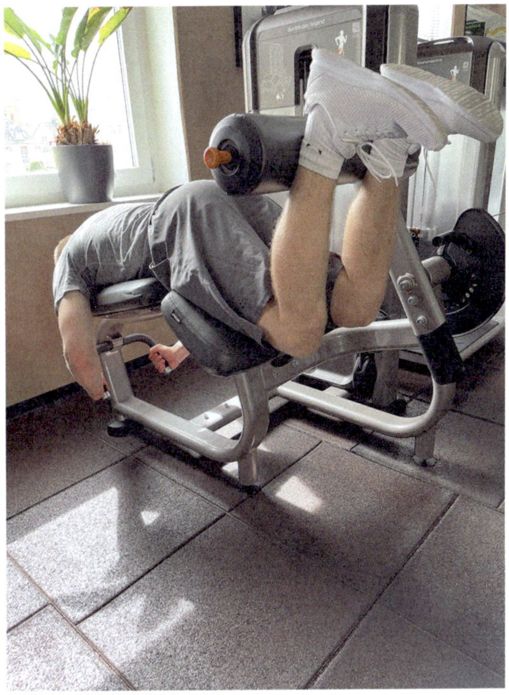

Fig. 5.47 MTT in Gonarthrosis—Knee Flexor

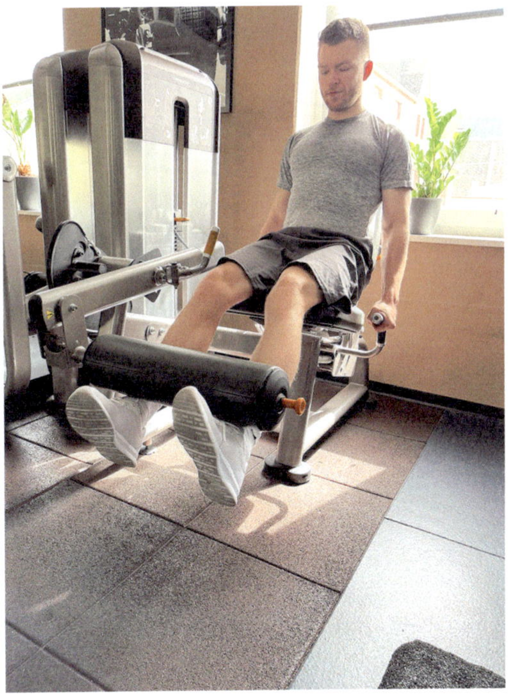

Fig. 5.46 MTT in Gonarthrosis—Knee Extender

sets per exercise varied between two and three, while the number of repetitions ranged between 12 and 20. In addition to proprioceptive training, the muscles surrounding the hip and knee were trained. The focus was on training the hip abductors and hip external rotators.

The exercises included single-leg stance training on various surfaces, squats on various surfaces, squats with a resistance band around the thighs, sidesteps with a resistance band around the ankles, hip abductor training on a step board in single-leg stance, lunge with medial pull through resistance band on the front thigh, Romanian deadlift in single-leg stance, and trunk or hip rotation training with a medicine ball (see Emamvirdi et al. 2019). Wall sitting and training of the gluteus maximus in the open chain can also be applied (see Hu et al. 2019).

In addition to improving the pain and strength situation, a reduction of the dynamic knee valgus angle by 59.48% was achieved. The described training approach is recommended for

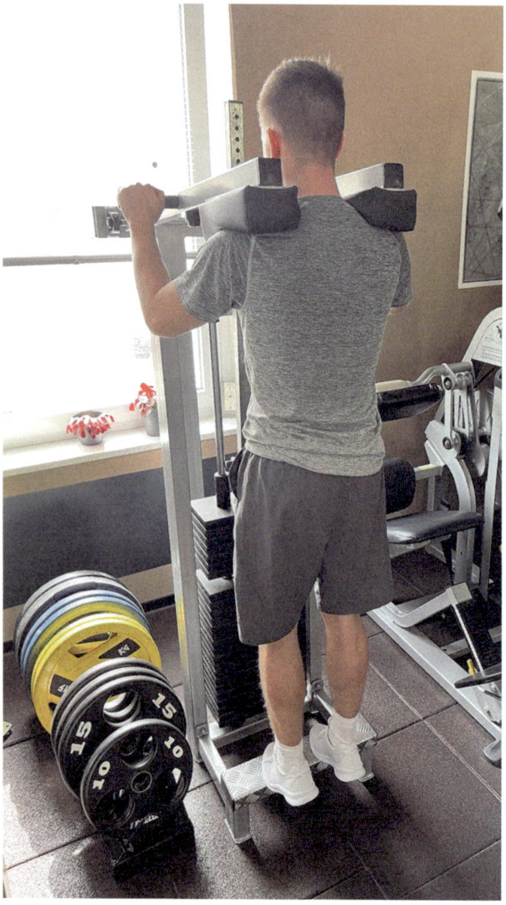

Fig. 5.48 MTT in Gonarthrosis—Calf Press

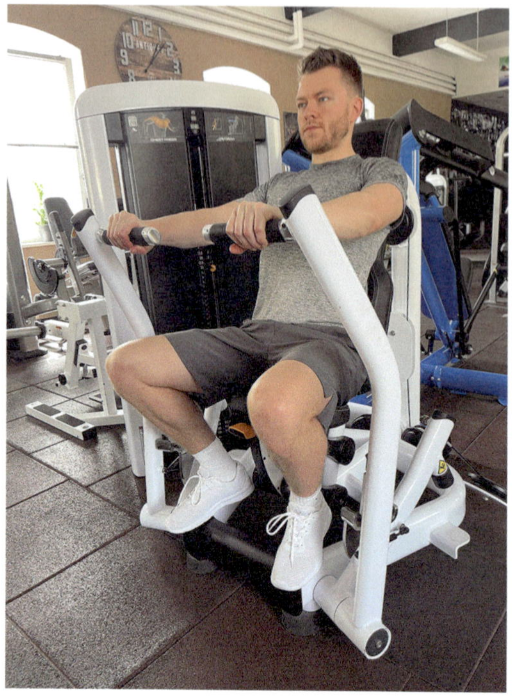

Fig. 5.49 MTT in Gonarthrosis—Chest Press

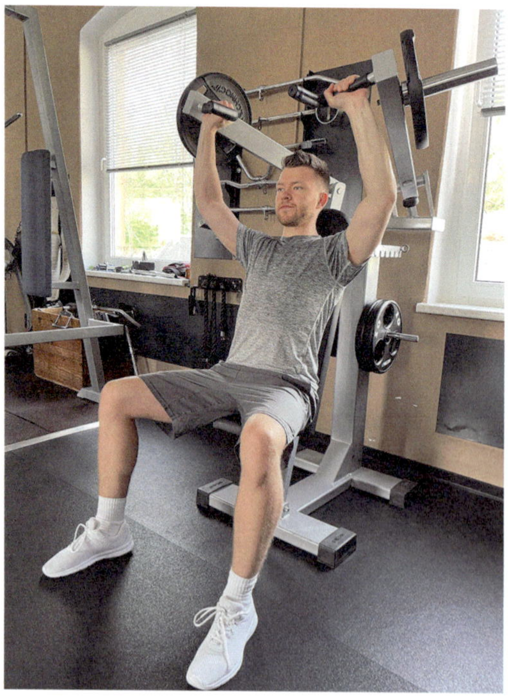

Fig. 5.50 MTT in Gonarthrosis—Shoulder Press

both therapy and prevention of patellofemoral pain syndrome (see Emamvirdi et al. 2019).

The focus of therapy should be on the muscles surrounding the knee. Due to additional positive effects such as improved pain reduction, the inclusion of the muscles surrounding the hip in the training program is recommended (see Fukuda et al. 2010; Ismail et al. 2013; Dolak et al. 2011; Alammari et al. 2023; Şahin et al. 2016).

Static and dynamic stretches of the quadriceps femoris muscle have an analgesic and function-improving effect (see Lee et al. September 2021). In addition, dynamic stretches of the hamstring muscles can represent another pain-relieving or function-improving therapy

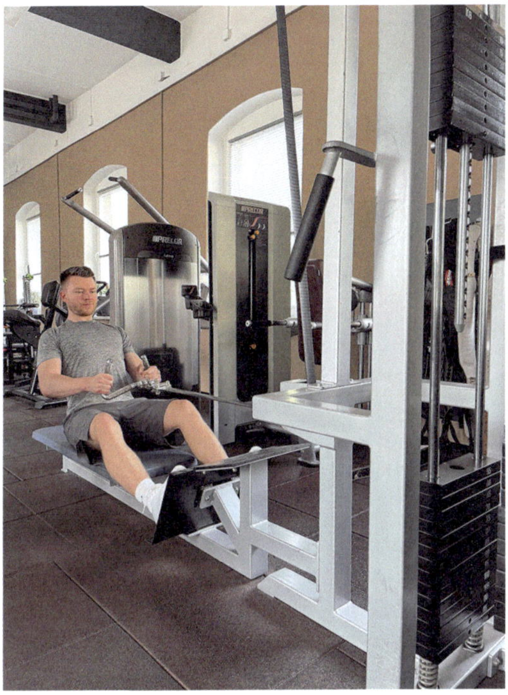

Fig. 5.51 MTT in Gonarthrosis—Rowing

component in patellofemoral pain syndrome (see Lee et al. January 2021).

Assessments include various hop tests (see Emamvirdi et al. 2019). More detailed information on the individual assessments can be taken from the assessment list in the appendix of this book.

Useful visualizations can be taken from Fig. 5.53, 5.54, 5.55, 5.56, 5.57, 5.58, 5.59, 5.60, 5.61, 5.62, 5.63 and Fig. 5.64.

Summary for Practice

Medical training therapy can correct the knee valgus angle in patellofemoral pain syndrome, alleviate pain, and improve the strength situation. The focus is on training the thigh muscles as well as the hip joint abductors and external rotators. In addition, proprioceptive training can positively influence the correction of the valgus position. Exercises that should be used in this context include single-leg stance and squats on various surfaces, as well as side-steps, single-leg stance or Romanian dead-lifts in single-leg stance. Also, stretching the quadriceps femoris muscle leads to pain relief and functional improvement.

These exercises not only have a rehabilitative-therapeutic effect but also a preventive one.

Fig. 5.52 provides an overview of the mentioned information.

5.2.3 Rupture of the Anterior Cruciate Ligament

The application of medical training therapy can be used for both prevention and conservative or postoperative therapy after rupture of the anterior cruciate ligament.

Training of the trunk muscles is recommended for the prevention of anterior cruciate ligament tears. In a randomized controlled study, the intervention group completed a prescribed trunk training three times a week over a period of ten weeks. After a 15-minute warm-up training, the exercises leg-raise, crunch, superman, plank-hip-twist, forearm support, side support, and bridging followed. The sets varied depending on the training exercise and week between 1–5. The repetition numbers between 12–20 and the holding times between 20–60 s. Finally, stretches of the lower and upper extremity were practiced. The training significantly improved trunk endurance performance. Both the valgus angle and the hip adduction angle decreased significantly. In addition, the coactivation of the erector spinae muscle and the rectus abdominis muscle, the ischiocrural muscles and the quadriceps femoris muscle, as well as between the vastus medialis muscle and the vastus lateralis muscle improved (see Jeong et al. 2021). Training of the pelvic floor muscles also contributes to the prevention of ruptures of the anterior cruciate ligament (see Ferri-Caruana et al. 2020). In addition, the muscles

Categories	Evidence-based training recommendation
Exercises	Strength training of the thigh muscles, hip joint abductors and external rotators / single-leg stand and squats on different surfaces / squats with resistance band around thigh / sidesteps with resistance band around ankle / abductor training on step board in single-leg stand / lunges with medial pull through resistance band on front thigh / Romanian deadlift in single-leg stand / trunk and hip rotation training with medicine ball / wall sits / strength training M. gluteus maximus in the open chain
Exercise parameters	2-3 sets of 12-20 repetitions
Elongation	Static and dynamic stretches of the quadriceps femoris muscle / dynamic stretches of the ischiocrural muscles

Fig. 5.52 Summary of MTT in patellofemoral pain syndrome

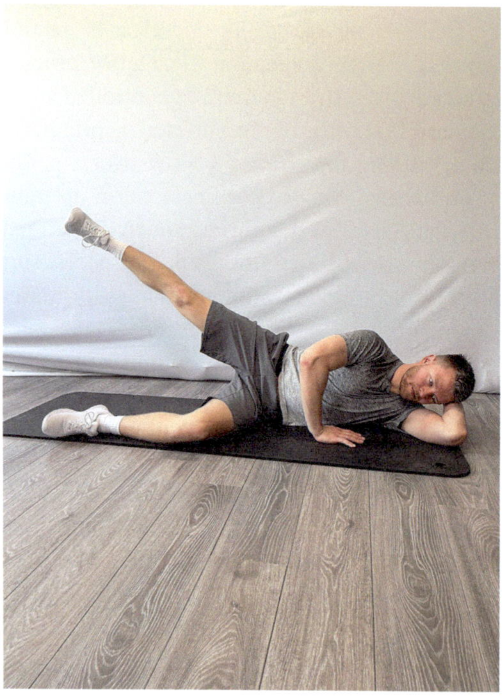

Fig. 5.53 MTT in patellofemoral pain syndrome—Strengthening hip abductors

of the lower extremity should be strengthened. Proprioceptive exercises also play a major role (see Olivares-Jabalera et al. 2021). To reduce the

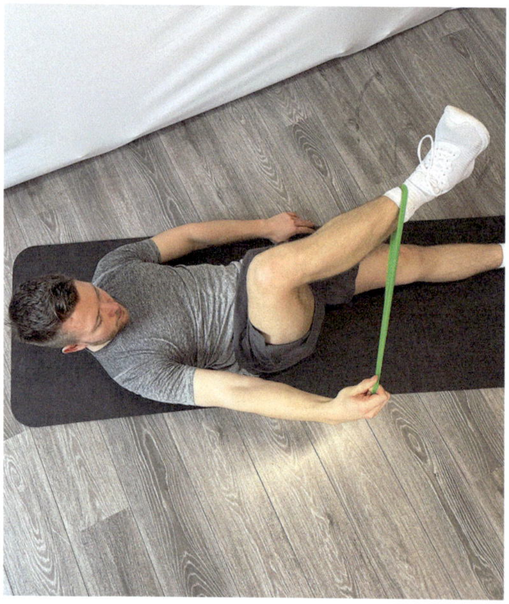

Fig. 5.54 MTT in patellofemoral pain syndrome—Strengthening hip external rotators

risk of injuries to the anterior cruciate ligament, plyometric exercises should also be integrated into preventive training concepts (see Attar et al. 2022). Prevention training programs are recommended in preparation for a season and during the season and should be carried out with a high

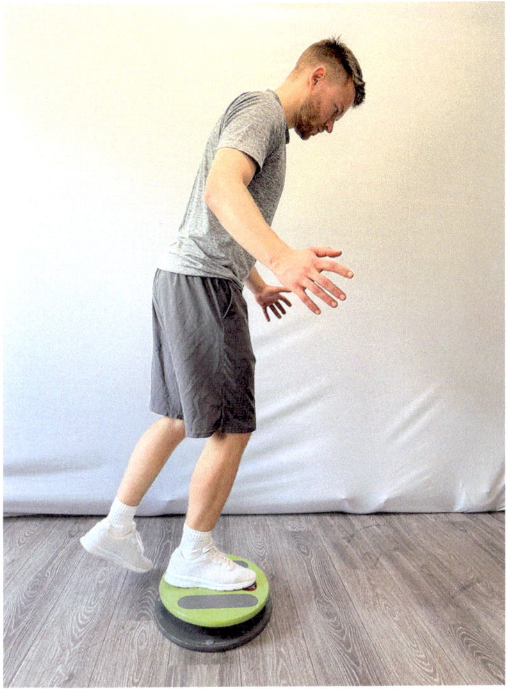

Fig. 5.55 MTT in patellofemoral pain syndrome—Single leg stance on various surfaces

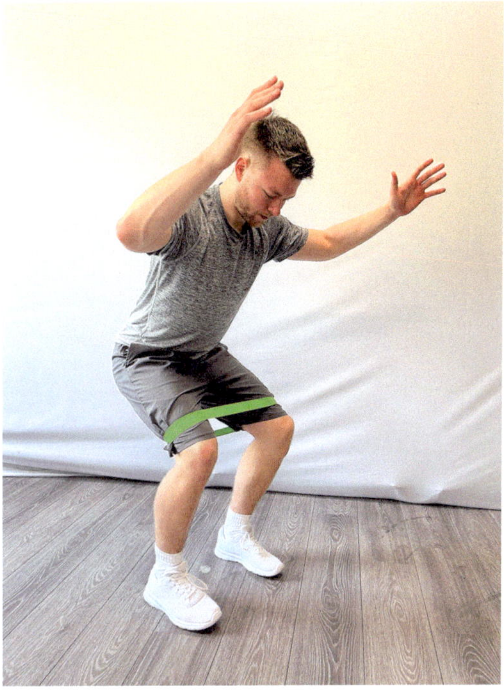

Fig. 5.57 MTT in patellofemoral pain syndrome—Squats with resistance band on the thigh

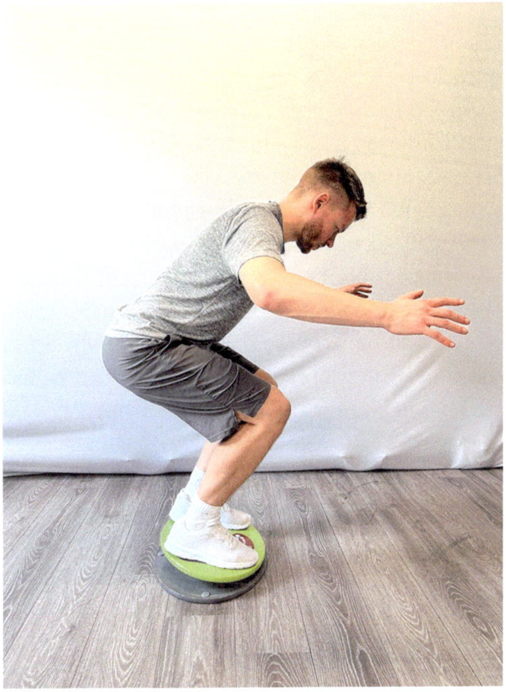

Fig. 5.56 MTT in patellofemoral pain syndrome—Squats on various surfaces

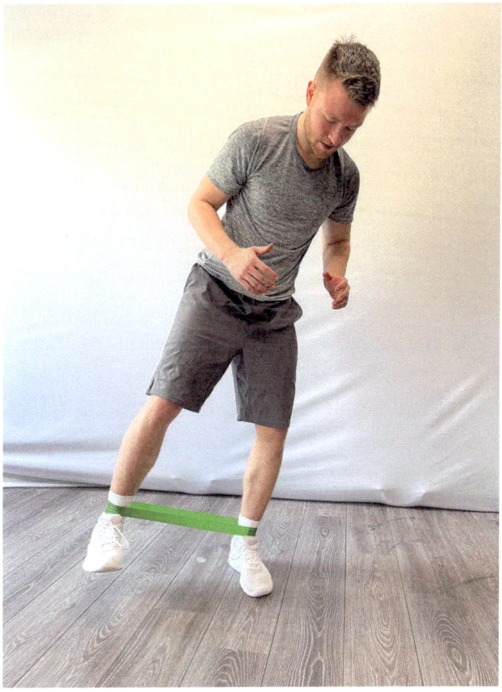

Fig. 5.58 MTT in patellofemoral pain syndrome—Sidesteps with resistance band around ankles

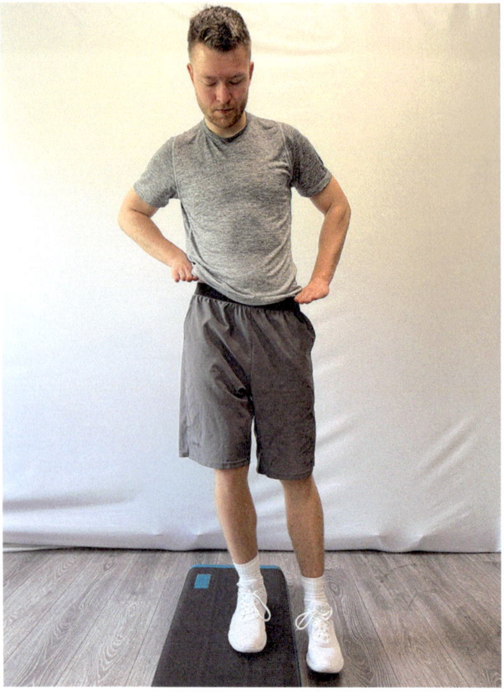

Fig. 5.59 MTT in patellofemoral pain syndrome—Strengthening hip abductors on step board in single leg stance

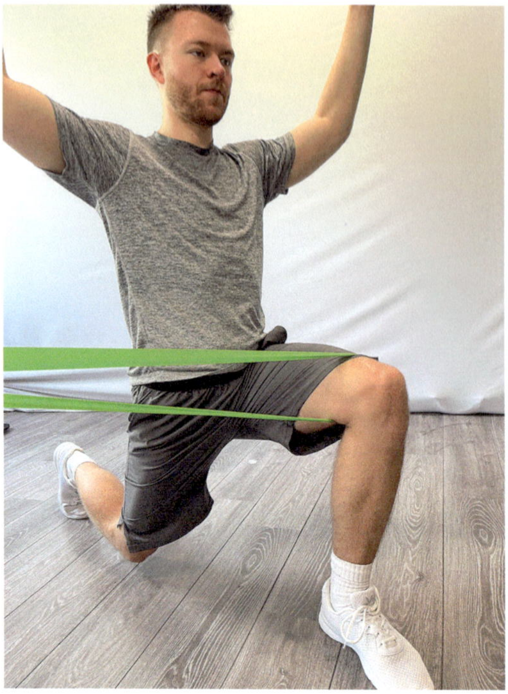

Fig. 5.60 MTT in patellofemoral pain syndrome—Lunge with medial pull through resistance band on the front standing thigh

degree of compliance (see Arundale et al. 2018). The FIFA 11+ prevention program includes, in addition to strength, plyometric and balance exercises, running exercises such as side gallop, hip rotation outward or inward, high and long jumps, changes of direction, and sprints forward and backward (see Silvers-Granelli et al. 2017). By practicing prevention programs, injury rates can be reduced by 53% (see Huang et al. 2020).

If an anterior cruciate ligament rupture is treated surgically, rehabilitation begins before the operation. By fully restoring mobility into the femorotibial extension, the postoperative risk of arthrofibrosis can be significantly reduced (see Månsson et al. 2013; McHugh et al. 2002). If the strength of the quadriceps femoris muscle on the affected side preoperatively falls by more than 20% compared to the unaffected side, this is an indicator that a strength deficit of the operated side can be expected even two years postoperatively (see Shaarani et al. 2013; de Jong et al. 2007). Therefore, a preoperative minimization of the loss of strength of the quadriceps femoris muscle is recommended.

In the first postoperative week, isometric tension exercises of the quadriceps femoris muscle are recommended. These can be supplemented with edema current (see Fitzgerald et al. 2003). From the second week, concentric training can take place within the closed system. If this does not provoke pain and swelling, external training weight can be used (see Tyler et al. 1998). From the start of the fourth week, training can be carried out in a range of 90–45° in the open system. In the case of patellar tendon plastic surgery, additional weight can be used, while in the case of ischiocrural plastic surgery, due to the risk of elongation, it should initially be done without additional weight (see van Melick et al. 2016; Heijne and Werner 2007). The range of motion can be increased to 90°–30° in the fifth week, to 90°–20° in the sixth week, and to 90°–10° in the seventh week. From the eighth week, the use of the full range of motion is advisable (see van

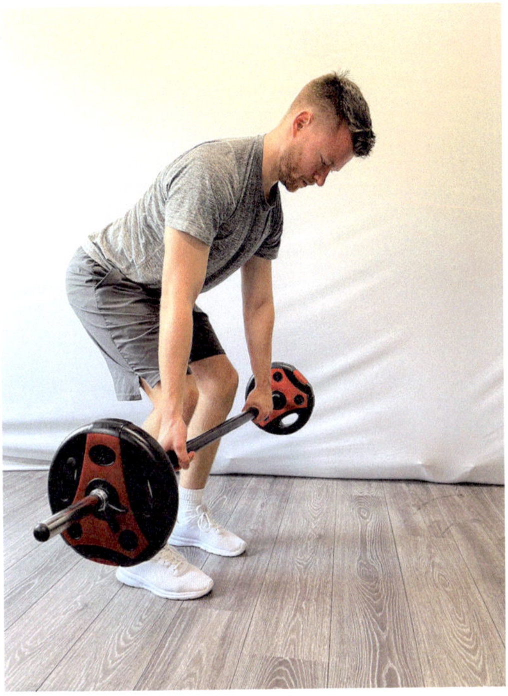

Fig. 5.61 MTT in patellofemoral pain syndrome—Romanian Deadlift with both legs or single leg

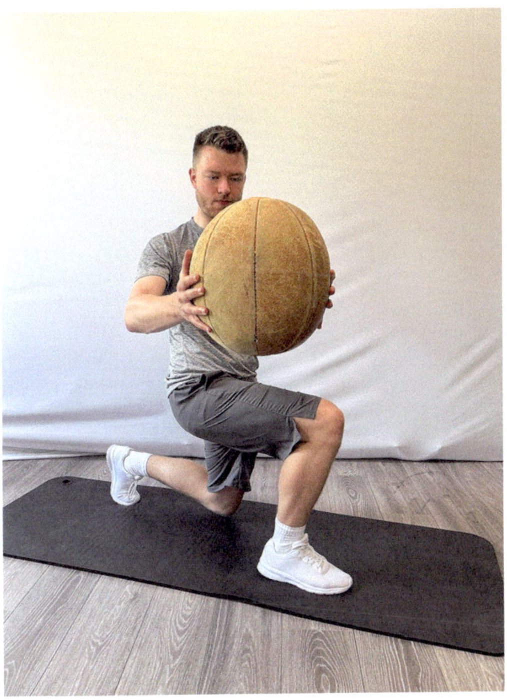

Fig. 5.62 MTT in patellofemoral pain syndrome—Trunk and hip rotation training

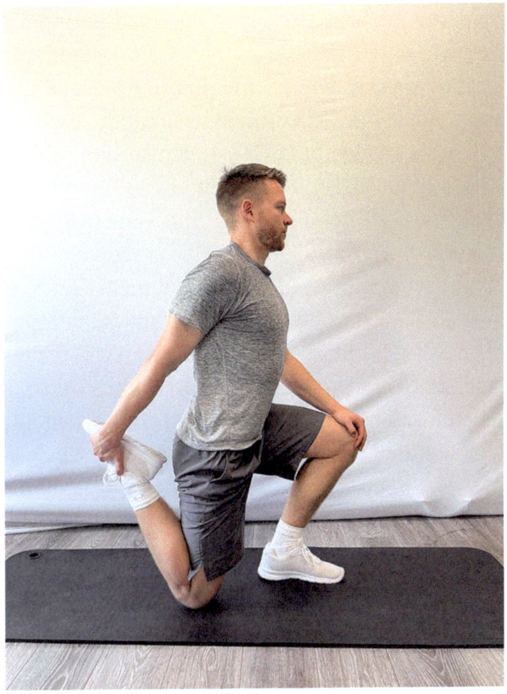

Fig. 5.63 MTT for patellofemoral pain syndrome—Stretching M. quadriceps femoris

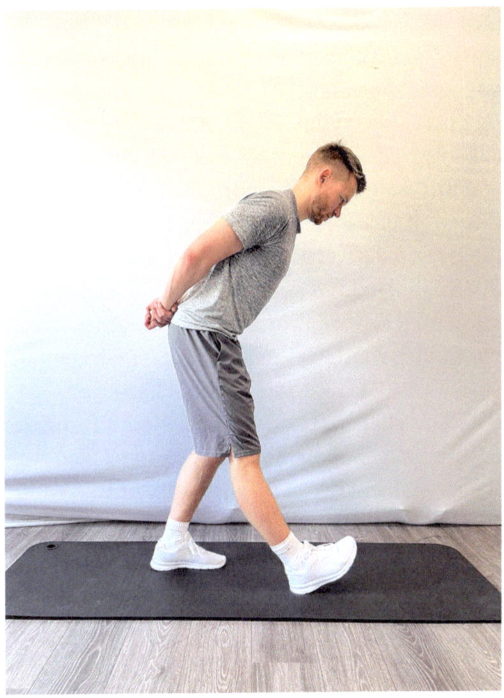

Fig. 5.64 MTT for patellofemoral pain syndrome—Stretching Mm. ischiocrurales

Grinsven et al. 2010). From the third postoperative week, eccentric training of the quadriceps femoris muscle within the closed system is recommended for maximizing strength capability (see Gokeler et al. 2014; Kruse et al. 2012; Bieler et al. 2014; Gerber et al. 2007). Vidmar et al. (2023) demonstrated the superiority of isokinetic eccentric training over conventional eccentric training of the quadriceps femoris muscle. The strength training should be complemented by proprioceptive training (see Berschin et al. 2014; Fu et al. 2013). During the course of rehabilitation, sport-specific load patterns should be integrated into the training plan.

The single-leg-landing-test can serve as an assessment for determining the dynamic valgus angle (see Ghanati et al. 2022). For the return-to-sport timing assessments, a postoperative period of at least eight months should have passed, at least two functional tests should have been passed, the strength of the anterior and posterior thigh muscles should be assessed, and additional information about psychological readiness should be obtained. Factors such as age and gender should also be taken into account (see Turk et al. 2023). The Y-Balance-Test shows a correlation to functionality and muscle strength after ruptures of the anterior cruciate ligament (see Kim et al. 2022). Functionality can also be assessed by the anterior-posterior-stability-index of the Biodex-Balance-System (see Kim et al. 2023). Another functional test is the single-leg-vertical-jump-test (see Lee et al. 2018). Subjective scoring systems include the subjective-international-knee-documentation-committee-score, lysholm-score, tegner-activity-scale, ACL-return-to-sports-after-injury-scale (see Lee et al. 2018). More detailed information on the individual assessments can be taken from the assessment list in the appendix of this book.

Useful visualizations can be found in Fig. 5.67, 5.68, 5.69, 5.70, 5.71, 5.72 and 5.73.

Summary for Practice

Both preventively and postoperatively, evidence-based medical training therapy can demonstrably help with injuries to the anterior cruciate ligament.

Preventively, the focus is on training the trunk muscles and reducing the knee valgus angle and hip adduction angle. At the same time, the coactivation of the M. erector spinae and the M. rectus abdominis, the Mm. ischiocrurales, and M. quadriceps femoris as well as the M. vastus medialis and lateralis is improved. Strengthening the pelvic floor muscles also serves to prevent ruptures of the anterior cruciate ligament, as well as stretches, proprioceptive exercises, balance exercises, running and strength exercises.

Fig. 5.65 provides an overview of the mentioned information.

The postoperative medical training therapy starts even before the operation with a focus on the fully restored knee extension in the femorotibial joint and the strengthening of the quadriceps femoris muscle. In general, proprioceptive training should complement strength training. Over time, it is advisable to incorporate sport-specific exercises.

Fig. 5.66 provides an overview of the mentioned information.

5.2.4 Rupture of the Posterior Cruciate Ligament

Kim et al. (2013) dealt with the postoperative specifications after treatment of ruptures of the posterior cruciate ligament. After evaluating the included studies, it was found that on average a range of motion of 90° in flexion is released in the sixth postoperative week. In 60% of the total 34 evaluated research works, full load was allowed from the sixth postoperative week. The active training of the ischiocrural muscles was prohibited until the postoperative weeks 6–24 depending on the study. Kim et al. (2013) mention that initial full load should be in extension position or slight flexion position and

Categories	Evidence-based training recommendation
Units	Three times a week / at least 10 weeks / both as preparation for the season and during the season
Exercises	15 minutes warm-up / leg-raise, crunch / superman / plank-hip-twist / forearm support / side support / bridging / pelvic floor training / running exercises such as side gallop / hip rotation to the outside/inside / high and long jumps / change of direction / sprints to the front and back
Exercise parameters	5 sets /12-20 repetitions / holding times between 20-60 seconds
Elongation	Stretching the muscles of the lower and upper extremities

Fig. 5.65 Summary of MTT for the prevention of anterior cruciate ligament rupture

Categories	Evidence-based training recommendation
Week 1	Isometric tension exercises of the quadriceps femoris muscle / supplementation with swelling current
Week 2	Concentric training in a closed system / possible with additional weight (if no pain/ swelling)
Week 3	As week 2 / eccentric training quadriceps femoris in closed chain (isokinetic eccentric before conventional eccentric)
Week 4	Training in the open chain at an angle of 90-45° / possible with additional weight for patellar tendon plastic surgery (ischiocrural plastic surgery without additional weight)
Week 5	Training in the open chain at 90-30°
Week 6	Training in the open chain in the 90-20° range
Week 7	Training in the open chain at 90-10°
Week 8	Full range of motion training

Fig. 5.66 Summary of MTT postoperatively after reconstruction of the anterior cruciate ligament

recommend initial exercises that cause a co-contraction between the quadriceps femoris muscle and the ischiocrural muscles.

Similarly, the postoperative training program by Pierce et al. (2013) is structured. It is divided into four time-limited phases. Phase 1 takes place from the time of surgery until the completion of the fifth postoperative week. During this time, hyperextension and posterior translation of the tibia should be prevented. These precautions, which prohibit isolated training of the hamstring muscles, should be maintained until about the twelfth week. In addition to increasing the load from initial partial load to full load, therapeutic value should be placed on improving the gait pattern.

In Phase 1, there should also be activation of the quadriceps femoris muscle. In addition to stretching and strengthening the calf muscles, strength training of the trunk and upper

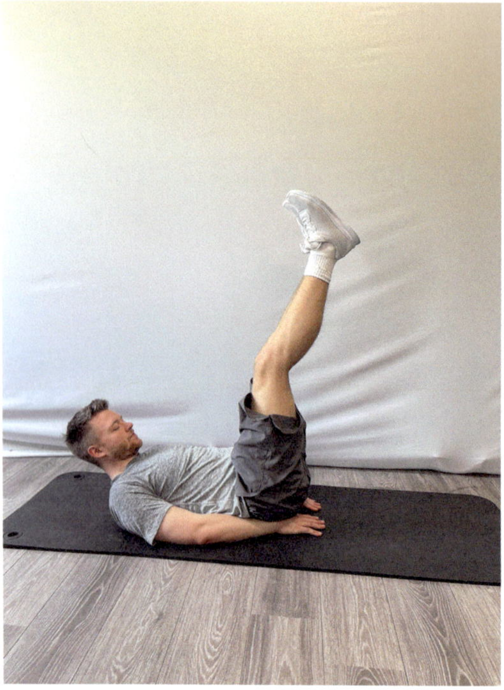

Fig. 5.67 MTT in case of rupture of the anterior cruciate ligament—Leg raise

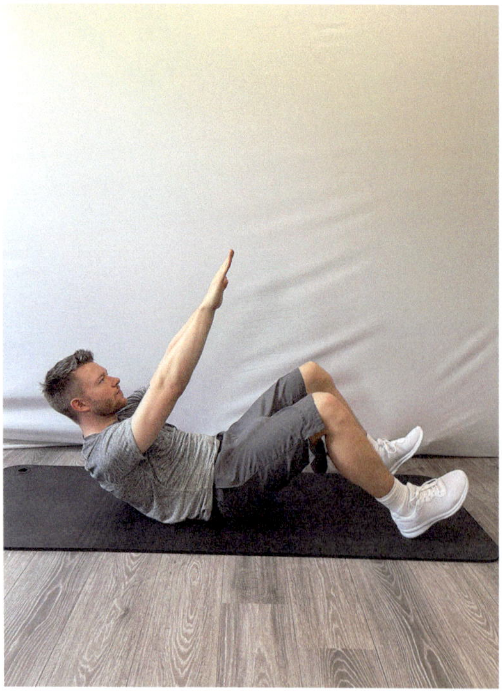

Fig. 5.68 MTT in case of rupture of the anterior cruciate ligament—Crunch

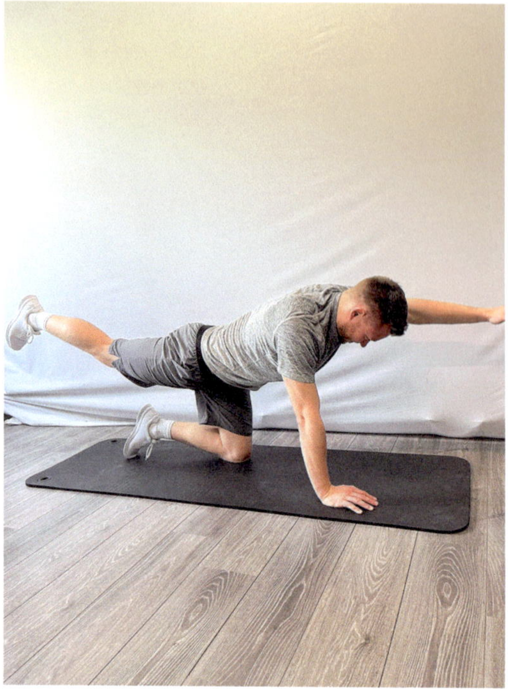

Fig. 5.69 MTT in case of rupture of the anterior cruciate ligament—Superman

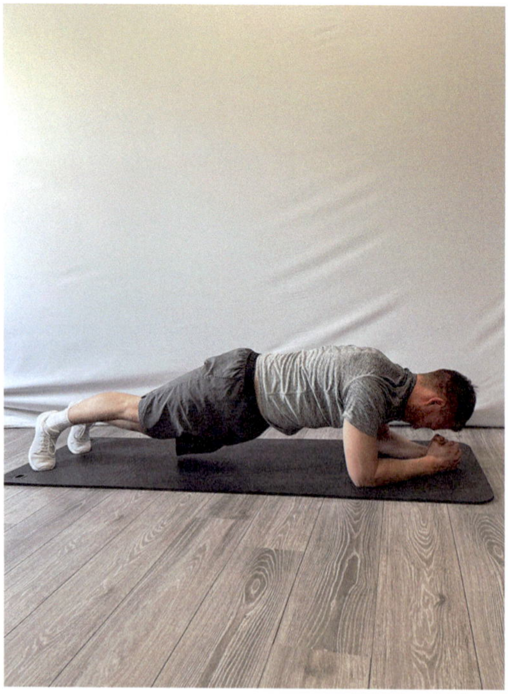

Fig. 5.70 MTT in case of rupture of the anterior cruciate ligament—Plank-hip-twist

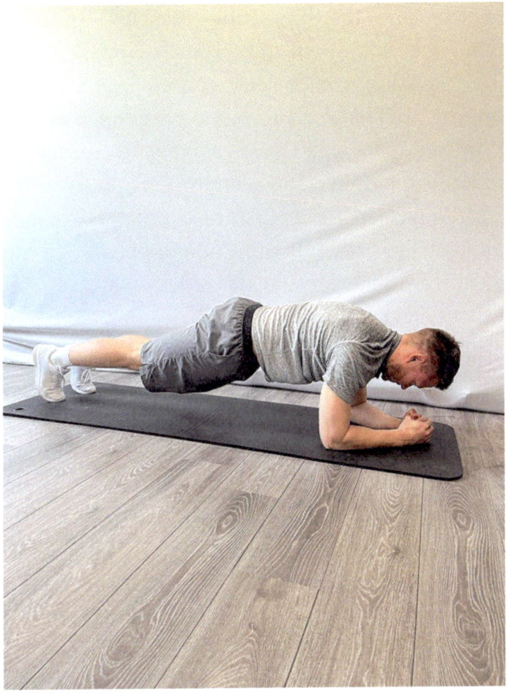

Fig. 5.71 MTT in case of rupture of the anterior cruciate ligament—Forearm support

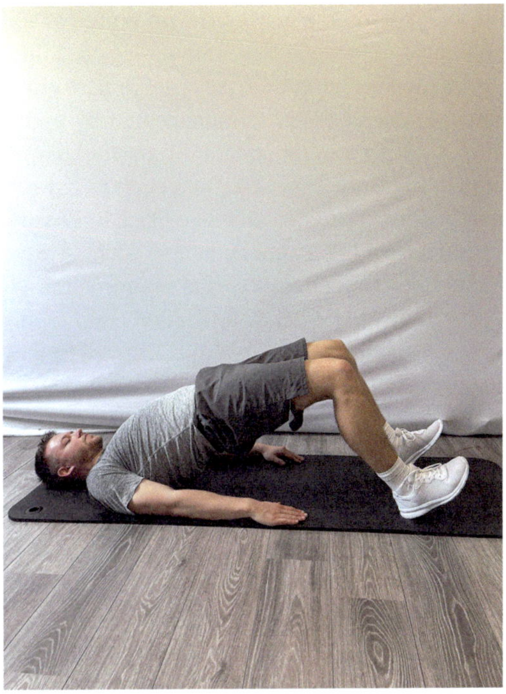

Fig. 5.73 MTT in case of rupture of the anterior cruciate ligament—Bridging

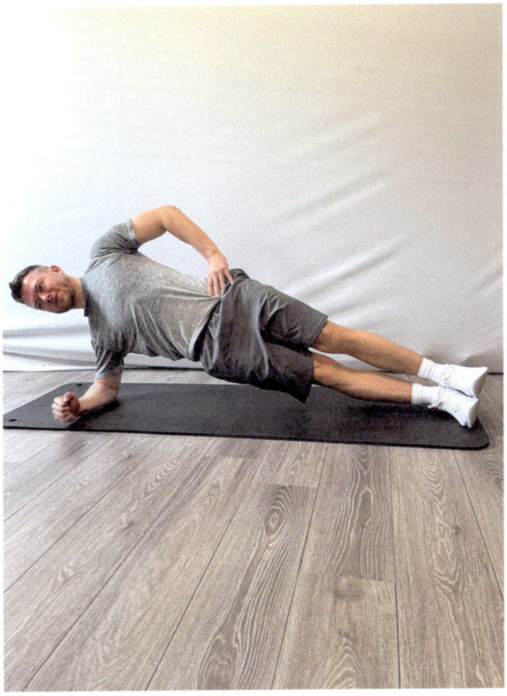

Fig. 5.72 MTT in case of rupture of the anterior cruciate ligament—Side support

extremity should also take place. Weight-shifting or balance-associated exercises can be used. If knee flexion ability is released and available, resistance-free training can be performed on the bicycle ergometer.

Phase 2 extends from week 6 to the end of week 12. In Phase 2, the contents from Phase 1 should be progressively adapted. In addition, work can be done on the leg press with a maximum flexion extent of 70°. Squats can also be used, which can be performed with weight shifts or on the toes. In Phase 2, static lunges with a flexion angle of 45° can also be performed. The hamstring muscles can be accentuated in the supine position through hip joint extension with the leg extended with the heel on a support or through single-leg deadlifts with the knee joint extended. As in Phase 1, Phase 2 should include balance exercises to achieve the goal of improving neuromuscular coordination.

Phase 3 fills the time frame between week 13–18. During this time, the main focus should be on improving muscle strength. Here, work can be done on the leg press with both legs and now also with one leg. Single-leg deadlifts, squats, and bridging exercises can be performed. Strength exercises are complemented by endurance training on the treadmill or the bicycle ergometer. If the functional status allows, a running training can gradually take place in Phase 3.

In Phase 4 (19 + weeks), factors such as maximum strength, endurance, and coordination are further developed and integrated into sport-specific training forms. At the time of return-to-sport, full active mobility, 85%–90% of the quadriceps strength compared to the opposite side, and no giving-way or instability feeling should be present. In addition, the psychological readiness to return to sport should be present (see Pierce et al. 2013).

Lu et al. (2021) deal with the conservative management of isolated ruptures of the posterior cruciate ligament using medical training therapy. A training program over a period of twelve weeks was researched. A training session was implemented twice a week with a respective time frame of one hour. Each training session was divided into a warm-up (10 min), strength training (20 min), balance training (15 min), and finally stretching exercises (10 min). The warm-up training was done on a bicycle ergometer. The balance training was performed on both sides of a half-sphere filled with air and the difficulty level was adjusted upwards on a monthly basis. The strength training includes the leg extensor and leg flexor machine and was practiced with two sets of twelve repetitions each. The training weight was 70% of the 1RM and was progressively adjusted during the study. The described training program led to an improvement in proprioceptive status, increased muscle strength, and thus equalized it to the uninjured leg. These results prevented a reconstruction surgery.

In a male sample aged between 18–35, the effect of medical training therapy on a conservatively treated and at least six months existing insufficiency of the posterior cruciate ligament was examined. It was found that a twelve-week eccentric training of the lower extremity in the closed system is capable of significantly increasing the strength of the quadriceps femoris muscle and the hamstring muscles. In addition, the values of the Tegner-Hop-Test and the Lysholm-knee-scale-score significantly improved. The used training program was performed daily and progressively increased in repetition number and weight. It included bilateral squats, in the course also unilateral squats as well as strengthening components of the gastrocnemius muscle or soleus muscle (see MacLean et al. 1999).

The proprioceptive status can be determined using the active-reproduction-of-a-passive-position-test as well as the passive-reproduction-of-a-passive-position-test using the Biodex-System-3-Pro. The ligamentous laxity of the femorotibial joint can be measured with the KT-1000-arthrometer (see Lu et al. 2021). More detailed information on the individual assessments can be taken from the assessment list in the appendix of this book.

Useful visualizations can be taken from Fig. 5.76, 5.77, 5.78 and 5.79, as well as Fig. 5.80, 5.81, 5.82, 5.83, 5.84, 5.85, 5.86, 5.87 and 5.88.

Summary for Practice

Medical training therapy can be beneficially used both postoperatively and in conservative care of posterior cruciate ligament ruptures. In summary, full load could be applied from the sixth week in a range of motion of 90°. At the beginning of rehabilitation, exercises with a co-contraction of the quadriceps femoris and the ischiocrural muscles are recommended.

Postoperatively, the training process can be divided into 4 phases.

Fig. 5.74 and 5.75 provide an overview of the mentioned information.

5.2.5 Meniscal Lesions

A meta-analysis from 2023 by Fernández-Matías et al. (2023) compared medical training therapy alone in people with degenerative

Categories	Evidence-based training recommendation
Phase 1 (surgery until completed week 5)	No hyperextension or posterior translation of the tibia / no isolated training of the ischiocrural muscles (until week 12) / slowly increase partial weight-bearing up to full weight-bearing with a view to a good gait pattern / strengthening of the quadriceps femoris and triceps surae muscles / strengthening of the trunk and upper extremities / balance exercises / stretching of the calf muscles
Phase 2 (week 6 to completed week 12)	Progressively increase phase 1 / leg press up to 70° / squat with weight shift to toes / static lunges with Flexion angle of 45° / strengthening of the ischiocrural muscles in a reclined position through hip extension with the leg extended or one-legged deadlifts with the knee joint extended / balance exercises
Phase 3 (week 13 to completed week 18)	Strengthening the leg muscles / two-legged and one-legged leg press / one-legged deadlifts / squats / bridging / gradual running training
Phase 4 (from week 19)	Maximum strength, endurance and coordination / sport-specific exercises / return-to-sport factors: full active mobility, 85-90% strength quadriceps femoris, no giving way or feeling of instability

Fig. 5.74 Summary of MTT postoperatively after reconstruction of the posterior cruciate ligament

Categories	Evidence-based training recommendation
Units	2 sessions per week of one hour each for the first 12 weeks
Exercises	Warm up 10 minutes (bike ergometer or similar) / strength training 20 minutes (leg extension + leg flexors / eccentric as well as one-legged and two-legged squats)
Exercise parameters	2 sets of 12 repetitions with 70% of 1RM / progressive increase

Fig. 5.75 Summary of MTT in conservative care of the rupture of the posterior cruciate ligament

meniscal tears to a combination of arthroscopic partial meniscectomy and medical training therapy. After statistical evaluation of the four included articles, it became clear that performing a partial arthroscopic meniscectomy does not provide any added value at a five-year follow-up. These results confirm the earlier findings of Ma et al. (2020). They concluded that the combination of arthroscopic partial meniscectomy and medical training therapy has a positive effect on pain and functionality in a six-month postoperative period. However, when longer follow-up periods are considered, no superiority can be determined compared to the sole implementation of medical training therapy without surgery (see Ma et al. 2020).

Kise et al. (2016) examined the effectiveness of a twelve-week training program, which

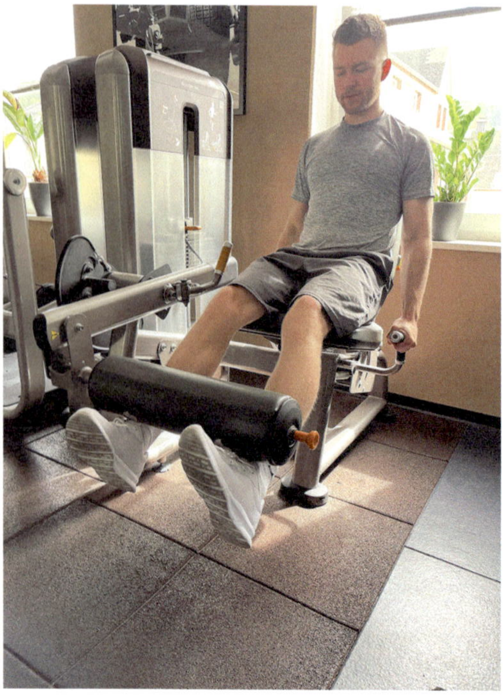

Fig. 5.76 MTT in rupture of the posterior cruciate ligament—leg extensor

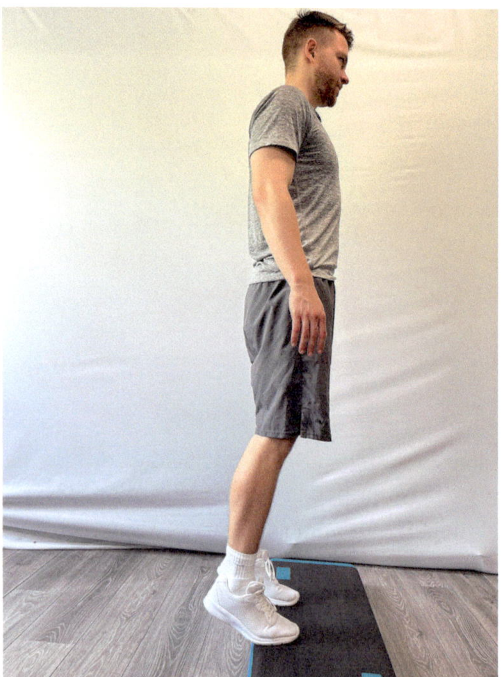

Fig. 5.77 MTT in rupture of the posterior cruciate ligament—stretching and strengthening of the calf muscles

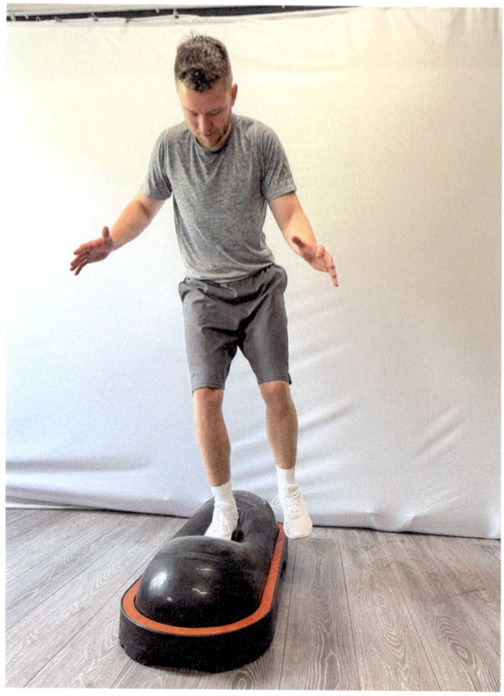

Fig. 5.78 MTT in rupture of the posterior cruciate ligament—balance exercise

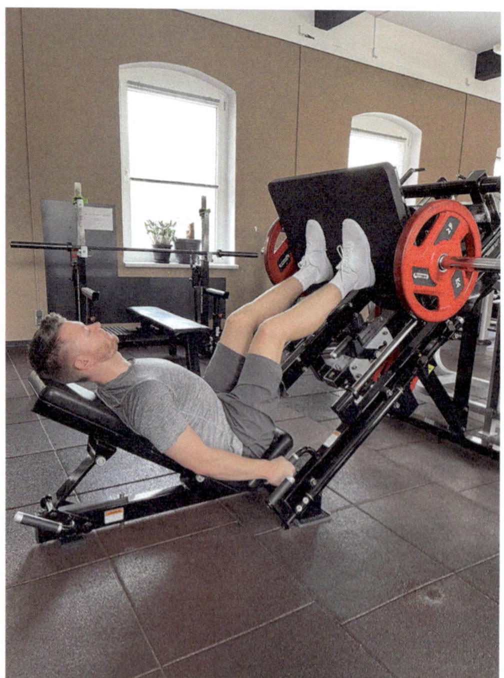

Fig. 5.79 MTT in rupture of the posterior cruciate ligament—leg press up to 70° flexion

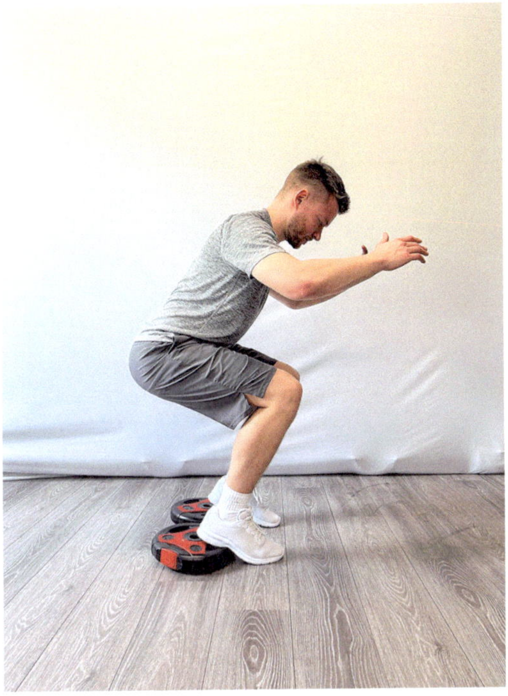

Fig. 5.80 MTT in rupture of the posterior cruciate ligament—squat with shift to tiptoes (weight plate under heel)

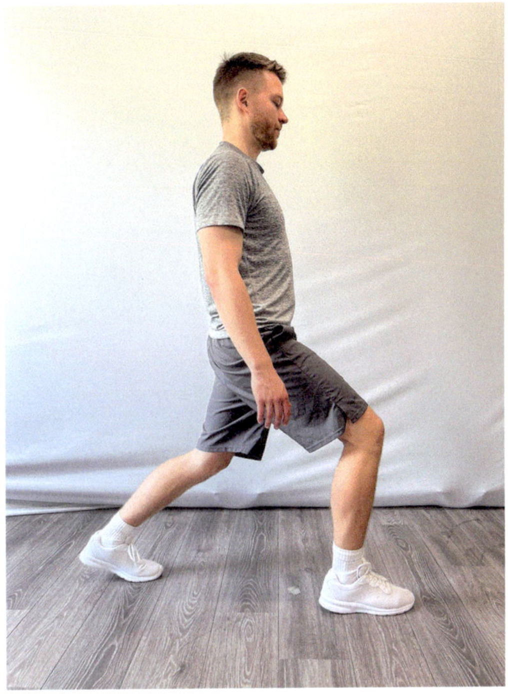

Fig. 5.81 MTT in rupture of the posterior cruciate ligament—lunges up to 45° flexion angle

includes both progressive proprioceptive components and progressive strength training. During the three-month period, two to three training sessions were held weekly. The training program begins with a 20-minute warm-up on the bicycle ergometer. This is followed by bilateral and unilateral squats. In addition, exercises on the step board, on the Pezziball, on an air cushion, as well as bilateral or unilateral plyometric exercises are used. In terms of strength machines, one-legged exercises are performed on the leg press up to a bending angle of 90°, one-legged on the leg extender, and one-legged on the leg curler while standing. The number of sets varies between 2 and 4 while the number of repetitions ranges from 6–15 (cf. Stensrud et al. 2012). The described training program is recommended for middle-aged people with degenerative meniscus lesions without radiographic evidence of gonarthrosis (cf. Kise et al. 2016).

In another publication, the effect of concentric isokinetic training on overweight women with degenerative meniscus tears was examined. It was found that a six-week training intervention, which consists of a combination of concentric isokinetic training and a conventional rehabilitation program, can achieve significant effects. These relate to improved mobility, increased functionality, reduced pain intensity, and improved quality of life (cf. Hammami et al. 2023). Luc-Harkey et al. (2018) confirmed an association between increased muscle strength of the quadriceps femoris and the ischiocrural muscles and reduced pain, improved feasibility of everyday activities, and increased mobility in people with gonarthrosis and accompanying meniscus tears.

To assess the functional status of people with degenerative meniscus tears, the maximum number of squats within 30 seconds (cf. Bremander et al. 2007), the one-leg-hop-for-distance test, and the 6 m-timed-up-and-hop test can be performed (cf. Noyes et al. 1991; Stensrud et al. 2015). Furthermore, the sit-to-stand test, the

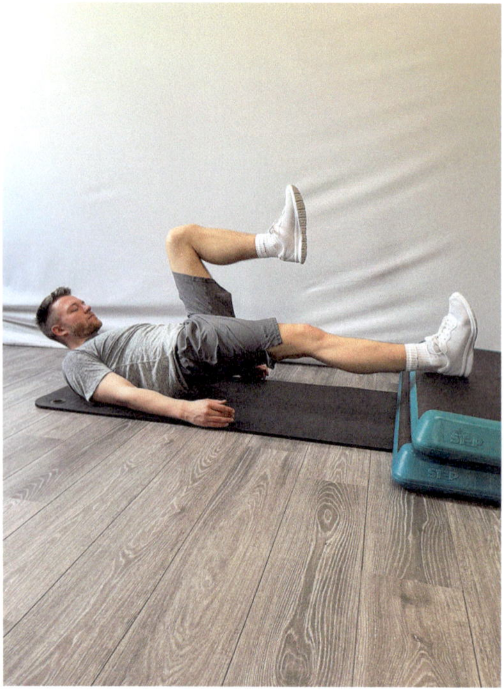

Fig. 5.82 MTT for rupture of the posterior cruciate ligament—Hip extension in supine position with extended leg and heel on support

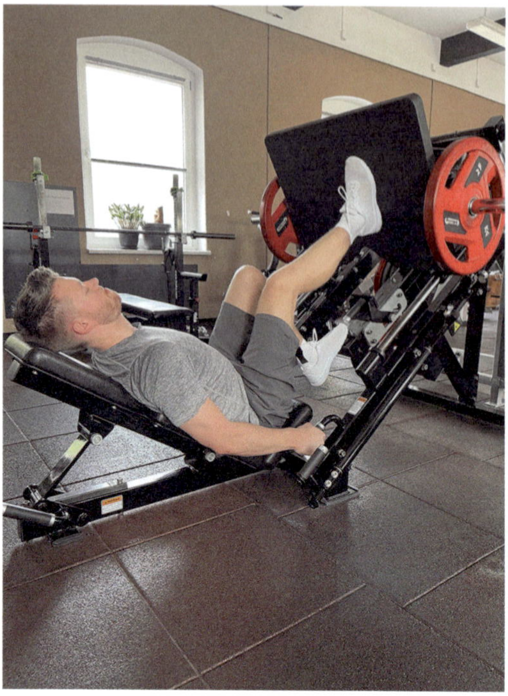

Fig. 5.84 MTT for rupture of the posterior cruciate ligament—Single or double leg press

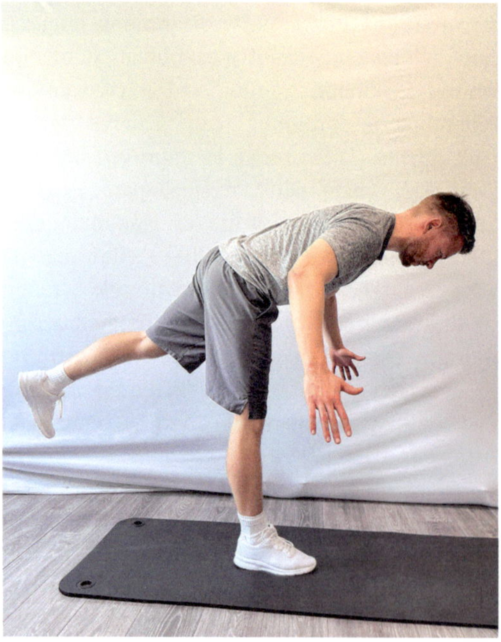

Fig. 5.83 MTT for rupture of the posterior cruciate ligament—Single-leg deadlifts with extended knee joint

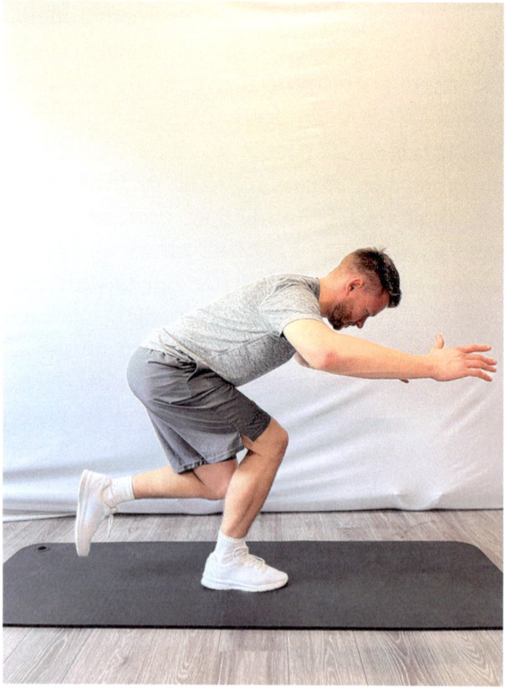

Fig. 5.85 MTT for rupture of the posterior cruciate ligament—Single or double leg squat

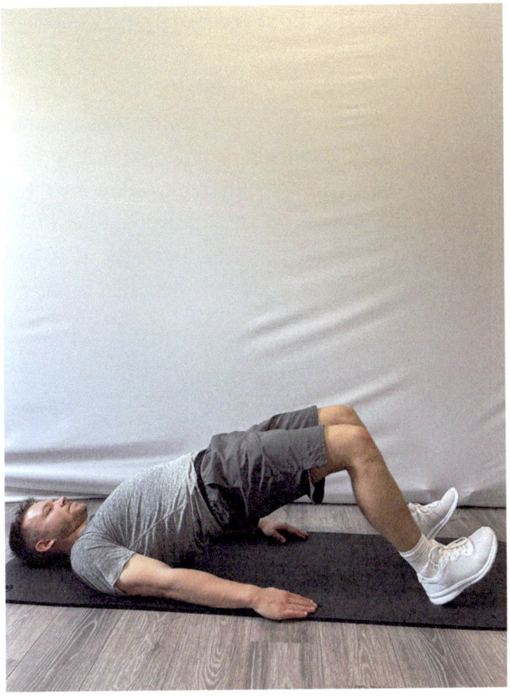

Fig. 5.86 MTT for rupture of the posterior cruciate ligament—Bridging

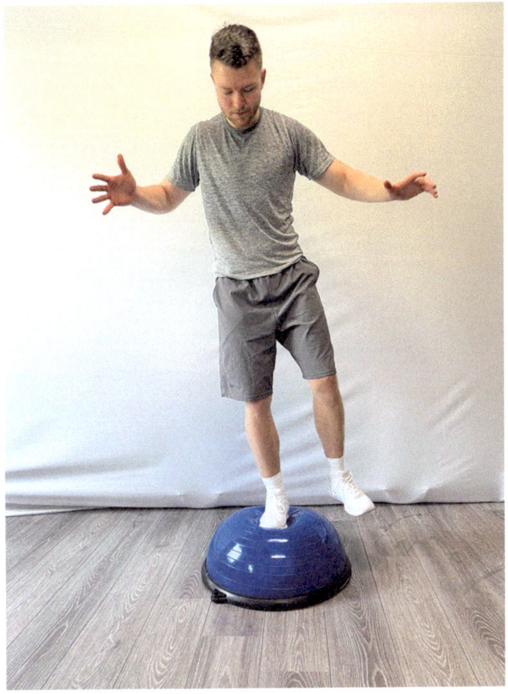

Fig. 5.88 MTT for rupture of the posterior cruciate ligament—Standing on an air-filled hemisphere

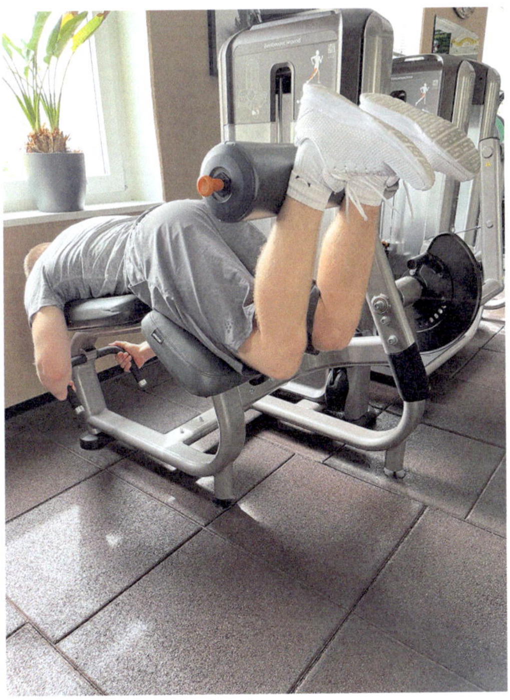

Fig. 5.87 MTT for rupture of the posterior cruciate ligament—Leg curl machine

stair-climb test, the heel-to-buttock test, and the KOOS-questionnaire-of-pain-and-quality-of-life can be used (cf. Hammami et al. 2023). More detailed information on the individual assessments can be taken from the assessment list in the appendix of this book.

Useful visualizations can be taken from Fig. 5.90, 5.91, 5.92, 5.93, 5.94, 5.95, 5.96 and 5.97.

Summary for Practice

Medical training therapy can be beneficially used in both conservatively and surgically treated meniscus lesions. Over a long period of time, surgery does not bring a better effect compared to training alone. The applicable training mainly involves progressive strength training with progressive proprioceptive components. Concentric isokinetic training in this context leads to an improvement in mobility and functionality, as well as pain reduction, and ultimately also to an improvement in quality of life. The focus is on strengthening the quadriceps femoris and the ischiocrural muscles.

Fig. 5.89 provides an overview of the mentioned information.

5.2.6 Patellar Dislocation

Regardless of whether a patellar dislocation is treated conservatively or surgically, Watson et al. (2022) recommend local and global strengthening of the knee and hip joint controlling muscles.

After the operation or femoropatellar dislocation, which usually occurs laterally, it is recommended to wear a motion-limiting brace for

Categories	Evidence-based training recommendation
Units	2-3 sessions per week á 45-60 minutes per session
Exercises	20-minute warm-up on the cycle ergometer / double-leg and single-leg squats / exercises on the step board, Pezziball, air cushion / double-leg and single-leg polymetric exercises / single-leg leg press up to 90° flexion / single-leg knee extensions / single-leg knee flexors in a standing position
Exercise parameters	2-4 sets, 6-15 repetitions

Fig. 5.89 Summary of MTT in Meniscus Lesion

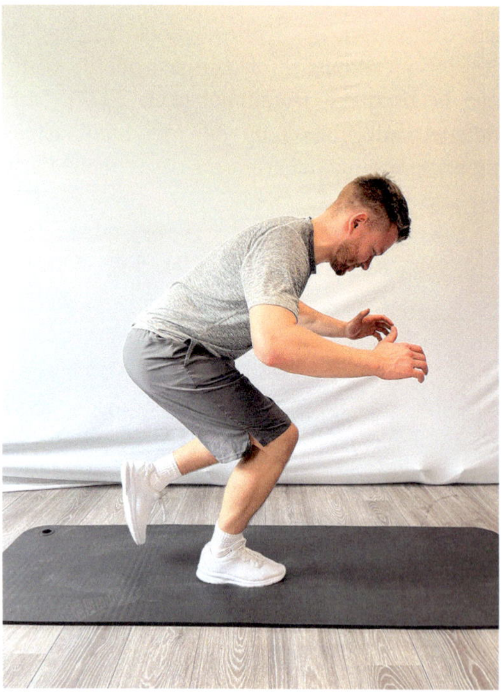

Fig. 5.90 MTT in Meniscus Lesion—Single and Double Leg Squat

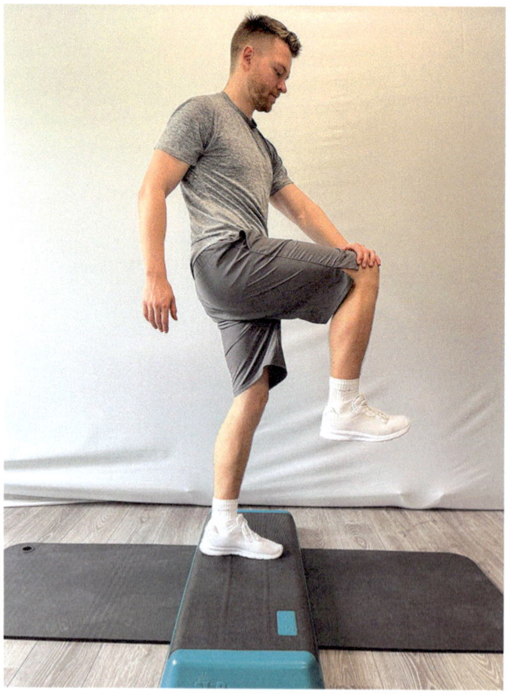

Fig. 5.91 MTT in Meniscus Lesion—Exercises on Step Board

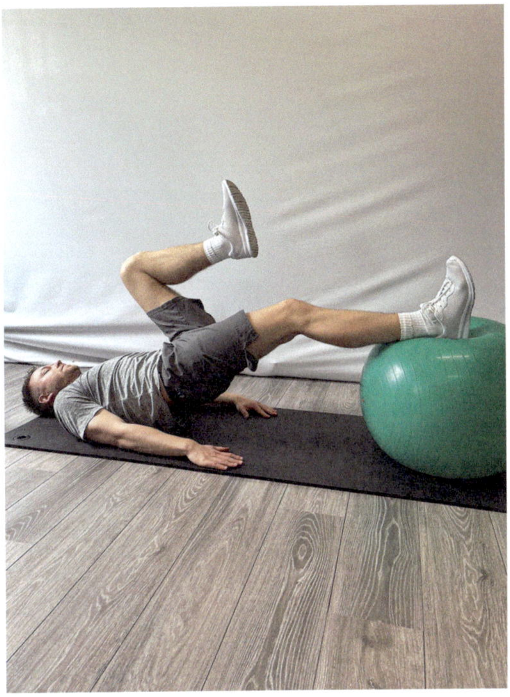

Fig. 5.92 MTT in Meniscus Lesion—Exercises on Pezzi Ball

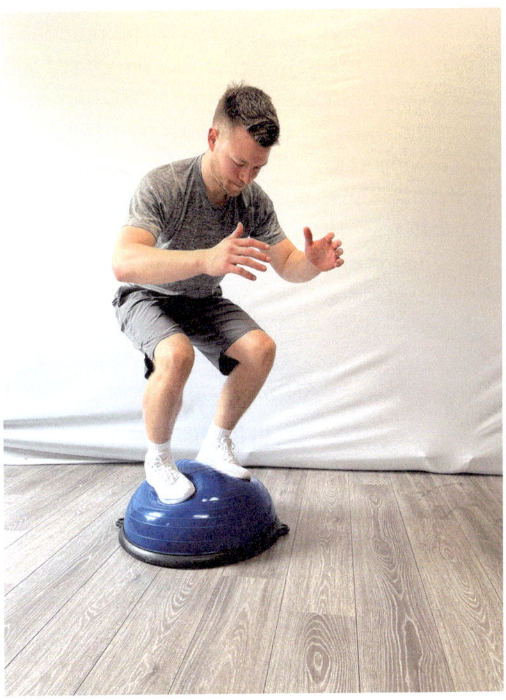

Fig. 5.93 MTT in Meniscus Lesion—Exercises on Air Cushion

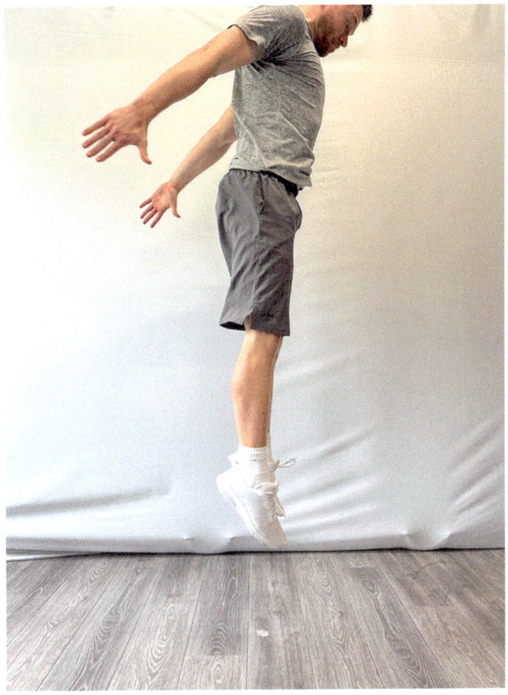

Fig. 5.94 MTT in Meniscus Lesion—Single and Double Leg Plyometric Exercise

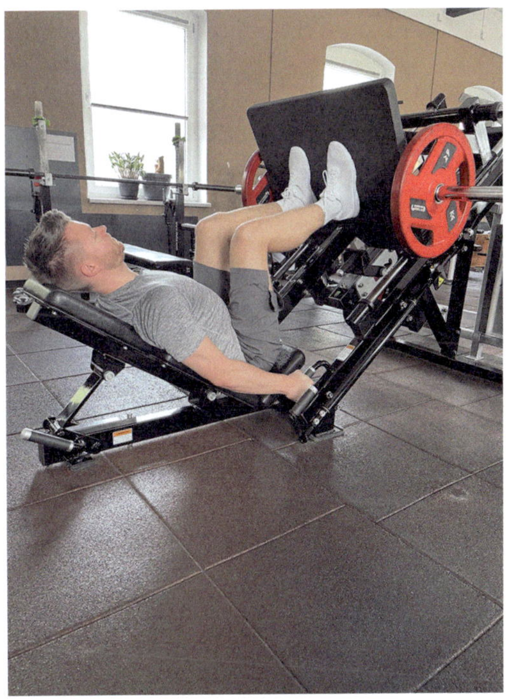

Fig. 5.95 MTT in Meniscus Lesion—Leg Press up to 90°

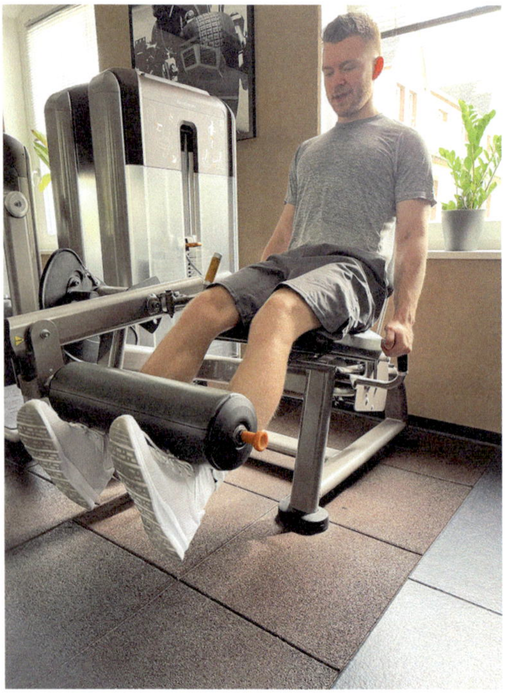

Fig. 5.96 MTT in Meniscus Lesion—Single and Double Leg Knee Extension

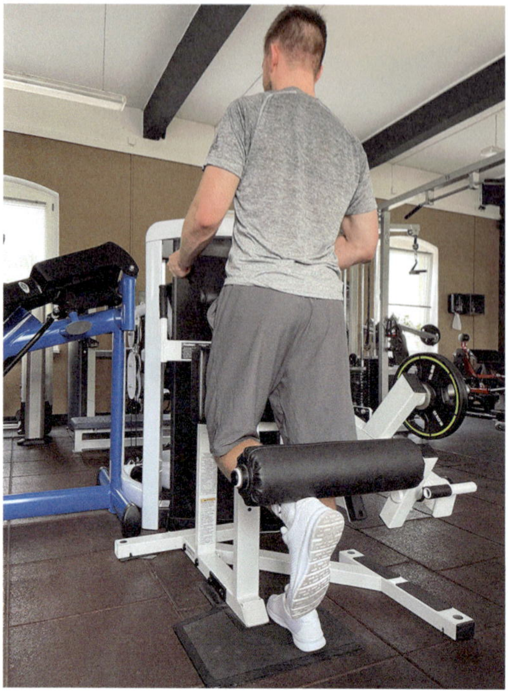

Fig. 5.97 MTT in Meniscus Lesion—Single Leg Knee Flexor in Standing Position

a period of about three weeks (see Flores et al. 2023). Postoperatively or post-traumatically, the affected leg can be progressively loaded pain-adapted or with a partial load of 15 kg over a period of about three weeks (see Honkonen et al. 2022; Petri et al. 2013). Regarding medical training therapy, emphasis should be placed on strengthening the quadriceps femoris muscle. In particular, the targeted activation of the vastus medialis muscle is the subject of existing literature (see Smith et al. 2015). Strengthening the ischiocrural muscles should also be part of the medical training therapy (see Straume-Næsheim et al. 2022). In people with recurring patellar dislocation, a significant weakness of the ischiocrural muscles was found (see Małecki et al. 2021). This underlines the relevance of training the knee flexors.

Bitar et al. (2012) recommend tension exercises for the quadriceps femoris muscle within the first three weeks of rehabilitation. Subsequently, resistance-free training on the bicycle ergometer can be practiced. In the course, proprioceptive training and strength training in the closed kinematic chain are well suited to prepare for training in the open kinematic chain (see Bitar et al. 2012). Xing et al. (2022) explicitly point out that the therapeutic response of the quadriceps femoris muscle as early as possible in the course of rehabilitation contributes to improved knee function and prophylaxis of atrophy.

Factors such as increased valgus position of the upper ankle joint or insufficiency of the hip abductors can force the knee joint into a valgus position and thus increase the risk of patellar (sub)luxations and should therefore be addressed therapeutically (see Han et al. 2017).

Assessments can include the Lysholm-knee-score and the Tegner-level-of-activity-score (see Smith et al. 2015). More detailed information on the individual assessments can be taken from the assessment list in the appendix of this book.

Useful visualizations can be taken from Fig. 5.99, 5.100, 5.101, 5.102, 5.103 and 5.104.

Summary for Practice

From the perspective of medical training therapy, after a patellar dislocation, the focus should be on strengthening the quadriceps femoris muscle, especially the vastus medialis muscle. Furthermore, it is important to train the ischiocrural muscles and to treat against a possible valgus position in the upper ankle joint and the insufficiency of the hip abductors. Directly after the dislocation or an operation, wearing a motion-limiting brace and the progressive and pain-adapted partial load of 15 kg for three weeks is recommended. The following strength training and proprioceptive training should initially be carried out in the closed and then open chain.

Fig. 5.98 provides an overview of the mentioned information.

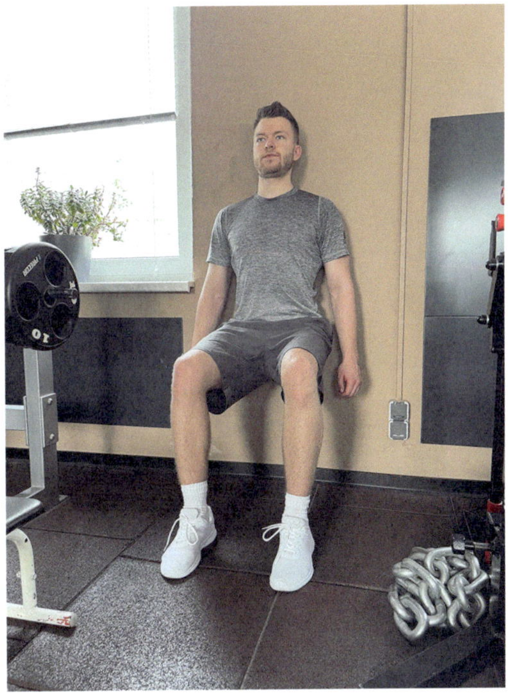

Fig. 5.99 MTT in Patellar Dislocation—Strengthening of M. quadriceps femoris in the closed chain with focus on the M. vastus medialis

5.3 Area Lower Leg/Foot

5.3.1 Supination Trauma/ Chronic Ankle Instability

Medical training therapy can not only be used in the aftercare of supination traumas, but also for the prevention of chronic instability of the ankles (see Doherty et al. 2017). In addition, the risk of recurrence can be reduced by training therapy (see Wagemans et al. 2022; Bleakley et al. 2019).

Hall et al. (2018) compared the influence of balance training and strength training in people with chronic ankle instability. Over a period of six weeks, three training sessions were

Categories	Evidence-based training recommendation
Exercises	Weeks 1-3 after dislocation or surgery: wearing a splint / partial weight bearing up to 15 kg / tension exercises for the quadriceps femoris muscle / resistance-free training with the bicycle ergometer / proprioceptive training in a closed chain / strength training in a closed chain From week 4: Increase exercises as above only progressively / also perform all exercises in an open chain

Fig. 5.98 Summary of MTT in Patellar Dislocation

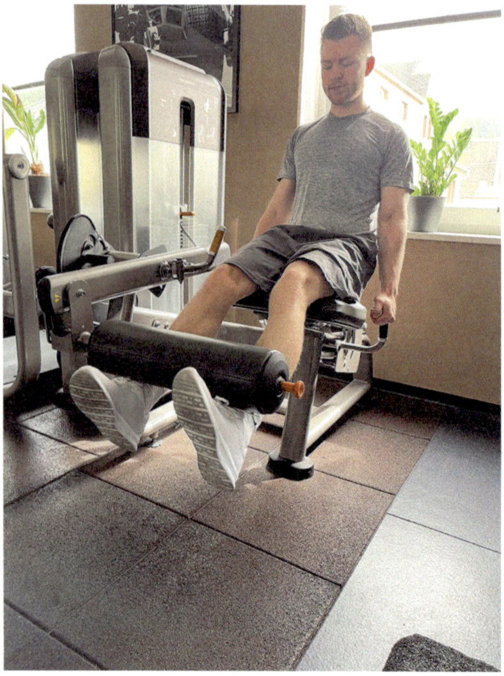

Fig. 5.100 MTT in Patellar Dislocation—Strengthening of M. quadriceps femoris in the open chain with focus on the M. vastus medialis

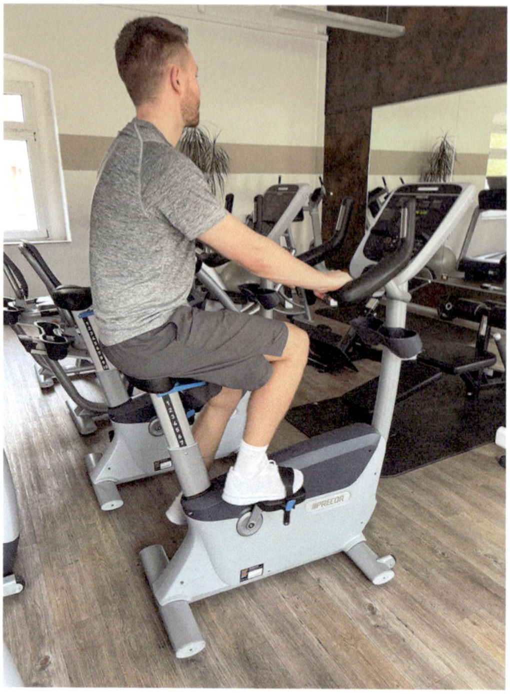

Fig. 5.102 MTT in Patellar Dislocation—Bicycle Ergometer

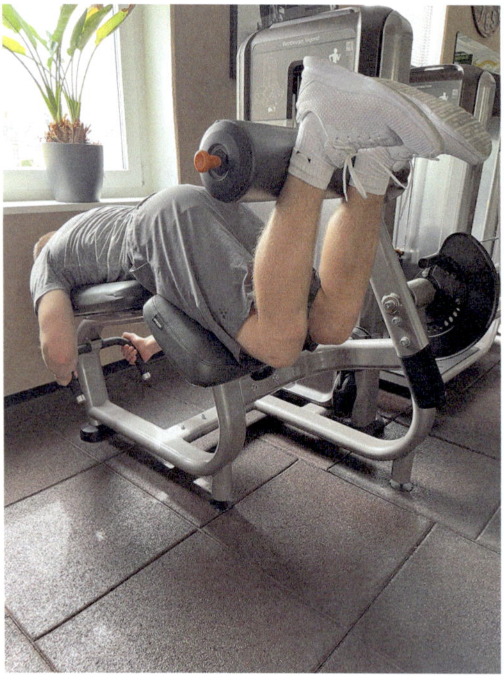

Fig. 5.101 MTT in Patellar Dislocation—Strengthening of Mm. ischiocrurales

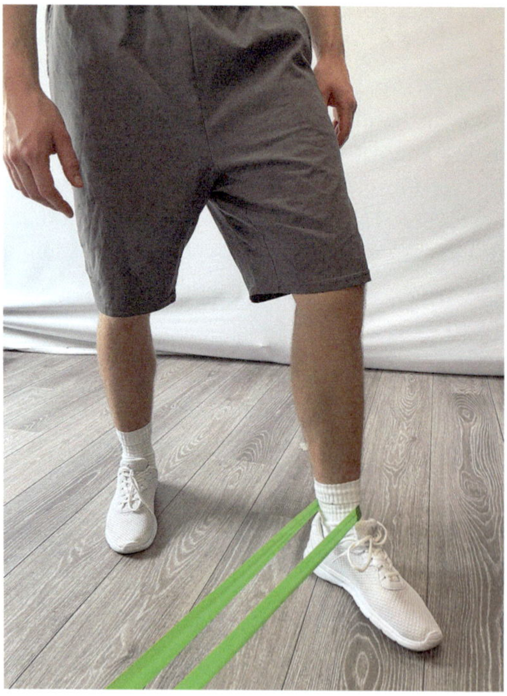

Fig. 5.103 MTT in Patellar Dislocation—Training against Valgus Position of the Foot

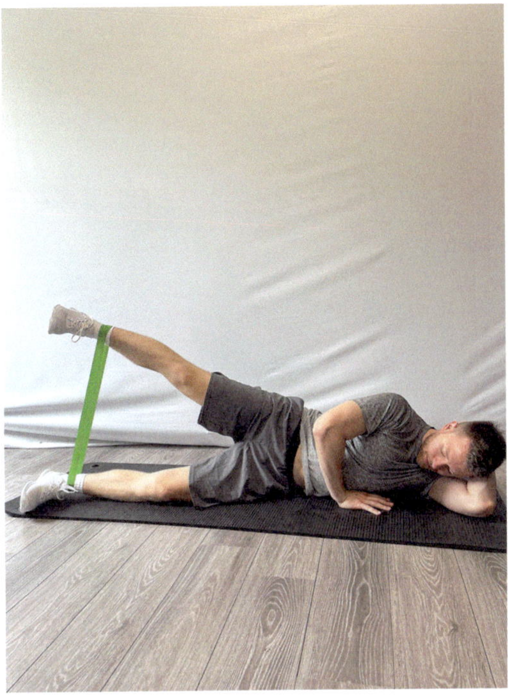

Fig. 5.104 MTT in Patellar Dislocation—Strengthening Hip Abductors

conducted weekly, each lasting 20 minutes. The balance training program was adopted from McKeon et al. (2008) and includes progressive training of single-leg stance. To increase intensity, altered arm positions, changed surfaces, longer holding times, and closing of the eyes are used. Additionally, jumps in various variations and directions are included. The strength training included training with Therabands in the movement directions of dorsiflexion, inversion, and eversion. With three sets and ten repetitions each, the resistance was progressively increased weekly. To strengthen the plantar flexors, heel raises were practiced on a stair step, utilizing the full range of motion. These were supplemented by the application of a proprioceptive neuromuscular facilitation diagonal. The number of sets increased from initially two to four in the last week of intervention. The number of repetitions varied between 10 and 15. Both balance and strength training led to a significant improvement in balance, strength, and functionality (see Hall et al. 2018). Similar training approaches also led to a reduction in pain intensity (see Hall et al. 2015).

Cain et al. (2020) compared a strength training program using Theraband in all directions of movement with balance training on a cone in people with chronic ankle instability. Both approaches significantly improved balance ability and functionality equally.

Lazarou et al. (2018) examined the influence of a balance training program in people aged 18–40 with post-acute supination traumas. Over a period of six weeks, ten training sessions were conducted. The training program included bilateral as well as single-leg exercises on a wobble board, a firm and a soft surface. The exercises included, for example, single-leg squats of the affected leg up to the tolerance limit, single-leg diagonal jumps, and jumps in the sagittal or frontal plane. After an eight-week follow-up period, a significant improvement in functionality, range of motion, and balance in the frontal plane was observed (see Lazarou et al. 2018).

Assessments include, among others, balance assessment tools such as stability index scores as well as functional tests such as the single-hop-for-distance-test and the single-leg-hops-for-time-test (see Lazarou et al. 2018). Furthermore, the side-hop functional performance test can be used (see Hall et al. 2018). Additionally, the foot-and-ankle-disability-index, time-to-boundery measurements, and the star-excursion-balance-test can be applied (see McKeon et al. 2008). Hall et al. (2015) used the figure-8-hop-test-for-time, the triple-crossover-hop-test-for-distance, and the y-balance-test. In addition, the time-in-balance-test, the foot-lift-test, the side-hop test, the foot-and-ankle-ability-measure, and the Cumberland-ankle-instability-tool can be used (see Cain et al. 2020). More detailed information on the individual assessments can be found in the assessment list in the appendix of this book.

Useful visualizations can be found in Fig. 5.106, 5.107, 5.108, 5.109, and 5.110.

Summary for Practice

Training therapy focusing on balance training and strength training can significantly improve the condition after a supination trauma in terms of functionality, balance, strength, and pain. A training period of at least six to eight weeks should be aimed for to produce a positive effect.

Fig. 5.105 provides an overview of the information mentioned.

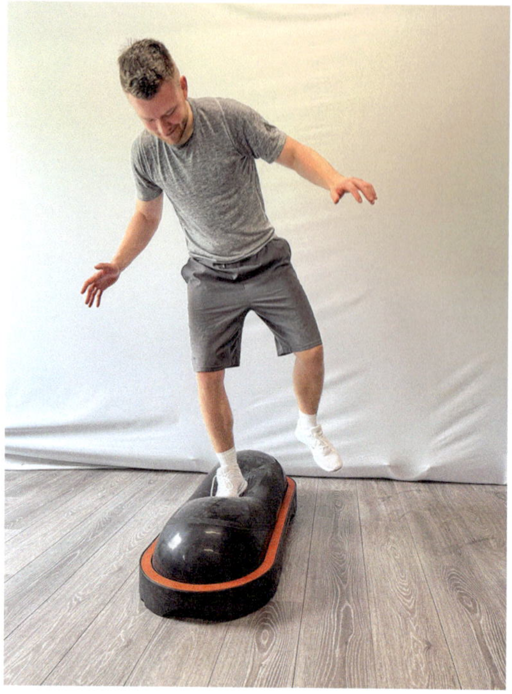

Fig. 5.106 MTT in supination trauma/chronic ankle instability—One-legged stance with possible variations

5.3.2 Achillodynia/Achilles Tendon Tendinopathy

In the medical training therapy of achillodynia, eccentric training plays an important role (see Silbernagel et al. 2001). Eccentric training is capable of significantly reducing pain intensity in Achilles tendon tendinopathy in the middle region of the tendon (see Prudêncio et al. 2023; Wilson et al. 2018).

At a stair step, the heel can be slowly lowered from the toe stand. If this exercise is practiced with an extended knee joint, the gastrocnemius muscle is accentuated. In addition, a slight bending of the knee joint can place increased strain on the soleus muscle. With increasing weight over time, two to three sets of 15 repetitions each

Categories	Evidence-based training recommendation
Units	6-8 weeks with 3 sessions of at least 20 minutes per session
Exercises	Progressive training of the one-legged stance (change of arm position, different surfaces, longer holding times, closed eyes) / jumps in different variations and directions, balance training on a cone and wobble board with one and two legs and on different surfaces / one-legged squat of the affected leg / one-legged diagonal jumps, jumps in sagittal and frontal plane Strength training with Theraband in dorsiflexion, eversion and inversion / heel raises on stairs in full range of motion / proprioceptive neuromuscular facilitation diagonals
Exercise parameters	3-4 sets of 10-15 repetitions each

Fig. 5.105 Summary of MTT in supination trauma/chronic ankle instability

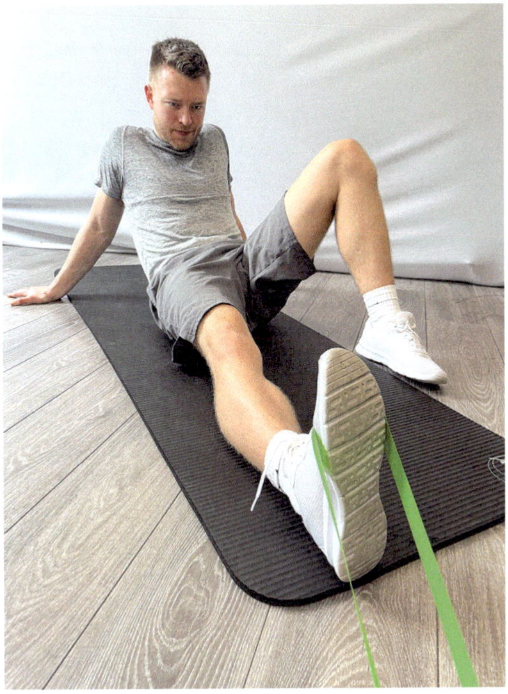

Fig. 5.107 MTT in supination trauma/chronic ankle instability—Training in dorsiflexion, eversion and inversion with Theraband

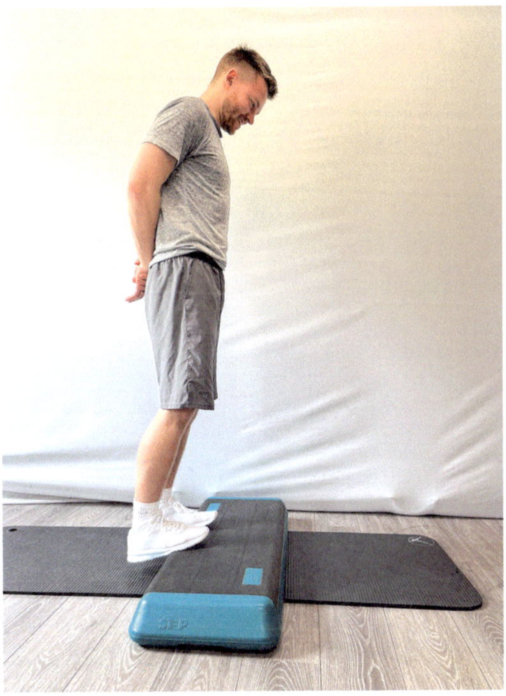

Fig. 5.108 MTT in supination trauma/chronic ankle instability—Heel-raises on stair step

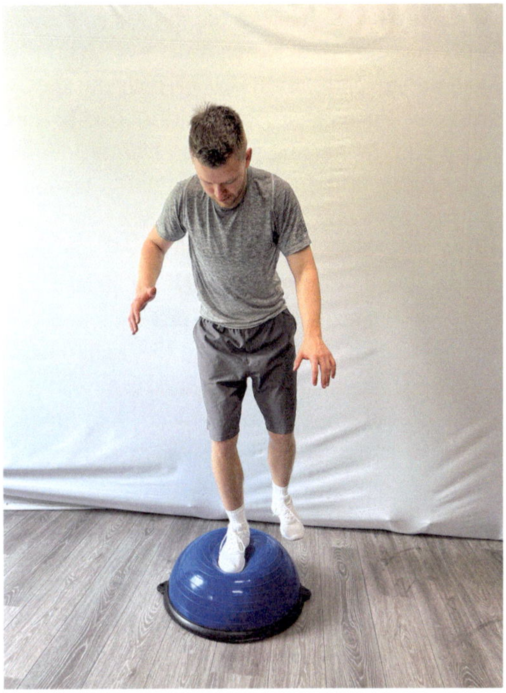

Fig. 5.109 MTT in supination trauma/chronic ankle instability—Balance training on cone

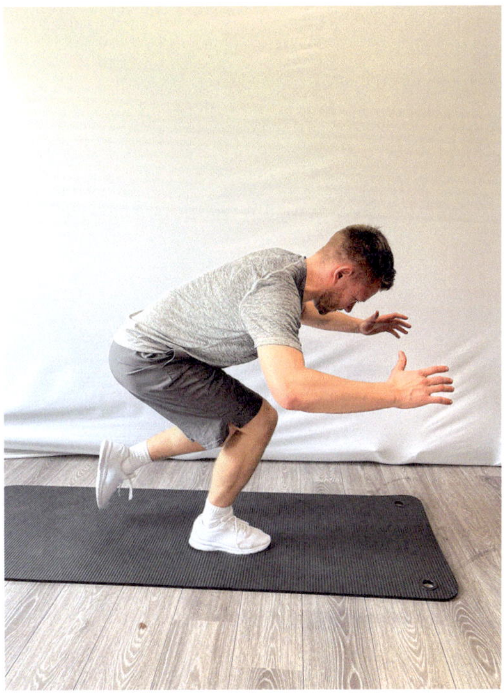

Fig. 5.110 MTT in supination trauma/chronic ankle instability—Single-leg squats

are recommended for both the gastrocnemius and soleus muscles (see Nørregaard et al. 2007). In addition, stretching exercises of both muscles of five times 30 seconds holding time can be integrated into the training program. During training, a slight pain in the area of the Achilles tendon is accepted. However, if the pain increases during the day or if increased morning stiffness is observed, this indicates overuse. The female gender and symptom localization in the distal area of the Achilles tendon seem to respond less well to medical training therapy (see Nørregaard et al. 2007).

Gatz et al. (2020) recognized that adding isometric training components to the classic eccentric approach does not bring any added value. Moreover, there seems to be no difference whether the eccentric training is performed isolated eccentrically or concentric-eccentrically (see Habets et al. 2021).

The pain-on-palpation-test serves as an assessment, for example (see Silbernagel et al. 2001). More detailed information on the individual assessments can be taken from the assessment list in the appendix of this book.

Useful visualizations can be found in Fig. 5.112, 5.113, 5.114 and 5.115.

Summary for Practice

Medical training therapy in the form of eccentric exercise can provide a significant improvement in pain symptoms in Achilles tendonitis. The focus here is on toe standing on a staircase with the slow lowering of the heel. Mild pain may occur during training. If the pain increases during the day or morning stiffness is added, the intensity is chosen too high.

Fig. 5.111 provides an overview of the mentioned information.

5.3.3 Flatfoot

A meta-analysis from 2022 advocates the use of training the short foot muscles and highlights a superiority to other therapy strategies (see Huang et al. 2022). The active form of therapy is superior to passive therapy strategies such as the sole provision of shoe inserts (see Hoang et al. 2021).

Brijwasi and Borkar (2023) examined the influence of a training program on people with flatfoot in a randomized controlled study. Over a period of six weeks, three training sessions were held each week, each lasting 30 minutes. The training program consisted of a warm-up phase, a training phase of the short foot muscles, and a training phase of the hip abductors and hip extensors. The exercises aimed at the short foot muscles included the extension of toes two to five, the extension of the hallux, the spreading of the toes, and the building of the foot arch

Categories	Evidence-based training recommendation
Units	Daily implementation
Exercises	Toe stand on step and slow eccentric lowering of the heel, if the heel is at the level of the step the intensity is lower, if the heel is below the level of the step the intensity is higher, if the knee is extended the focus is on the gastrocnemius muscle, if the knee is flexed the focus is on the soleus muscle.
Exercise parameters	2-3 sets of 15 repetitions
Elongation	Stretching the gastrocnemius and soleus muscles 5 times for 30 seconds each

Fig. 5.111 Summary MTT in Achilles tendonitis/Achilles tendon tendinopathy

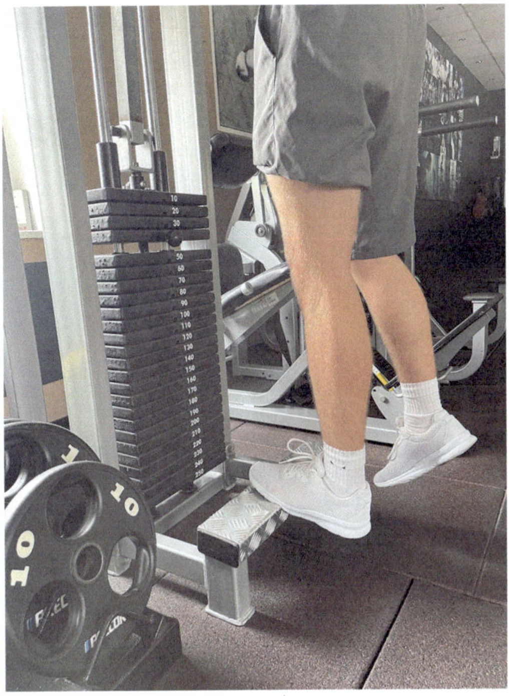

Fig. 5.112 MTT in Achilles tendonitis/Achilles tendon tendinopathy—Toe standing on step with lowering of the heel with extended knee joint

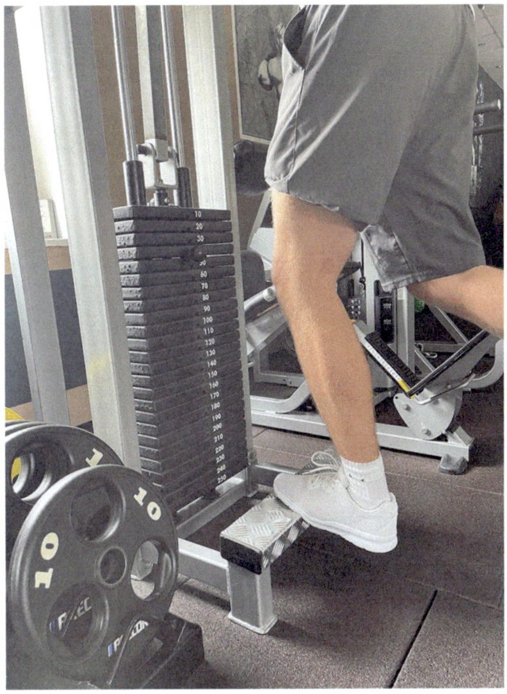

Fig. 5.113 MTT in Achilles tendonitis/Achilles tendon tendinopathy—Toe standing on step with lowering of the heel with bent knee joint

by bringing the big and little toe balls and the heel closer together. The exercises were progressively increased during the course of the study by varying the starting position and the contraction time from initially 5 to 15 seconds. The initially sitting position was followed by standing and finally one-legged standing. The exercises were each performed with two sets of 15 repetitions. The hip abductors and hip extensors were trained in side or prone position with 2 sets and 10-12 repetitions each. Progression was achieved by extending the contraction time from 0 to 10 seconds. The described training program was able to increase the distance between the ground and the tuberosity of the navicular bone. In addition, the longitudinal arch angle was improved by 16° (see Brijwasi and Borkar 2023).

As another therapy exercise, the instruction can also be given to pull the head of the Os metatarsale I towards the heel without bending the toes and maintaining the tension. Elsayed et al. (2023) chose three sets of 10 repetitions and 5 seconds holding time for this. A one-minute break was taken between sets. This exercise was practiced daily over a period of six weeks. Within the six weeks, progression was achieved by modifying the starting position from sitting to standing and finally to single-leg standing (see Elsayed et al. 2023). Namsawang et al. (2019) chose a similar exercise execution as Elsayed et al. (2023) and added a swelling current to the muscle belly of the Musculus abductor hallucis during the exercise execution. This resulted in increased muscle activity of the Musculus abductor hallucis compared to training therapy alone without electricity.

Alam et al. (2019) chose a similar approach with the difference that they had a towel grasped by toe flexion. In addition, specific training of the Musculus tibialis posterior and stretching exercises of the Musculus iliopsoas are

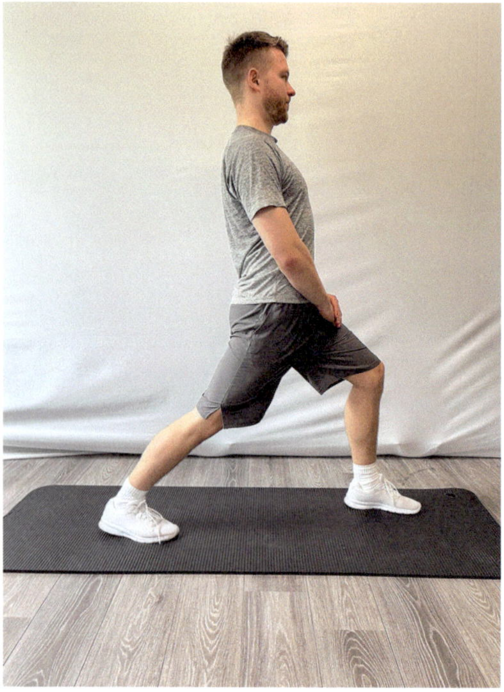

Fig. 5.114 MTT in Achilles tendonitis/Achilles tendon tendinopathy—Stretching M. gastrocnemius

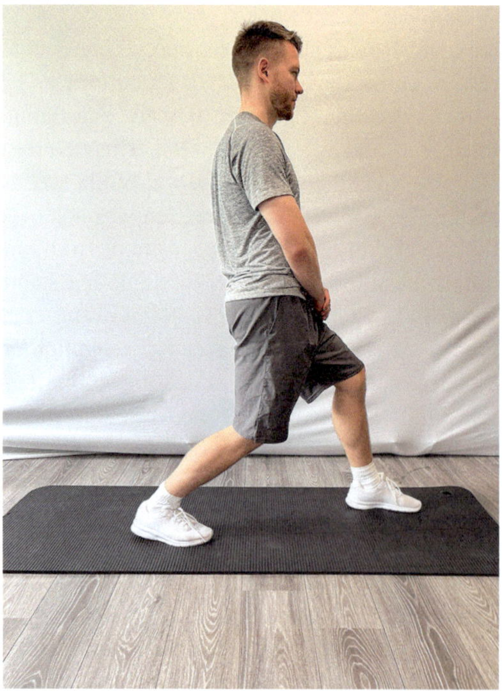

Fig. 5.115 MTT in Achilles tendonitis/Achilles tendon tendinopathy—Stretching M. soleus

recommended. The combination of these measures is capable of positively influencing the position of the Os naviculare and also leads to improved muscular activity and a harmonization of dynamic balance (see Alam et al. 2019). The training of the Musculus tibialis posterior can be realized, for example, by walking on tiptoes.

In this context, Utsahachant et al. (2023) recognized that specific training of the short foot muscles in combination with global training of the lower extremity has a positive effect on the medial longitudinal arch during the stance phase of walking.

Useful visualizations can be taken from Fig. 5.117, 5.118, 5.119, 5.120, 5.121 and 5.122.

Summary for Practice

Active evidence-based training therapy is significantly superior to passive care alone, such as the use of shoe inserts to correct a flatfoot.

The focus is on the progressive strengthening of the short foot muscles as well as the hip abductors and hip extensors. As a supplement, a swelling current can be applied to the M. abductor hallucis during training.

Fig. 5.116 provides an overview of the mentioned information.

5.4 Lumbar Spine Area

5.4.1 Lumbar Radiculopathy/Lumbar Disc Herniation/Discectomy

Both conservative and postoperative therapy for symptomatic lumbar disc herniations recommend medical training programs aimed at stabilizing the lumbar spine (see Pourahmadi et al. 2022). This statement is confirmed by Choo and Chang (2023), who also mention that in addition to stabilization exercises, strengthening exercises for the trunk muscles can make a significant contribution to reducing pain intensity and

Categories	Evidence-based training recommendation
Units	6 weeks, 3-7 training sessions per week, 30 minutes per session
Exercises	Active extension of the toes 2-5, extension of the hallux, spreading the toes, building up the arch of the foot by bringing the ball of the big and smal toes and the heel closer together (increase the exercise progressively, first sitting then standing then standing on one leg and extending the holding time) / Train hip abductors and hip extensors in lateral position and abdomen by spreading the leg (progression is the extension of the holding time from 0-10 seconds) / Pause time between exercises no longer than one minute / In addition, swelling current can be applied to the abductor hallucis muscle during the exercises. In addition, the toe flexors can be exercised by wrapping a towel around them and the posterior tibialis muscle by walking on tiptoe
Exercise parameters	2 sets of 10-15 repetitions
Elongation	Stretching exercises of the iliopsoas muscle are recommended

Fig. 5.116 Summary of MTT for Flatfoot

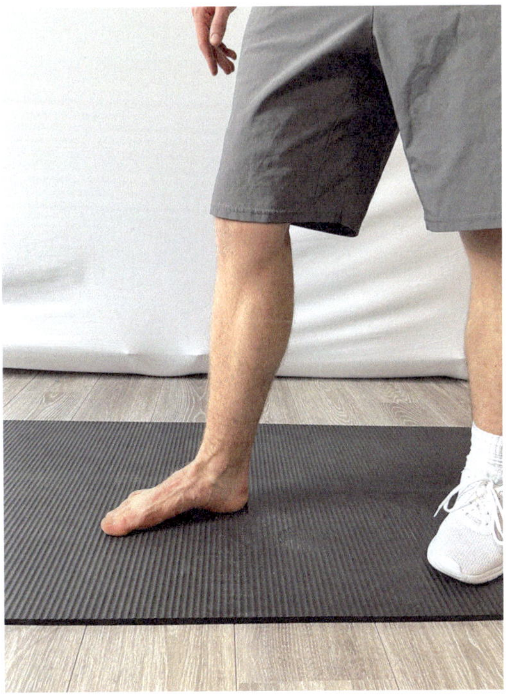

Fig. 5.117 MTT for Flatfoot—Arch Construction (Sitting, Standing, Single Leg Stand)

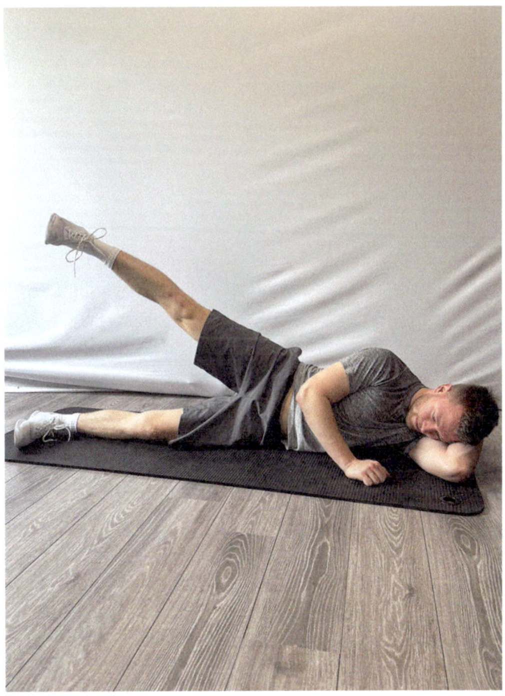

Fig. 5.118 MTT for Flatfoot—Strengthening of the Hip Abductors in Lateral Position

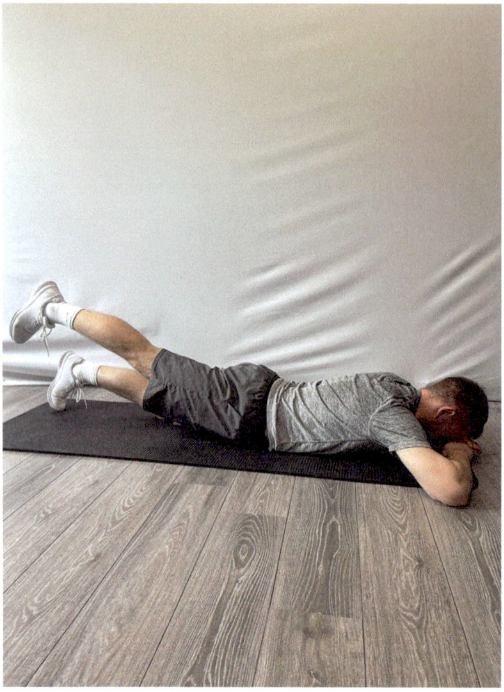

Fig. 5.119 MTT for Flatfoot—Strengthening of the Hip Extensors in Prone Position

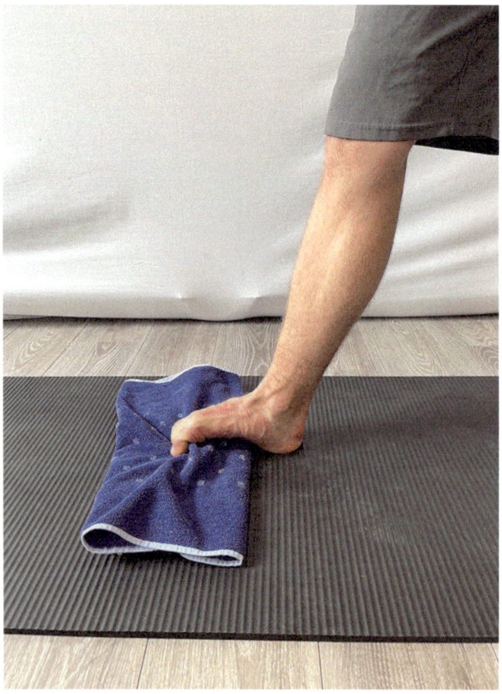

Fig. 5.120 MTT for Flatfoot—Toe Flexion by Grabbing a Towel

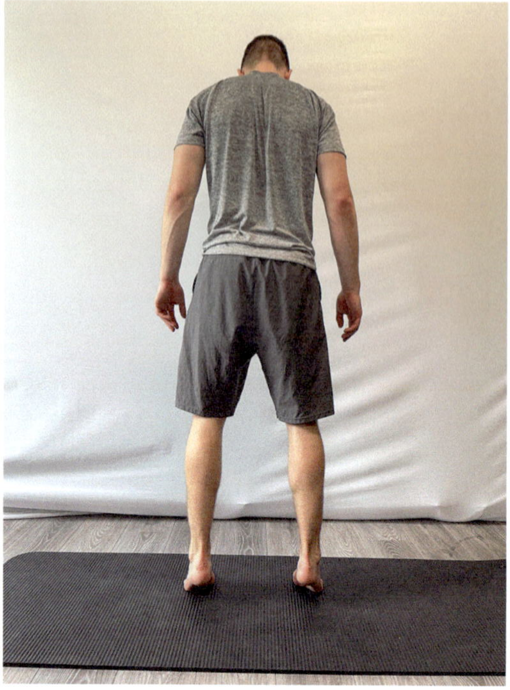

Fig. 5.121 MTT for Flatfoot—Strengthening of the M. tibialis posterior through Toe Walking

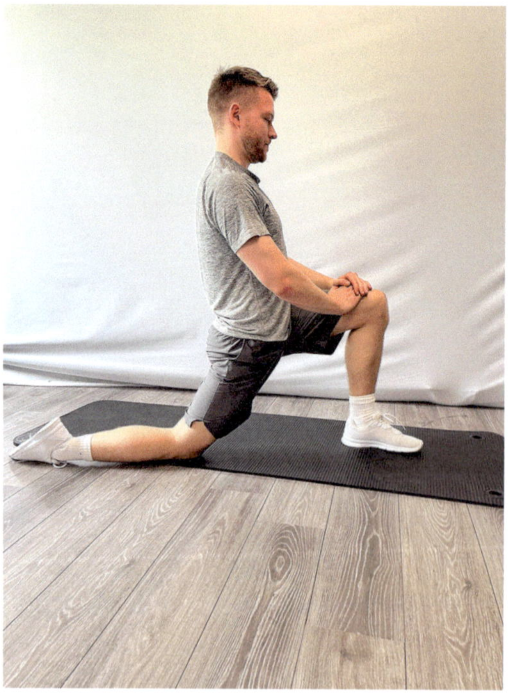

Fig. 5.122 MTT for Flatfoot—Stretching M. iliopsoas

reducing functional disability. Whether a stabilization program is carried out on land or in water seems to make no difference. Both approaches are effective (see Bayraktar et al. 2016). In the aftercare of discectomy patients, both local stabilization exercises of the multifidus muscles and the transversus abdominis muscle as well as general strengthening exercises of the trunk can be used (see Hebert et al. 2015).

In a randomized controlled study, which included 80 people with chronic lumbar back pain with lumbar radiculopathy, a lumbar stabilization program in the open or closed chain was compared to a lumbar stabilization program with mobilizing contents of the thoracic spine in the closed system. Both groups carried out the training program assigned to them over a period of eight weeks. In terms of reducing pain intensity or reducing the degree of functional disability, the lumbar stabilization program with mobilizing contents of the thoracic spine in the closed system was significantly superior. This exercise program included a weight shift in standing at the ladder bar towards the posterior with simultaneous flexion movement of the thoracic spine and return, a flexion movement of the thoracic spine in the lunge with return and simultaneous continuous gripping of the ladder bar, an alternating flexion and extension mobilization of the thoracic spine in the quadruped position, as well as an alternating extension and flexion mobilization of the thoracic spine in the wall sit at approx. 45° hip flexion (cf. Kostadinović et al. 2020).

Renovato França et al. (2019) recognized that the implementation of a motor control training is beneficial for people with a lumbar disc herniation and accompanying radiculopathy. The training program used focused on the activation of the transversus abdominis muscle and the multifidus muscles. In standing, a co-contraction was initiated under palpation of the mentioned muscles. In addition, the transversus abdominis muscle was specifically targeted in the supine position as well as in the quadruped position. In the prone position, a contraction of the multifidus muscles was facilitated by palpation impulses (cf. Bauer and Wolfram 2022). In addition, using a pressure biofeedback device in the prone position, the activation of the transversus abdominis muscle was made visible by a decrease in pressure. Over a period of eight weeks, two training sessions were conducted weekly. In addition to reduced pain intensity, this approach led to a reduction in functional disability and an increased activation of the transversus abdominis muscle (cf. Renovato França et al. 2019). These results confirm earlier research findings by Ramos et al. (2018). This information matches the data from Ramos et al. (2016) who found that people with a lumbar disc herniation have a weakness of the lumbar multifidus muscles and a reduced recruitment ability of the transversus abdominis muscle (cf. Ramos et al. 2016). A targeted stabilization of lumbar disc herniations with radiculopathy using medical training therapy also corresponds to the findings of the systematic review by Hahne et al. (2010).

Recently, the effectiveness of a Pilates program was demonstrated in a population with symptomatic disc herniations. The implementation of this program was carried out three times a week over a period of six weeks. Each training session lasted 45–60 minutes. The training program included auto-mobilizations of the extremities and the trunk as well as strengthening exercises for the trunk muscles and the muscles close to the trunk. Through implementation, the population benefited from a reduction in pain intensity, a reduction in the degree of disability, improved static and dynamic endurance, and in some cases improved quality of life (cf. Taşpınar et al. 2023).

In people with postoperative lumbar discectomy, the implementation of an extension-based or flexion-based training program is possible from the sixth postoperative week. While both approaches are capable of relieving pain intensity, the extension-based training program can significantly better train the extent of functional disability and endurance ability of the trunk muscles (cf. Abdi et al. 2023; Choi et al. 2005).

The Oswestry Disability Index can be used as an assessment, among other things (cf. Kostadinović et al. 2020). In addition, the modified Biering-Sorensen test and the trunk flexion endurance test can be used (cf. Abdi et al. 2023). More detailed information on the individual assessments can be taken from the assessment list in the appendix of this book.

Useful visualizations can be taken from Fig. 5.124, 5.125, 5.126, 5.127 and 5.128.

Summary for Practice

Medical training therapy can lead to pain relief and functional improvement in both conservatively and postoperatively treated findings. The focus is on stabilization, strengthening, and mobilization exercises. The muscles that should be given the most attention are the M. transversus abdominis and the Mm. multifidii. With the help of the described training units and a pressure biofeedback device, the training can be optimally designed.

A 45–60 minute Pilates program, performed three times a week, can also improve pain intensity as well as static and dynamic endurance.

For postoperative lumbar discectomies, extension and flexion-based implementations should only be carried out from the sixth postoperative week onwards.

Fig. 5.123 provides an overview of the information mentioned.

5.4.2 Low back Pain

A meta-analysis from 2022 addressed the question of which medical training programs are best suited for pain relief or improvement of disability in people with chronic lower back pain. A total of 118 randomized controlled studies with a total population of 9710 people aged 18–65

Categories	Evidence-based training recommendation
Units	8 weeks, 2-3 training sessions per week á 45-60 minutes per session
Exercises	Stabilization exercises and strengthening exercises for the core muscles with a focus on the transversus abdominis and multifidius muscles / mobilization exercises for the lumbar spine and thoracic spine multifidii / mobilization exercises of the lumbar spine and thoracic spine / weight shift in a standing position on the wall bars to the posterior with simultaneous flexion movement of the thoracic spine and return / flexion movement of the thoracic spine in a lunge with return and simultaneous continuous gripping of the wall bars / alternating flexion and extension mobilization of the thoracic spine in a four-footed position / alternating extension and flexion mobilization of the thoracic spine in a seated position on the wall with approx. 45° hip flexion / cocontraction of the transversu abdominis muscle and the multifidii muscles while standing, lying on the back, standing on four feet and lying on the back with pressure biofeedback device (mechanical blood pressure monitor) / Pilates programme with mobilization of the extremities and trunk and strengthening of the trunk and trunk-related muscles

Fig. 5.123 Summary of MTT in lumbar radiculopathy/lumbar disc herniation/discectomy

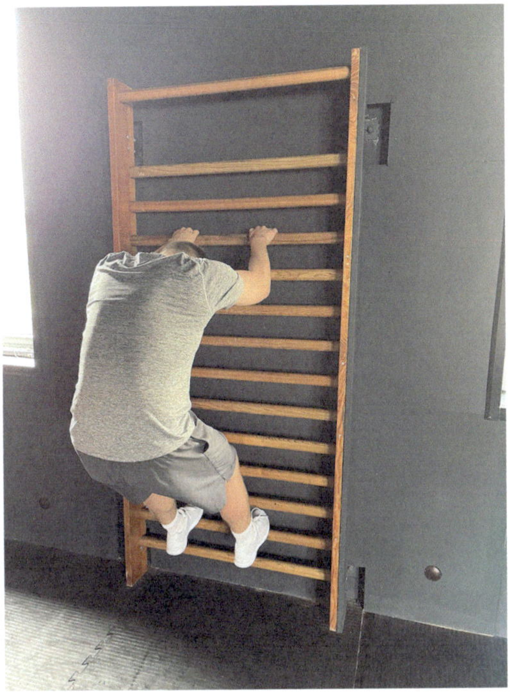

Fig. 5.124 MTT in lumbar radiculopathy/lumbar disc herniation/discectomy—Weight shifting in standing at the ladder bar posteriorly with simultaneous flexion movement of the thoracic spine and return

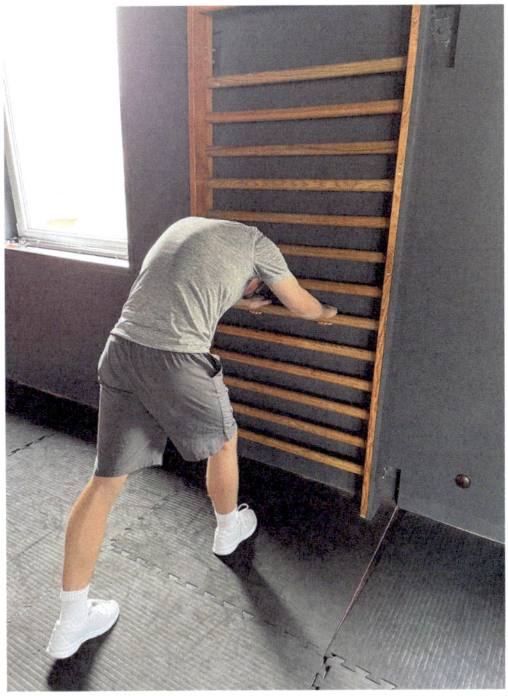

Fig. 5.125 MTT in lumbar radiculopathy/lumbar disc herniation/discectomy—Flexion movement of the thoracic spine in lunge with return and simultaneous continuous gripping of the ladder bar

years were included. It was found that almost any form of physical activity is capable of positively affecting the aforementioned outcomes. The research group recommends at least one to two training sessions per week. First significant improvements are to be expected within a period of three to nine weeks. Evidence-based training approaches include Pilates, core stability training, mind-body programs, and strength training (see Fernández-Rodríguez et al. 2022). Owen et al. (2020) supplement the use of stabilization programs, which aim to improve motor control. In addition, there is evidence of the effectiveness of aerobic training (see Owen et al. 2020).

Home training programs are a viable way to combat nonspecific lower back pain. To achieve optimal pain relief, guidance under therapeutic supervision is suggested (see Quentin et al. 2021). Hayden et al. (2021) point out that individual preferences of the person to be treated in terms of the choice of training form can enhance therapy success.

In a randomized controlled study, the effectiveness of a stabilization program was demonstrated in people with subacute chronic lower back pain. During an intervention period of one month, training was conducted three times a week for 30 minutes each. The stabilization program aimed at specific training of the transversus abdominis muscle and the lumbar multifidus muscles. Among other things, a pressure biofeedback device was used. This was placed in the prone position with a pressure of 70 mmHg under the abdomen of the trainees. Through targeted recruitment of the transversus abdominis muscle, the pressure was supposed to reduce in a range between 6–10 mmHg. By lifting the contralateral arm while simultaneously tensing the transversus abdominis muscle, the activity of the lumbar multifidus muscles was facilitated. An additional palpation stimulus in

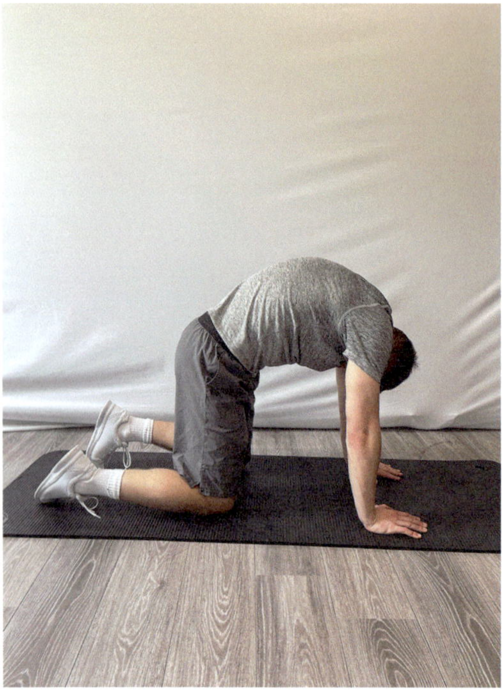

Fig. 5.126 MTT in lumbar radiculopathy/lumbar disc herniation/discectomy—Alternating flexion and extension mobilization of the thoracic spine in quadruped position

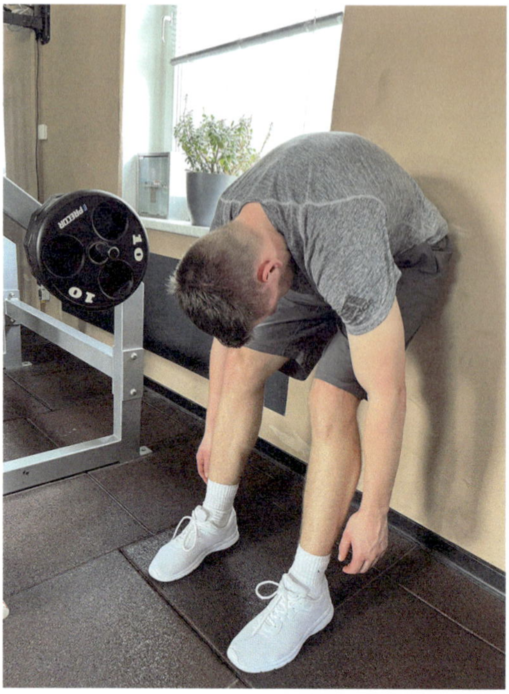

Fig. 5.127 MTT in lumbar radiculopathy/lumbar disc herniation/discectomy—Alternating extension and flexion mobilization of the thoracic spine in wall sit at approx. 45° hip flexion

the paravertebral area was supportive. During the course of the study, a co-contraction of the mentioned muscles was practiced in different starting positions. As soon as this was possible, movements of the extremities were practiced with maintained recruitment of the stabilizing musculature. After statistical evaluation of the collected data, it could be shown that this form of medical training therapy is capable of significantly improving balance, the cross-section of the transversus abdominis muscle and the lumbar multifidus muscles, pain intensity, functional disability, and the extent of kinesiophobia (see Hlaing et al. 2021).

Narouei et al. (2020) added general strengthening exercises of the hip surrounding musculature to a specific strengthening of the transversus abdominis muscle and the lumbar multifidus muscles. These included, among other things, strengthening exercises of the straight and oblique abdominal muscles via sit-ups as well as general strengthening exercises of the spine and hip extensors. Furthermore, bridging exercises as well as the side support and exercises in the quadruped position were used. As a result, the degree of disability in people with nonspecific chronic lower back pain could be reduced after a training period of four weeks (see Narouei et al. 2020). In addition to strengthening exercises, stretching exercises of the hip surrounding musculature can also make a positive contribution to quality of life, pain relief, balance, and degree of disability (see Kim and Yim et al. 2020).

Gibbs et al. (2022) compared strength training with one's own body weight to training with external weights in people with chronic lower back pain. Both groups also received the same professional education. It was calculated that both interventions are equally capable of evoking significant improvements in terms of pain, degree of disability, anxiety, and self-efficacy.

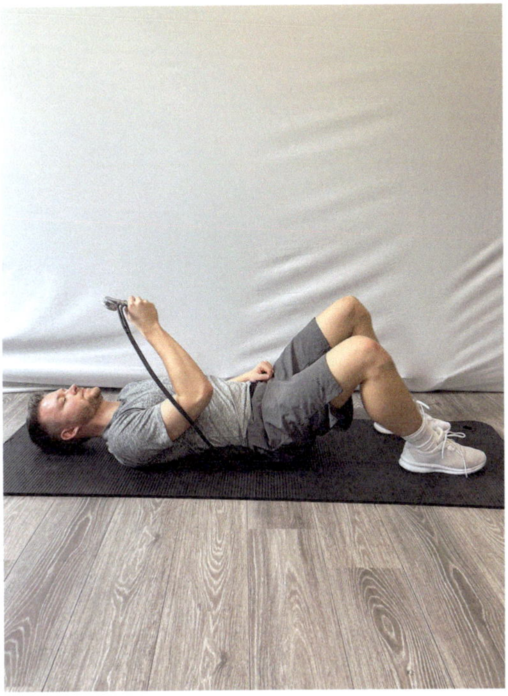

Fig. 5.128 MTT in lumbar radiculopathy/lumbar disc herniation/discectomy—Co-contraction of the M. transversus abdominis and the Mm. multifidii in standing, in supine position, in quadruped position and in supine position with pressure biofeedback device

The relevance of therapeutic transparency becomes clear (see Gibbs et al. 2022).

Assessments include the visual analog scale or the numerical analog scale, the roland-morris-disability-questionnaire, and the oswestry-disability-index (see Nava-Bringas et al. 2021). More detailed information on the individual assessments can be taken from the assessment list in the appendix of this book.

Useful visualizations can be taken from Fig. 5.130, 5.131, 5.132, 5.133, 5.134 and 5.135.

Summary for Practice

Evidence-based medical training therapy provides a good opportunity to improve pain and the degree of disability in chronic lower back pain. The focus here is on physical activity in the form of strength training, stabilization training, mind-body programs, Pilates, stretching, and perception through a pressure biofeedback device or direct palpation. The training focuses on the M. transversus abdominis and the Mm. multifidii. Furthermore, emphasis should be placed on strengthening the muscles surrounding the hip as well as the straight and oblique abdominal muscles and spinal extensors.

Fig. 5.129 provides an overview of the information mentioned.

5.4.3 Spondylolisthesis/Lumbar Spondylosis

In the case of predominant degenerative spondylolisthesis, the performance of trunk flexion strengthening exercises is recommended from a training therapy perspective (see Kalichman and Hunter 2008).

Nava-Bringas et al. (2021) pursued the scientific question of whether a trunk-stabilizing exercise program in people with degenerative spondylolisthesis is more efficient than a therapeutic approach consisting of flexion exercises. The stabilizing exercise program began with a 15-minute lumbosacral warm-up through the application of a heat pad. This was followed by stretching exercises of the thoracolumbar fascia, the hip flexors, and the ischiocrural muscles. The next step was to work on a neutral spinal position and the targeted recruitment ability of the transversus abdominis muscle, the internal oblique muscle of the abdomen, the multifidus muscles, the respiratory diaphragm, and the pelvic floor muscles. Progression during the study was achieved through anterior and lateral bridging components and exercises in the quadruped position. The flexion program included components of the williams-back-exercises and was carried out with the identical warm-up part (cf. Dydyk and Sapra 2023). This is a conglomerate of exercises that induce a flexion or delordosis of the lumbar spine. These include, for example, sit-up variations and knee-to-chest variations.

Categories	Evidence-based training recommendation
Units	3 - 9 weeks, 1-3 times a week, at least 30 minutes per session
Exercises	Pilates / mind-body programs / prone position pressure biofeedback device under abdomen to 70mmHg - tension of the transversus abdominis muscle to reduce by 6-10mmHg / same exercise with additional lifting of the contralateral arm, this can be supported by a paravertebral palpation stimulus of the multifidii muscles / same exercise with additional movement of the extremities in different starting positions / sit-ups, bridging exercises, side support, exercises in the four-footed position
Elongation	Stretching the muscles surrounding the hips

Fig. 5.129 Summary of MTT in Low-back-pain

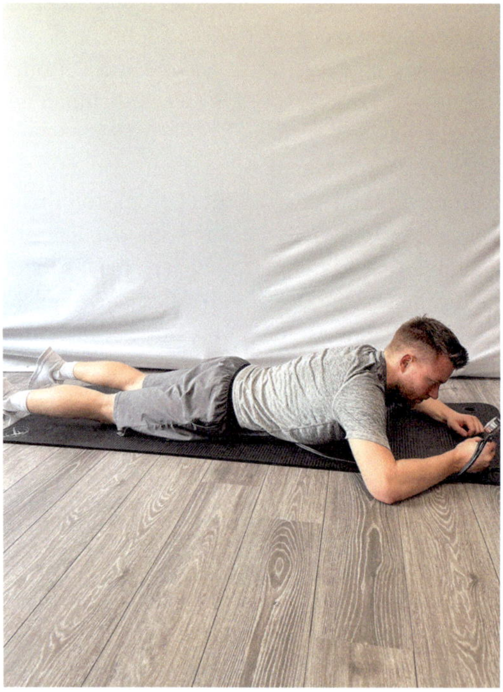

Fig. 5.130 MTT in Low-back-pain—Pressure biofeedback device under stomach at 70 mmHg—Tension of the M. transversus abdominis to achieve a reduction of 6–10 mmHg

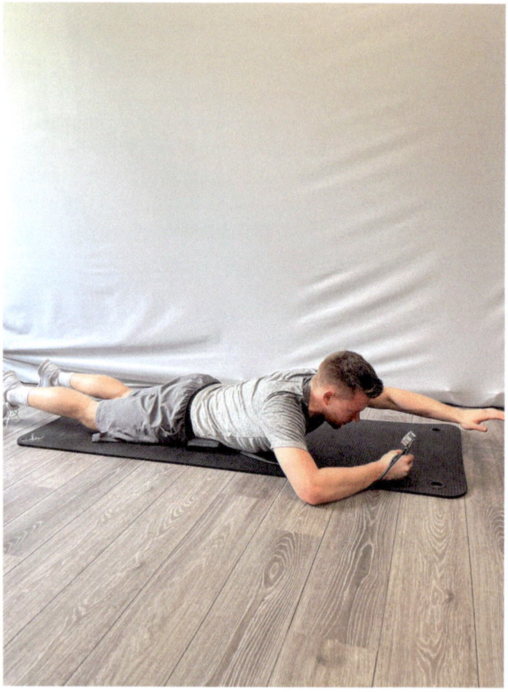

Fig. 5.131 MTT in Low-back-pain—Pressure biofeedback device under stomach at 70 mmHg—Tension of the M. transversus abdominis to achieve a reduction of 6–10 mmHg with additional lifting of the contralateral arm

The intervention period was six months, during which the groups trained daily. Six supervised training sessions were held each month. After evaluating the collected data, it can be concluded that both therapy interventions have a positive effect on pain and disability in people

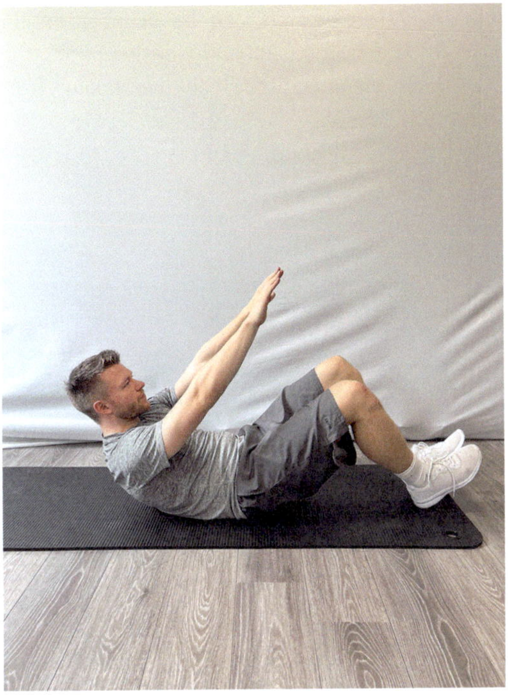

Fig. 5.132 MTT in Low-back-pain—Sit-ups

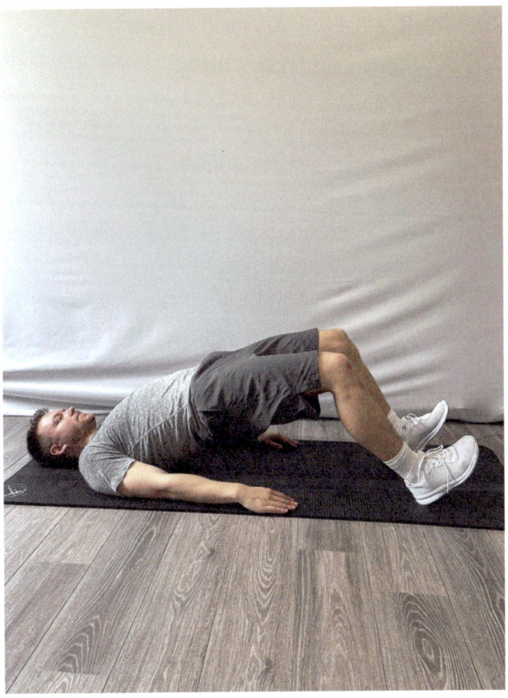

Fig. 5.133 MTT in Low-back-pain—Bridging

with degenerative spondylolisthesis. There is no significant difference between the interventions (cf. Nava-Bringas et al. 2021).

These results confirm the research work of O'Sullivan et al. (1997). This research group already demonstrated the effectiveness of a specific lumbar stability program in people with spondylosis or spondylolisthesis in 1997. The focus of the training program was on learning the targeted recruitment of the transversus abdominis muscle and the lumbar multifidus muscles. Subsequently, the co-contraction of the mentioned muscles was integrated into activities and movement sequences. After a ten-week intervention period, a significant reduction in pain intensity and an improved disability level were observed. These results were also maintained in a follow-up period after 30 months (cf. O'Sullivan et al. 1997).

Another randomized controlled study compared the effectiveness between a global and segmental stabilization program in a sample of 26 individuals with grade I spondylolisthesis. The segmental stabilization program focused on learning targeted recruitment of the transversus abdominis muscle and the lumbar multifidus muscles. This was followed by a progressive implementation in various starting positions and exercises. The exercises of global stabilization included the single-knee-to-chest and the double-knee-to-chest exercise execution. Furthermore, stretches of the iliopsoas muscle, the ischiocrural muscles, and the piriformis muscle were performed. The heel-slide exercise in supine position was completed by bridging, straight and oblique sit-ups, and "bicycling" of both legs in supine position. Both approaches were able to reduce pain intensity and decrease the level of disability. In terms of intervertebral mobility and the extent of kinesiophobia, the segmental stabilization group produced better results (cf. Mohammadimajd et al. 2020).

In addition to the visual analog scale or the numerical analog scale, the roland-morris-disability-questionnaire and the oswestry-disability-index serve as assessments (cf. Nava-Bringas et al. 2021). More detailed information on the

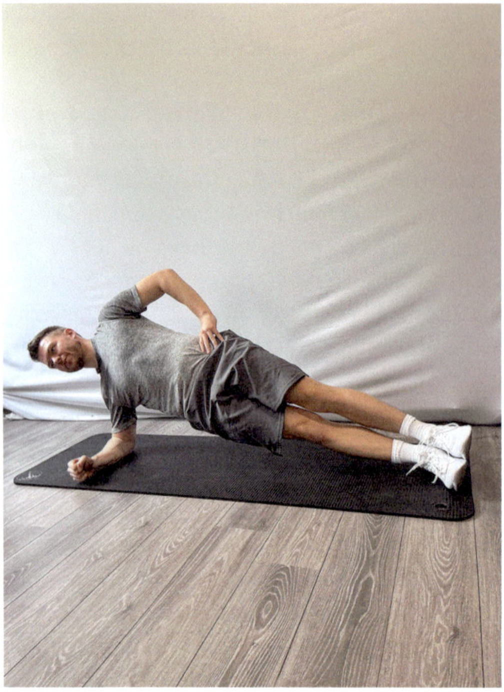

Fig. 5.134 MTT in Low-back-pain—Side support

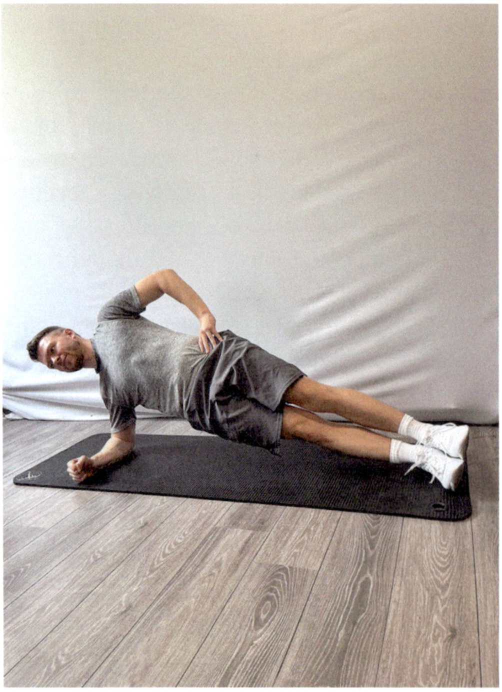

Fig. 5.135 MTT in Low-back-pain—Exercises in quadruped position

individual assessments can be taken from the assessment list in the appendix of this book.

Useful visualizations can be taken from Fig. 5.137, 5.138, 5.139, 5.140, 5.141, 5.142, 5.143, 5.144, 5.145 and 5.146.

Summary for Practice

The targeted evidence-based medical exercise therapy provides the opportunity to reduce pain in spondylolisthesis and lumbar spondylosis, lower the degree of disability, and improve intervertebral mobility. The training consists of a specific sequence of various exercises and targets the thoracolumbar fascia, the hip flexors, the ischiocrural muscles, as well as the transversus abdominis muscle, the internal oblique muscle of the abdomen, the multifidus muscles, the respiratory diaphragm, and the pelvic muscles.

Fig. 5.136 provides an overview of the mentioned information.

5.4.4 Lumbar Instability

Puntumetakul et al. (2021) investigated whether, in the presence of instability, training of the superficial trunk muscles or the deep stabilizing muscles is recommended. Both interventions were compared over a period of ten weeks. The results of the treated study recommend specific training of the deep stabilizing muscles. The following will explain this approach in more detail. The abdominal-drawing-in-maneuver-technique was used to learn the recruitment of the transversus abdominis muscle. In addition, a pressure biofeedback device was used. This was placed with a pressure of 70 mmHg in the prone position at the level of the lower abdomen on a line between the anterior superior iliac spines. The command "pull the navel in and up without moving the lumbar spine or pelvis" was intended to reduce the pressure between 4–10 mmHg. At the same time, the recruitment or co-activation of the lumbar multifidus muscles was

Categories	Evidence-based training recommendation
Units	6 months with daily training, recommendation between 45 and 60 minutes per session
Stabilizing exercise program	Step 1: 15 minutes of warming the lumbosacral area with a heating pad Step 2: Stretching the thoracolumbar fascia, the hip flexors and the ischiocrural muscles Step 3: Targeted recruitment of the transversus abdominis muscle, the. M. obliquus internus abdominis, the Mm. multifidii. of the respiratory diaphragm, the pelvic floor muscles in a neutral spinal position Step 4: Progression in the course of training through bridging components and exercises in the quadruped position
Inflection program	Step 1: 15 minutes of warming the lumbosacral area with a heating pad Step 2: Stretching the thoracolumbar fascia, the hip flexors and the ischiocrural muscles Step 3: targeted recruitment of the transversus abdominis muscle, the. M. obliquus internus abdominis, the Mm. multifidii. of the respiratory diaphragm, the pelvic floor muscles in a neutral spinal position Step 4: Sit-up variations, knee-to-chest variations, William-back exercises Step 5: Progression through the implementation of movements, Bridging, heel-slide exercises, cycling in supine position
Elongation	Stretching of the muscles mentioned (hip flexors, ischiocrural muscles, piriformis muscle, thoracolumbar fascia)

Fig. 5.136 Summary of MTT in Spondylolisthesis/Lumbar Spondylosis

trained. During the course of the study, movements of the extremities or activities were carried out with existing recruitment of the deep stabilizing muscles. Over a period of ten weeks, training was carried out twice a week for 20 minutes each time. By practicing this training, a significant decrease in pain intensity, improved recruitment ability of the transversus abdominis muscle, and reduced sagittal translation in the L4–L5 and L5–S1 segments were observed in people with lumbar instability after ten weeks (see Puntumetakul et al. 2021). These findings are consistent with previous research results (see Javadian et al. 2012).

In another research work, it was investigated whether a training program for lumbar instability benefits from a combination with a respiratory resistance device or the implementation on a whole-body vibration device. Training was carried out three times a week over an intervention period of five weeks. Squats, forearm support, sit-ups, lunges, bridging, and bridging with knee extension were used. The coupling of these exercises with a respiratory resistance device and/or the execution on a whole-body vibration device can contribute to optimizing functionality or the degree of disability (see Park et al. 2022).

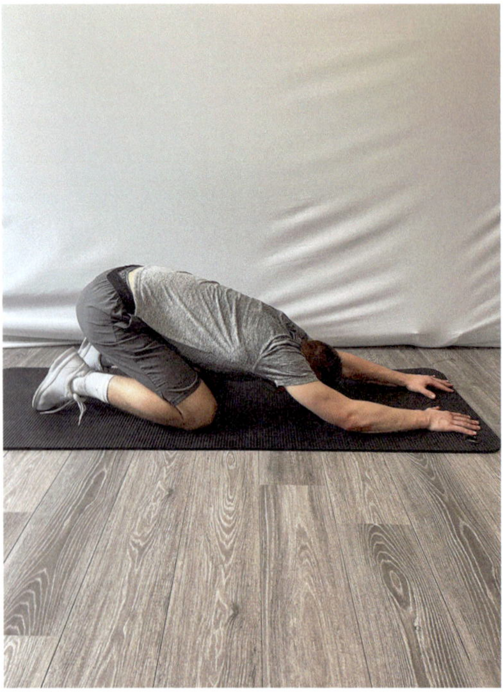

Fig. 5.137 MTT in Spondylolisthesis/Lumbar Spondylosis—Stretching of the Thoracolumbar Fascia

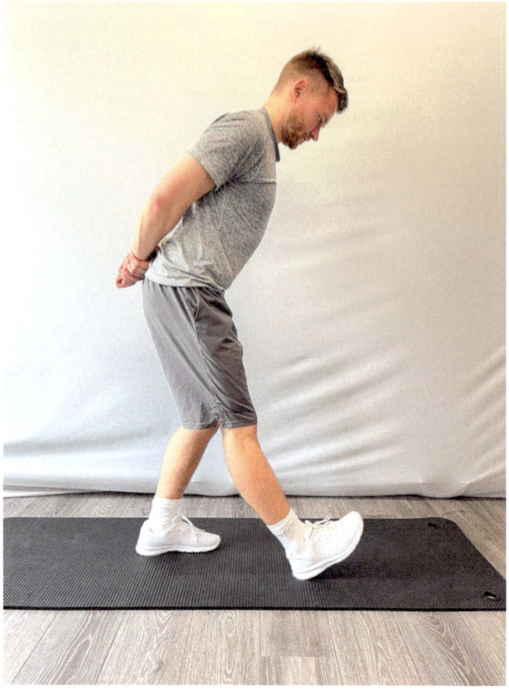

Fig. 5.139 MTT in Spondylolisthesis/Lumbar Spondylosis—Stretching of the Hamstrings

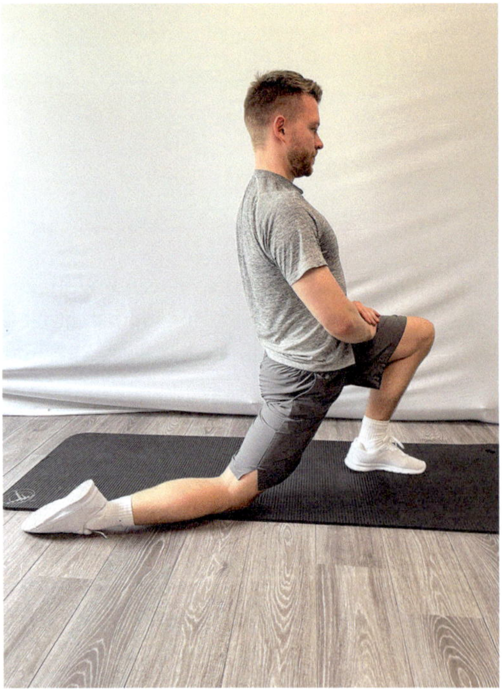

Fig. 5.138 MTT in Spondylolisthesis/Lumbar Spondylosis—Stretching of the Hip Flexors

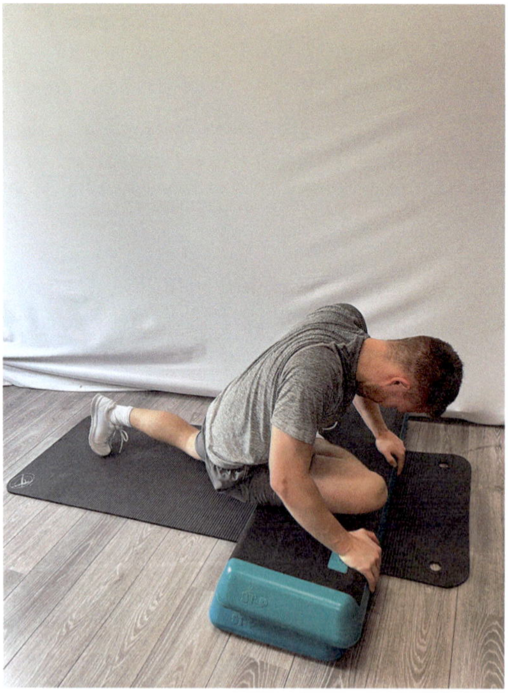

Fig. 5.140 MTT in Spondylolisthesis/Lumbar Spondylosis—Stretching of the Piriformis Muscle

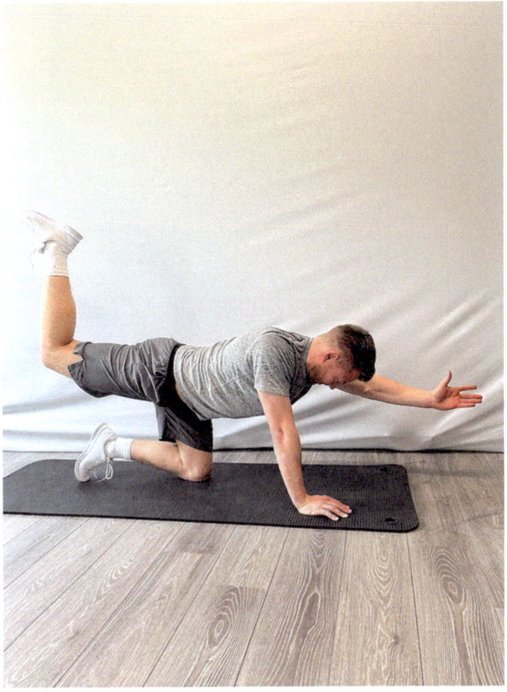

Fig. 5.141 MTT in Spondylolisthesis/Lumbar Spondylosis—Exercises in Quadruped Position

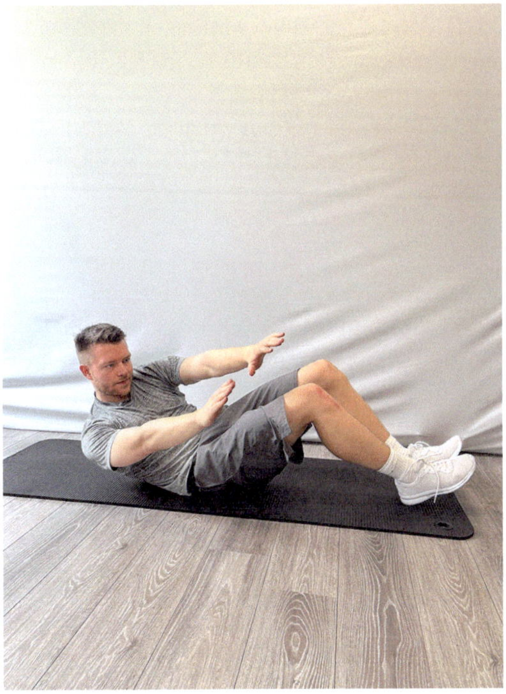

Fig. 5.142 MTT in Spondylolisthesis/Lumbar Spondylosis—Sit-up Variations

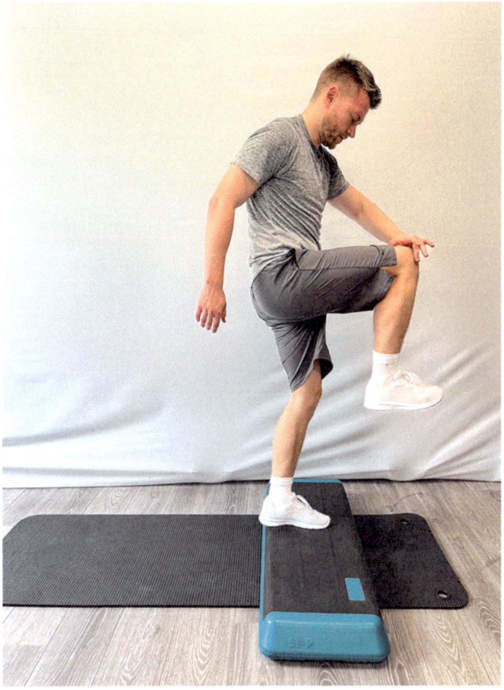

Fig. 5.143 MTT in Spondylolisthesis/Lumbar Spondylosis—Knee-to-chest Variations (single/double)

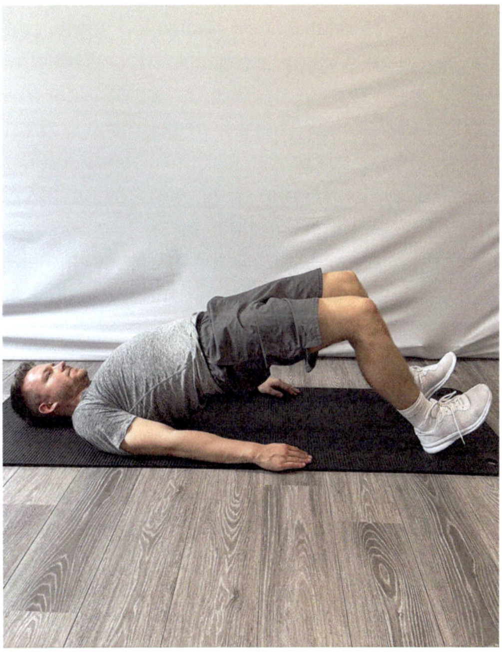

Fig. 5.144 MTT in Spondylolisthesis/Lumbar Spondylosis —Bridging

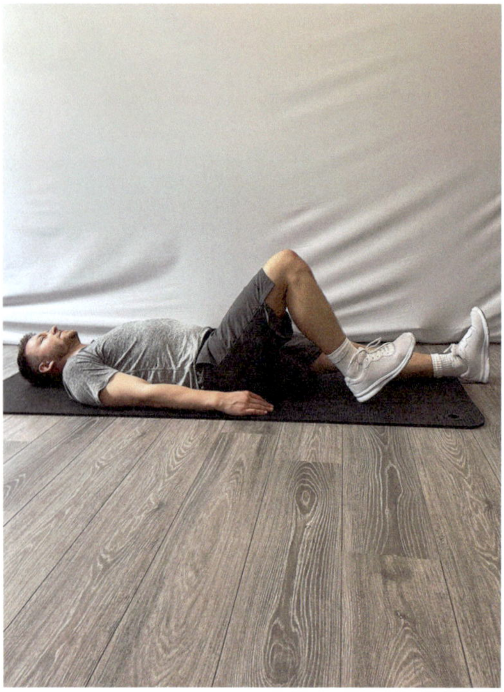

Fig. 5.145 MTT in Spondylolisthesis/Lumbar Spondylosis—Heel Slide Exercises

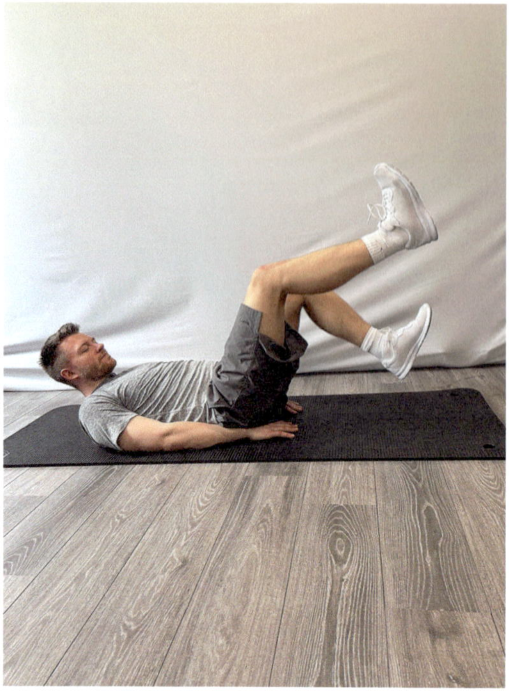

Fig. 5.146 MTT in Spondylolisthesis/Lumbar Spondylosis—Cycling in Supine Position

In another randomized controlled study, progressively increasing exercises in combination with a respiratory resistance device also contributed to therapeutic success in people with lumbar instability over a four-week study period. The exercise program was carried out three times a week for 40 minutes each. The exercises included sit-ups, dead-bugs, Superman, and side support with knee flexion (see Park and Lee 2019).

Exercise execution with elastic bands in the sling table is also conceivable (see Kim et al. 2018).

Assessments can include the Roland-Morris-low-back-pain-and-disability-questionnaire and the Korean-version-of-fear-avoidance-beliefs-questionnaire (see Park et al. 2022). In addition, the Oswestry-Disability-Index can be used (see Kim et al. 2018).

Furthermore, the Lumbar-spine-instability-questionnaire can be used (see Macedo et al. 2021). More detailed information on the individual assessments can be taken from the assessment list in the appendix of this book.

Useful visualizations can be taken from Fig. 5.148, 5.149, 5.150, 5.151, 5.152, 5.153, 5.154 and 5.155.

Summary for Practice

A targeted and evidence-based medical training therapy can relieve pain in patients with lumbar instability and reduce sagittal translation in the L4–L5 and L5–S1 segments. The focus is on learning the conscious recruitment of the M. transversus abdominis and the Mm. multifidii. This is best achieved with a pressure biofeedback device or a blood pressure cuff.

Fig. 5.147 provides an overview of the information mentioned.

Categories	Evidence-based training recommendation
Units	10 weeks, 2-3 sessions per week á 20-40 minutes per session
Exercises	Abdominal-drawing-in-maneuver-technique / pressure biofeedback device in prone position at the height of the line between the right and left SIAS, pressure at 70mmHg, instruction "draw the navel inwards and upwards without moving the lumbar spine or pelvis". The pressure should be reduced to between 4-10mmHg / support can be provided by palpatory stimuli / progression via movements of the extremities while maintaining tension / combination of squats, forearm support, sit-ups, lunges, bridging variations, dead bugs, superman, side support with breathing resistance device or a whole-body vibration device

Fig. 5.147 Summary of MTT in lumbar instability

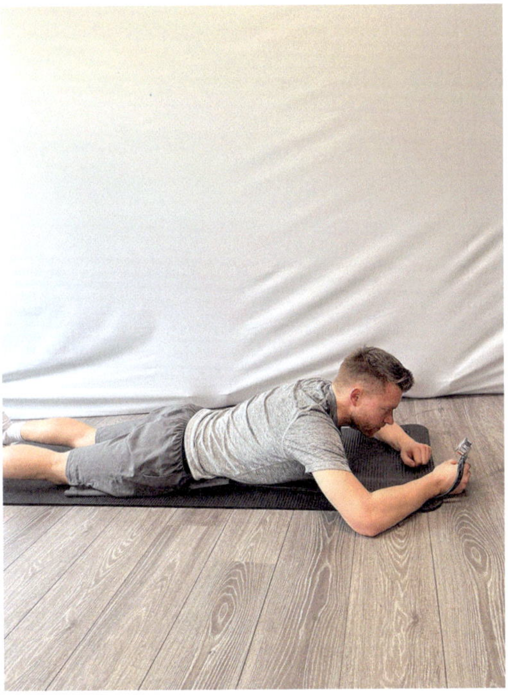

Fig. 5.148 MTT in lumbar instability—Pressure biofeedback device in prone position at the level of the line between the right and left SIAS, pressure at 70 mmHg, instruction "pull navel inward upward without moving the lumbar spine or the pelvis", the pressure should be reduced between 4–10 mmHg

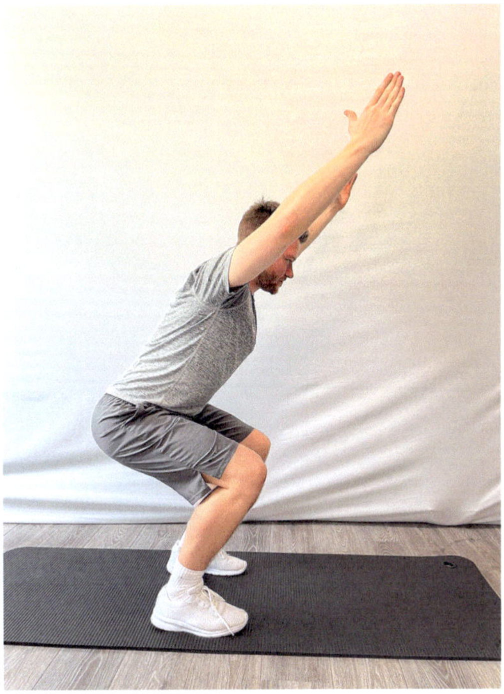

Fig. 5.149 MTT in lumbar instability—Squats

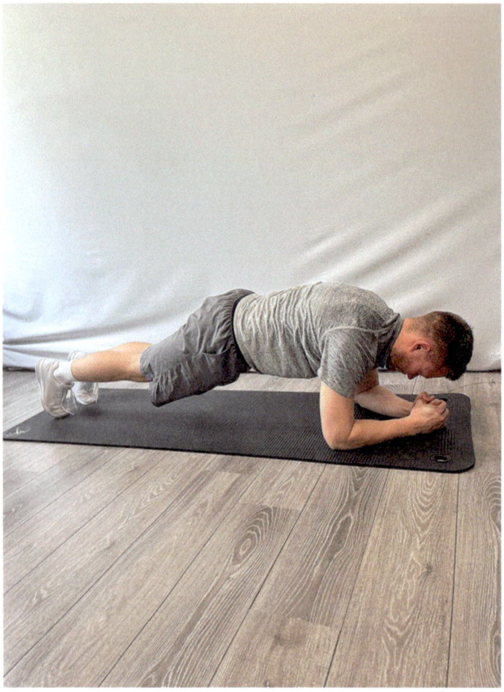

Fig. 5.150 MTT in lumbar instability—Forearm support

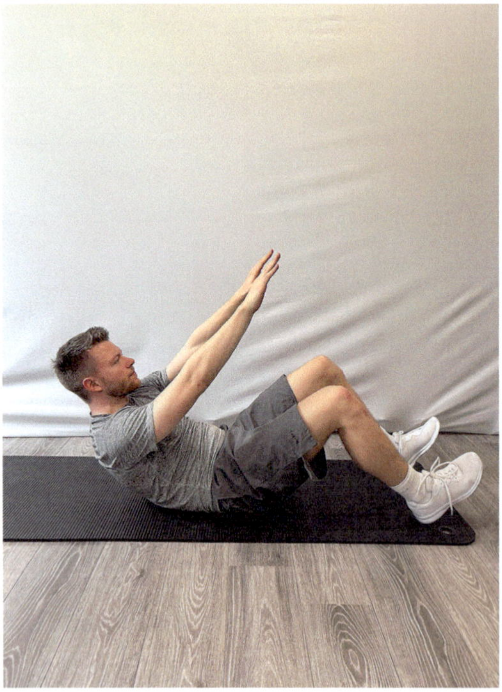

Fig. 5.151 MTT in lumbar instability—Sit-ups

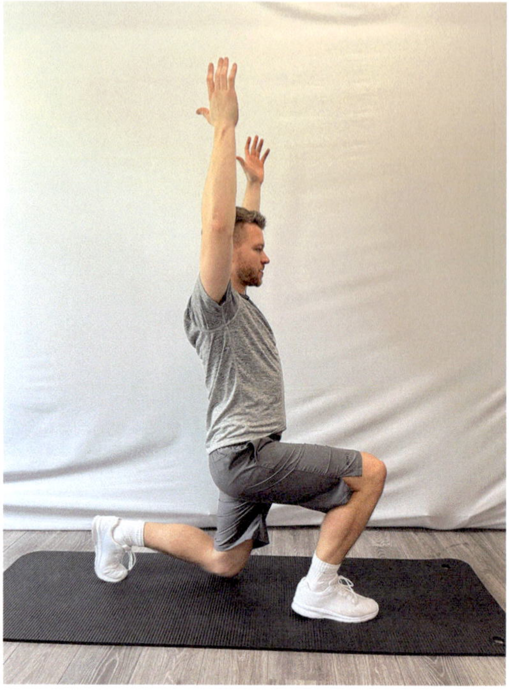

Fig. 5.152 MTT in lumbar instability—Lunges

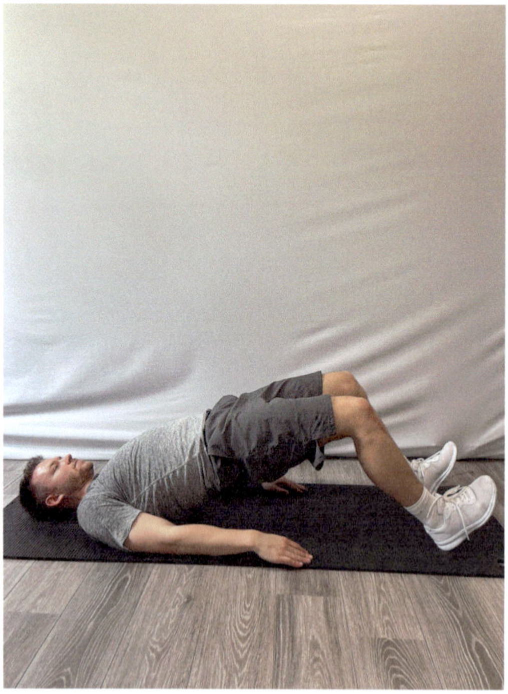

Fig. 5.153 MTT in lumbar instability—Bridging

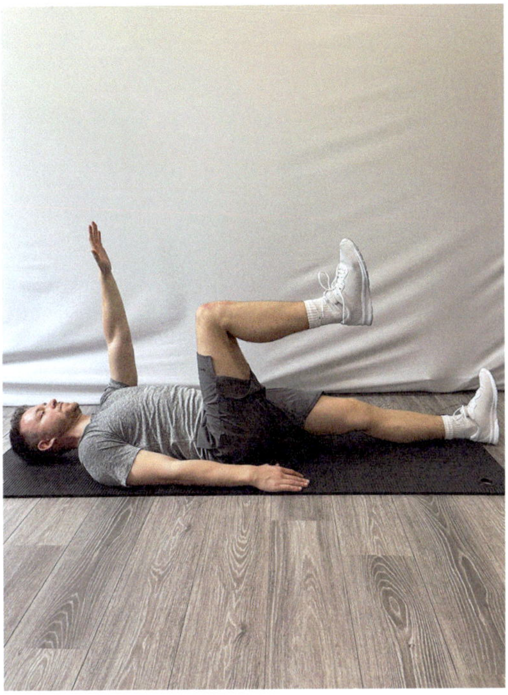

Fig. 5.154 MTT in lumbar instability—Dead-bugs

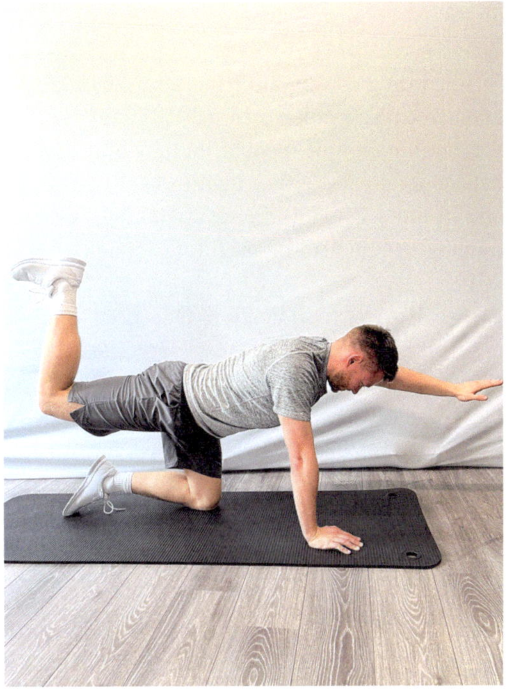

Fig. 5.155 MTT in lumbar instability—Superman

5.4.5 Spinal Stenosis

In a systematic review, Ammendolia et al. (2022) attribute moderate evidence of applicability to medical training therapy in spinal stenosis with accompanying neurogenic claudication.

A meta-analysis comparing surgical decompression by laminectomy with the conservative approach of medical training therapy concludes that both therapy options produce simultaneous results. At the same time, the small sample sizes and low study quality of the three included articles are discussed (see Mo et al. 2018).

The meta-analysis by Comer et al. (2023) summarizes the already researched training approaches for spinal stenosis. In most studies, flexion-based exercises are practiced under supervision. Successful measures also include stretching and core strength training, as well as cycling. The heterogeneity of the data situation currently does not allow a conclusion on an optimal evidence-based medical training program (cf. Comer et al. 2023).

Low to moderate evidence suggests that the combination of manual therapy and supervised exercise therapy is capable of improving walking ability and pain intensity in people with degenerative lumbar spinal stenosis in the short term (cf. Jacobi et al. 2021).

In addition to relieving pain intensity, medical exercise therapy is able to positively influence the degree of disability, the intake of analgesics, depression, and anger in people with lumbar spinal stenosis (cf. Slater et al. 2015).

Zhong et al. (2023) found in the postoperative stage in people with previous lumbar spinal stenosis that it is therapeutically valuable to adapt the therapy measures to the patient's gait pattern. This can significantly better influence factors such as pain intensity, the quality and symmetry of the gait pattern, and the degree of disability compared to empirical exercises (cf. Zhong et al. 2023).

Regarding conservative therapy, the data situation from Schneider et al. (2019) suggests that the combination of manual therapy and individualized medical exercise therapy is the best therapy option. In addition to stretching, strength training should also be used (cf. Schneider et al. 2019).

The Zurich Claudication Questionnaire and the self-paced walking test serve as assessments (cf. Minetama et al. 2019). In addition, the Oswestry Disability Index can be used (cf. Zhong et al. 2023). More detailed information on the individual assessments can be taken from the assessment list in the appendix of this book.

Useful visualizations can be taken from Fig. 5.157 and 5.158.

Summary for Practice

Medical exercise therapy can relieve pain in patients with spinal stenosis, as well as positively influence the degree of disability, the intake of analgesics, depression, and anger. It should be noted here that there is only low to moderate evidence due to small sample sizes in individual studies. The combination of manual therapy with medical exercise therapy is effective. The focus during training is on flexion-based exercises as well as stretching and core strength exercises. High value is attributed to the optimization of the gait pattern.

Fig. 5.156 provides an overview of the mentioned information.

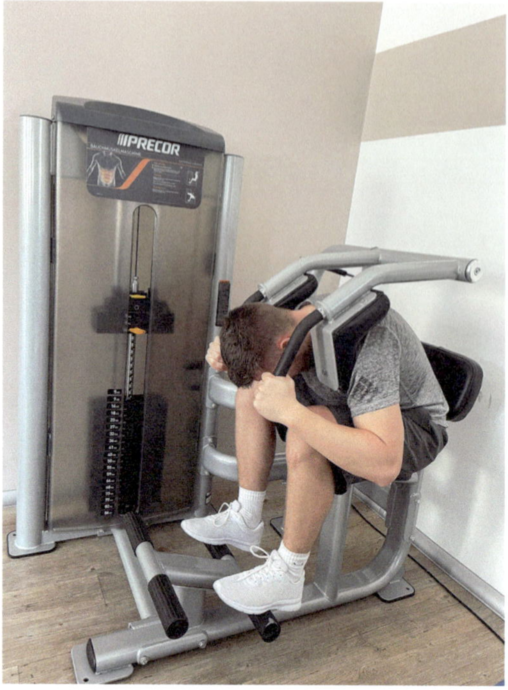

Fig. 5.157 MTT in Spinal Stenosis—Flexion-based exercises of the lumbar spine

5.5 Thoracic Spine Area

5.5.1 Ankylosing Spondylitis/Spondylitis Ankylosans

Medical training programs for people with ankylosing spondylitis are capable of alleviating pain intensity, improving functionality, and dampening disease activity (see Hu et al. 2020). Regardless of the specific training program, a combination of flexibility exercises, strength

Categories	Evidence-based training recommendation
Exercises	Flexion-based exercises for the lumbar spine / stretching the muscles of the lumbar spine / strength training for the muscles of the lumbar spine / combination of exercise therapy with manual therapy

Fig. 5.156 Summary MTT in Spinal Stenosis

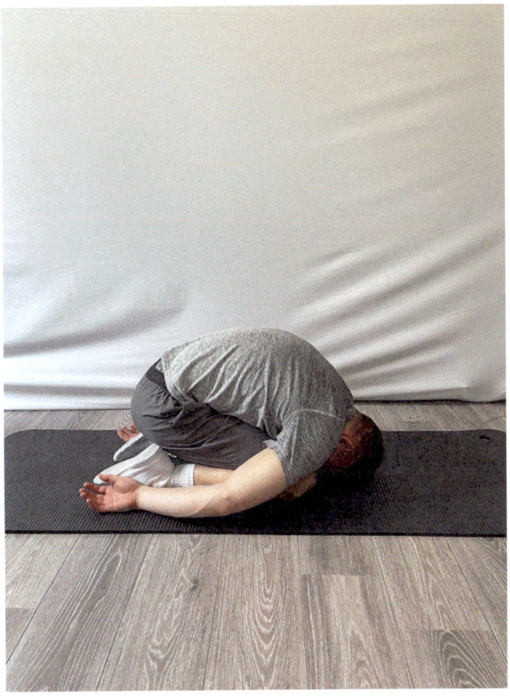

Fig. 5.158 MTT in Spinal Stenosis—Package position lumbar spine

training, and aerobic endurance training can achieve both an improvement in spinal mobility and functional improvement (see Boudjani et al. 2023).

The research group led by Pécourneau et al. () found that exercise therapy for ankylosing spondylitis is applied in the form of home exercise programs, Pilates, swimming, or supervised training sessions. The summary of the data situation in the meta-analysis prepared in this regard recognizes the therapeutic potential of these applications, but points out the numerically low total sample and the existing heterogeneity of the collected data (see Pécourneau et al. 2018).

After meta-analytical evaluation of eight included studies, it was shown that water-based therapy for people with ankylosing spondylitis is capable of positively influencing the pain situation and disease activity. However, no evidence was found that water therapy improves spinal mobility and functional capacity (see Liang et al. 2021).

Group therapies performed better in terms of improvements in depression and anxiety as well as mental health than home exercise programs. However, the practice of home exercise programs for improving depression is better than no intervention (see Lane et al. 2022).

Harpham et al. (2022) describe that various aerobic endurance sports such as running, walking, and swimming lead to a reduction in C-reactive protein and thus positively influence the pathophysiology. This positive change corresponded to the subjective perception of the affected individuals regarding disease activity.

In a randomized controlled study, a sample of 32 people was divided into a conventional training group and a conventional training group with additional strengthening of the inspiratory muscles. After the eight-week intervention period, it was found that additional training of the inspiratory auxiliary muscles with a respiratory resistance device strengthens the inspiratory muscles, increases functional capacity during training, and dampens disease activity (see Calik et al. 2018).

The bath-ankylosing-spondylitis-disease-activity-index and the bath-ankylosing-spondylitis-functional-index serve as assessments (see Pécourneau et al. 2018). In addition, the bath-ankylosing-spondylitis-metrology-index can be used (see Martins et al. 2014). Furthermore, the ankylosing-spondylitis-quality-of-life-questionnaire can be used (see Acar et al. 2023). More detailed information on the individual assessments can be taken from the assessment list in the appendix of this book.

Useful visualizations can be found in Fig. 5.160 and 5.161.

Summary for Practice

Medical exercise therapy is capable of alleviating pain, improving functionality, and dampening disease activity in patients with ankylosing spondylitis. The focus is on flexibility exercises, aerobic endurance training, Pilates, swimming, and water therapy. Furthermore, training of the inspiratory auxiliary muscles with a respiratory resistance device leads to a dampening of disease activity and increases functional capacity.

Group therapies can have a positive effect on additional depression.

Fig. 5.159 provides an overview of the mentioned information.

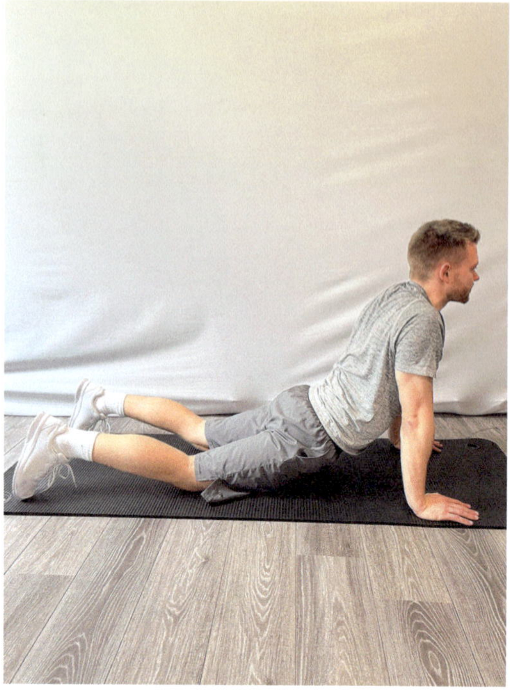

Fig. 5.160 MTT in Ankylosing Spondylitis/Spondylitis ankylosans—Spine Flexibility Exercises

5.5.2 Adolescent Idiopathic Scoliosis

A meta-analysis, which includes information from eight randomized controlled studies, advocates for the use of medical training therapy in people with mild to moderate adolescent idiopathic scoliosis. Regular training can achieve both a reduction in spinal deformity and improved quality of life (see Gámiz-Bermúdez et al. 2022). Furthermore, medical training therapy is also considered a tool for prevention against adolescent idiopathic scoliosis (see Qi et al. 2023).

There is moderate evidence that training therapy can positively influence the Cobb angle, the angle of trunk rotation, thoracic trunk rotation, and lumbar lordosis. However, there is only low evidence for the reduction of the average lateral deviation through training interventions (see Anwer et al. 2015). Ceballos-Laita et al. (2023) add that quality of life can be positively influenced by Schroth therapy. They mention in the same breath that the change in the Cobb angle through Schroth therapy has no clinical relevance (see Ceballos-Laita et al. 2023). A recommendation of Schroth therapy can be made for people with a Cobb angle between 10–30°. A training period of at least one month is advised. Regular and targeted application of Schroth therapy can achieve both an improvement in structural deformity and an increase in trunk strength (see Park et al. 2018). There is evidence that postural control and balance can be improved through the application of Schroth therapy (see Kastrinis et al. 2023).

The research group around Chen et al. (2023) mention yoga, trunk strength training, Schroth therapy, and sling table training. The mentioned

Categories	Evidence-based training recommendation
Exercises	Flexibility exercises / strength training (focus on the trunk in the largest possible ROM) / Endurance training / swimming, Pilates, running, walking / mobilization exercises in the water / training the inspiratory auxiliary respiratory muscles with a breathing resistance device

Fig. 5.159 Summary of MTT in Ankylosing Spondylitis/Spondylitis ankylosans

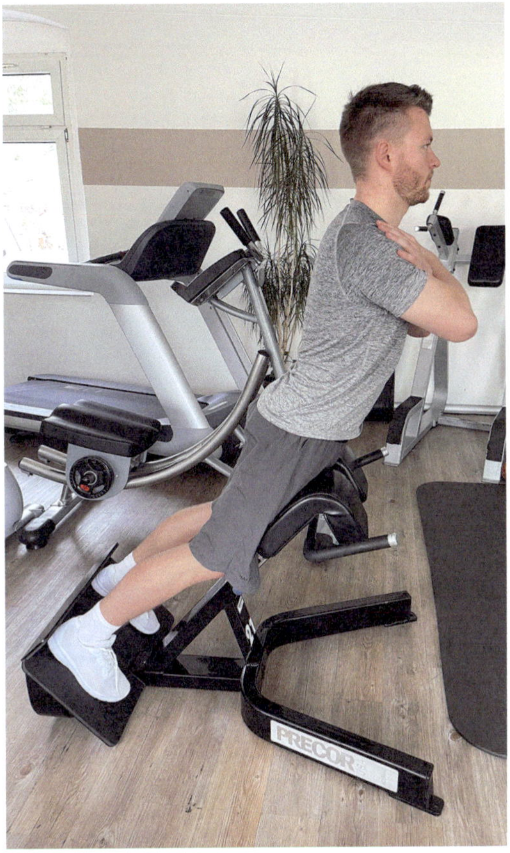

Fig. 5.161 MTT in Ankylosing Spondylitis/Spondylitis ankylosans—Strength Training (Focus on Trunk with as Large a Range of Motion as Possible)

order is from the strongest to the weakest recommendation (see Chen et al. 2023).

Lung volumes in people with adolescent idiopathic scoliosis can also be positively influenced by training therapy (see Rafferty et al. 2023).

In a randomized controlled study, a trunk stability training was compared to the Schroth therapy method using a 28-person sample. The trunk stability training focused on learning and activity integration of the recruitment of the transversus abdominis muscle using the abdominal-drawing-in maneuver. The Schroth therapy included rotation-related breathing, spinal elongation exercises, deflection exercises, derotation exercises, stretching exercises of the concave side, strengthening exercises, and endurance exercises of the postural muscles. Over a period of 10 weeks, training was conducted three times a week for 90 minutes each. It was calculated that the Schroth group achieved significantly better results in terms of a change in the Cobb angle, thoracic trunk rotation, cosmetic trunk deformity, spinal deformity, and quality of life. Therefore, Schroth therapy is considered more effective than trunk stability training in terms of scoliosis correction (see Kocaman et al. 2021).

According to the results of a recently conducted randomized controlled study, the addition of strengthening the inspiratory muscles to a specific training program seems helpful. Basbug et al. (2023) were able to demonstrate improved respiratory function, improved inspiratory muscle strength, and functional capacity of the respiratory system by using a breathing resistance device twice daily for 15 minutes over a period of eight weeks.

The six-week combination of Schroth therapy and balance training is superior to Schroth therapy alone. To ensure optimal improvement of the trunk rotation angle, the Cobb angle, the Scoliosis Research Society-22 scale, and balance, the coupling of the interventions is therefore recommended (see Shen et al. 2023).

The Cobb angle, the angle of trunk rotation, the strength of the trunk extensors and flexors, the expansion of the chest, pulmonary function, and quality of life serve as assessments (see Park et al. 2018). The Adam's test is used to assess trunk rotation. The cosmetic trunk rotation can be assessed by the Walter Reed Visual Assessment Scale. The Scoliosis Research Society-22 questionnaire is used to assess quality of life. The Cobb angle can be determined radiologically (see Kocaman et al. 2021). More detailed information on the individual assessments can be found in the assessment list in the appendix of this book.

Useful visualizations can be found in Fig. 5.163 and 5.164.

Summary for Practice

The evidence-based treatment of choice for adolescent idiopathic scoliosis is the combination of Schroth therapy with balance exercises. Breathing exercises with a breathing resistance device and trunk stability training can further positively influence the results.

At the center of Schroth therapy is rotation-related breathing, spinal elongation exercises, deflection exercises, derotation exercises, stretching of the concave side, strengthening exercises, and endurance exercises of the postural muscles.

As a result, a reduction in spinal deformity, improved quality of life, and improved balance can be expected. There is moderate evidence that targeted training therapy can positively influence the Cobb angle, the angle of trunk rotation, thoracic trunk rotation, and lumbar lordosis.

Fig. 5.162 provides an overview of the mentioned infwormation.

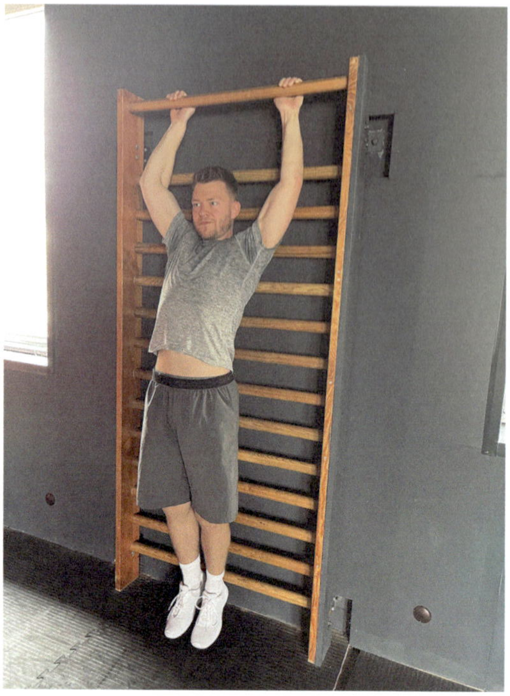

Fig. 5.163 MTT in adolescent idiopathic scoliosis—Spinal elongation exercise

5.6 Cervical Spine Area

5.6.1 Cervical Radiculopathy/ Cervical Disc Herniation

The meta-analysis by Liang et al. (2019) confirms the use of medical training therapy in people with cervical radiculopathy.

In a randomized controlled study, the effect of a cervical spine stabilization program was examined in 50 people with cervical disc herniation. In a second group, the identical stabilization program was supplemented by additional

Categories	Evidence-based training recommendation
Units	10 weeks, 3x per week á 90 minutes per unit
Exercises	Schroth therapy (rotation-related breathing, spinal elongation exercises, deflection exercises, derotation exercises, stretching of the concave side, strengthening exercises, endurance exercises for the postural muscles / balance training / yoga / strength training, trunk stability with a focus on the transversus abdominis muscle / training in the sling table / inspiratory breathing training with a breathing resistance device (15 minutes twice a day)
Elongation	Stretching the muscles of the concave side

Fig. 5.162 Summary MTT in adolescent idiopathic scoliosis

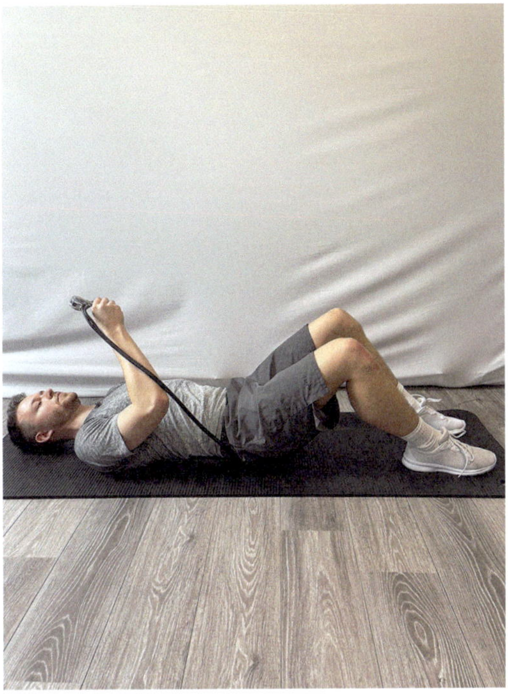

Fig. 5.164 MTT in adolescent idiopathic scoliosis—Strengthening of the transversus abdominis muscle

trunk muscle training. The intervention period was two months. During this time, training was conducted three times a week. The cervical spine stabilization program was carried out in three phases. Initially, the local recruitment of the longus capitis muscle, the longus colli muscle, and the extensor-acting short neck muscles was trained. In the second phase, emphasis was placed on improving the endurance and strength performance of the corresponding muscles. In the third phase, the strength of the muscles was further developed. The exercises of the stabilization program include the execution of cranio-cervical flexion in the supine position, standing with a ball between the back of the head and the wall, and with combined movements of the upper extremity. Furthermore, stabilization of the cervical spine is carried out in forearm support as well as in the quadruped position. The exercises with a Theraband include wall sitting with simultaneous resistance exercises of the upper extremity, bilateral resistance-overcoming external rotation of the shoulder joints with simultaneous rotation of the cervical spine, and resistance overcoming against the Theraband in the direction of lateral flexion or cranio-cervical flexion of the cervical spine (cf. Buyukturan et al. 2017). The cervical spine stabilization program was able to produce a significant effect on pain intensity, recruitment ability and static endurance of the deep cervical spine flexors, the cross-section of the longus colli muscle, the degree of disability, and the extent of kinesiophobia. The addition of the trunk stabilization program did not bring any additional significances (cf. Buyukturan et al. 2017).

Yaşa et al. (2021) investigated the influence of balance training in people with a herniation of the cervical disc. Based on a total sample of 30 people aged between 18-55 years, two groups were formed. Both groups received three therapy units over a six-week period. The control group initially received a cervicothoracic hot pack followed by an interference current, strengthening and posture exercises, as well as stretches of the trapezius muscle and the scalene muscles. The intervention group additionally carried out balance training. Both groups benefited from a highly significant reduction in pain intensity. With regard to the outcomes of balance, the intervention group performed better compared to the control group. Therefore, the implementation of balance training in medical training therapy for people with cervical disc herniation is recommended (cf. Yaşa et al. 2021).

Akkan and Gelecek (2018) also advocate the practice of stabilizing exercises of the cervical spine in patients with cervical radiculopathy.

The Cranio-cervical-flexion-test, the Visual analog scale, the Neck-disability-scale, the Tampa-scale-of-kinesiophobia, and the Neck-flexors-endurance-test can be used as assessments (cf. Buyukturan et al. 2017). Furthermore, the Activity-Specific-Balance-Confidence scale can be used (cf. Yaşa et al. 2021). The Neck Disability Index and the Corbin-postural-assessment-scale can also be used (cf. Akkan and Gelecek 2018). More detailed information on the individual assessments can be taken from the assessment list in the appendix of this book.

Useful visualizations can be taken from Fig. 5.166, 5.167, 5.168, 5.169, 5.170, 5.171 and 5.172.

Summary for Practice

Through evidence-based medical training therapy, a significant effect on pain intensity, recruitment ability and static endurance of the deep cervical spine flexors, the degree of disability, and the extent of kinesiophobia can be achieved in patients with cervical radiculopathy. The focus is on cervical spine stabilization programs, particularly those of the M. longus capitis, the M. longus colli, and the extensor-acting short neck muscles. Targeted interference currents, cervicothoracic hot packs, and especially balance exercises can further positively influence the result.

Fig. 5.165 provides an overview of the mentioned information.

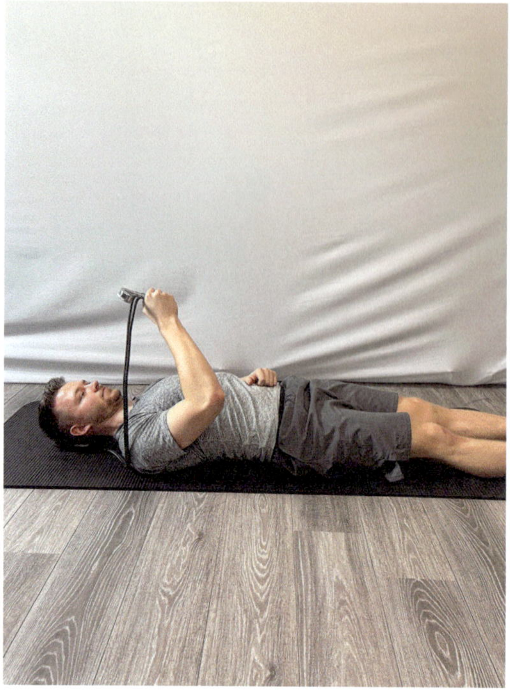

Fig. 5.166 MTT in cervical radiculopathy/cervical disc herniation—Cranio-cervical flexion in supine position

Categories	Evidence-based training recommendation
Units	6-9 weeks, 3 times a week, 45-60 minutes per session is recommended
Exercises	Hot pack in the cervicothoracic region at the start of therapy / craniocervical flexion in supine position, standing with a ball between the back of the head and the wall, as well as with combined movements of the upper extremity / stabilization exercises of the cervical spine in forearm support and quadruped position / wall sitting with Theraband exercises of the upper extremity / wall sitting with resistance overcoming Theraband exercises of the shoulder joint in external rotation with simultaneous rotation of the cervical spine / resistance exercises with Theraband in lateral flexion and craniocervical flexion of the cervical spine / balance training / interference current after hot pack possible
Elongation	Stretching the trapezius muscle and the scaleni muscles

Fig. 5.165 Summary of MTT in cervical radiculopathy/cervical disc herniation

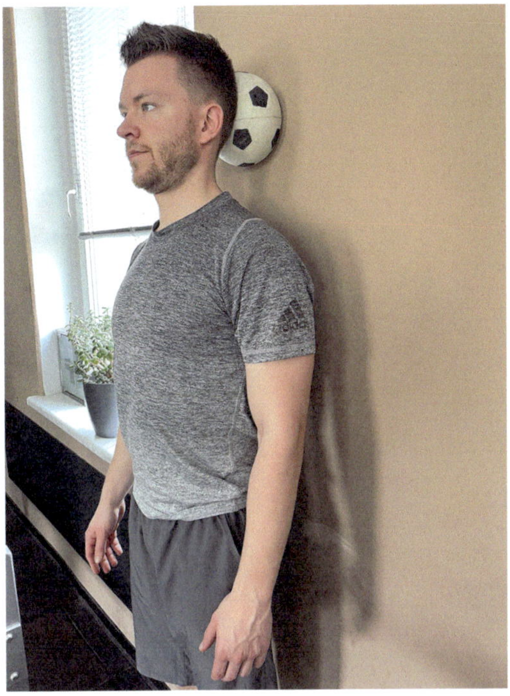

Fig. 5.167 MTT in cervical radiculopathy/cervical disc herniation—Cranio-cervical flexion standing with a ball between the back of the head and the wall

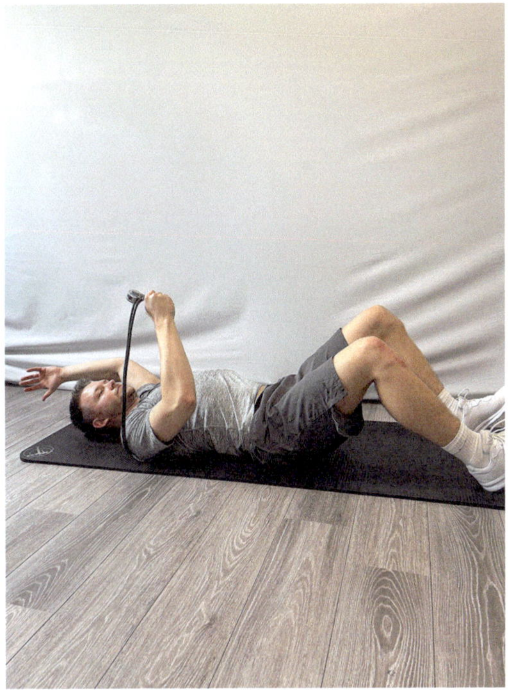

Fig. 5.168 MTT in cervical radiculopathy/cervical disc herniation—Cranio-cervical flexion with combined movements of the upper extremity

5.6.2 Neck Pain

A meta-analysis from the year 2023 summarizes the effect of various training therapeutic interventions in people with chronic neck pain (see Rasmussen-Barr et al. 2023). It is found that the practice of medical training therapy is not superior to any application. A short-term effect on pain and the degree of disability is proven. The work includes data from 25 systematic reviews and meta-analyses with a total population of 17,321 subjects. The interventions where an effect is proven include motor control training, Pilates, strength training, traditional Chinese exercise programs, and yoga. All mentioned forms of training are capable of producing a pain-reducing effect and, with the exception of strength training, reducing the degree of disability (see Rasmussen-Barr et al. 2023).

Over a period of 4–6 weeks, a cervical spine stabilization program can alleviate the intensity of neck pain (see Wu et al. 2020).

The use of biofeedback can positively affect the degree of disability in neck pain, but less so the intensity of pain (see Campo et al. 2021). In contrast, the results of Tsiringakis et al. (2020) were able to demonstrate a biofeedback-associated effect on pain.

Cho et al. (2023) confirm the effect of medical training therapy for chronic neck pain. In addition, it is mentioned that the data situation regarding training therapeutic effects for acute and subacute neck pain is insufficient.

Mueller et al. (2023) point out that an increased frequency and a longer duration of training sessions have a positive effect on training programs aimed at motor control. The exploration of an optimal dosage of medical training

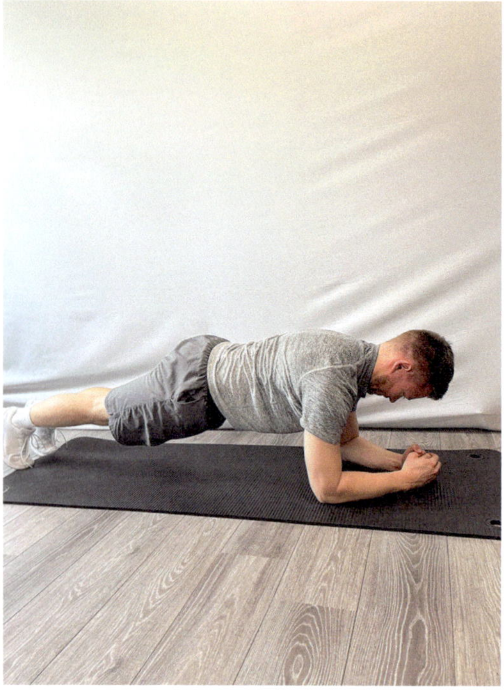

Fig. 5.169 MTT in cervical radiculopathy/cervical disc herniation—Stabilization exercises of the cervical spine in forearm support or quadruped position

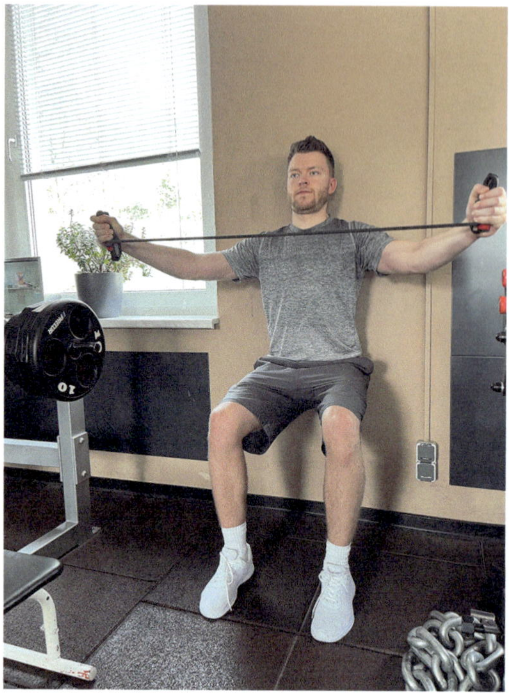

Fig. 5.170 MTT in cervical radiculopathy/cervical disc herniation—Wall sit with Theraband exercises of the upper extremity

therapy for neck pain has so far been unsuccessful (see Wilhelm et al. 2020).

Kang and Kim (2022) researched the influence of a training program focusing on the scapular surrounding musculature in a randomized controlled study. The training program was applied to people with chronic neck pain. Over a period of one month, five training sessions were conducted each week. In addition to the chin-in exercise, rowing exercises were performed in various starting positions such as long sitting, bent standing, upright standing, and sitting. In addition, bilateral retraction of the shoulder blades was practiced with a resistance band. The training program was completed with lat pull-down training and the standing chest press. Each training session practiced each exercise with three sets, a repetition number of 10–20, and a rest period of 30 seconds between sets. The application of these exercises achieved a significant reduction in pain intensity with improved mobility of the cervical spine. In addition, the tone of the trapezius muscle pars descendens, the degree of disability, and the quality of life could be significantly positively influenced. Application in people with chronic neck pain is therefore recommended (see Kang and Kim 2022).

In a sample of 50 women with nonspecific chronic neck pain, the effect of posture training was compared to a specific neck training program. During the four-week intervention period, training was conducted twice a week for 40 minutes each time. As part of the posture training, which was aimed at optimizing joint alignment, posture exercises were practiced in supine and standing positions under guidance. The specific neck training included strengthening of the deep neck extensors and a biofeedback-associated strengthening of the deep neck flexors. In addition, sensorimotor exercises were practiced with a visual feedback rehab laser. Both interventions

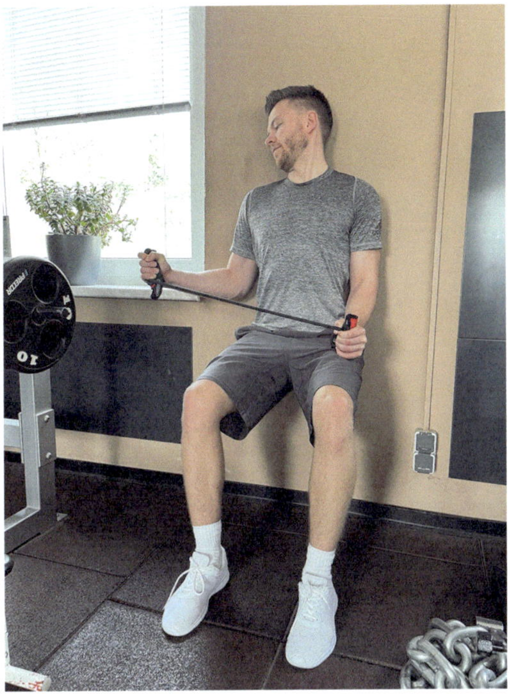

Fig. 5.171 MTT in cervical radiculopathy/cervical disc herniation—Wall sit with resistance overcoming Theraband exercises of the shoulder joint in external rotation with simultaneous rotation of the cervical spine

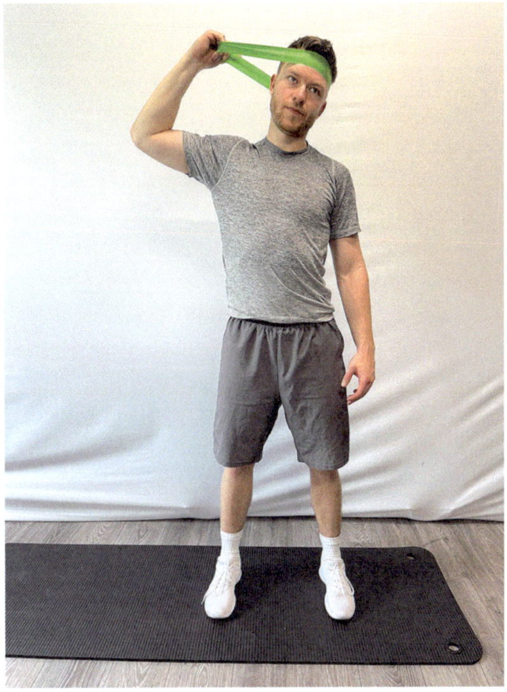

Fig. 5.172 MTT in cervical radiculopathy/cervical disc herniation—Resistance exercises with Theraband in lateral flexion or cranio-cervical flexion of the cervical spine

were equally able to significantly improve pain intensity, degree of disability, and mobility. In addition, the activity of the superficial neck flexors was reduced (see Fernandes et al. 2023).

Another randomized controlled study recognizes that the combination of medical training therapy and a neuroscience education of the affected individuals has a better effect than the sole implementation of the medical training therapy (see Javdaneh et al. 2021).

Among other things, the neck disability index serves as an assessment (see Kang and Kim 2022) as well as the Neck-Pain-and-Disability-Scale (see Javdaneh et al. 2021). Furthermore, the activation of the superficially located neck flexors during the cranio-cervical flexion test can be used (see Fernandes et al. 2023). Other assessments used in connection with neck pain are the Pain-Catastrophizing-Scale, the Pain-Self-Efficacy-Questionnaire, and the Fear–Avoidance-Beliefs-Questionnaire (see Javdaneh et al. 2021). The previously quoted training program integrated a strengthening of the deep neck flexors through the performance of a cranio-cervical flexion. In addition to this, various exercises were used to train the musculature of the shoulder joint and the shoulder girdle. More detailed information on the individual assessments can be taken from the assessment list in the appendix of this book.

Useful visualizations can be found in Fig. 5.174, 5.175, 5.176, 5.177, 5.178 and 5.179.

Summary for Practice

The different results of numerous randomized controlled studies and meta-analyses suggest that targeted training can have a positive effect on the degree of disability, pain intensity, mobility, and quality of life in nonspecific neck pain. Motor control training, Pilates, strength training, traditional Chinese exercise programs, and yoga produce a positive effect on pain and the degree of disability.

The focus is on general and specific stabilization and mobilization programs. Scientific evidence is attributed to the training of the scapular muscles, posture training, and a specific neck training program. A further positive effect is achieved by the neuroscientific education of the affected person.

Fig. 5.173 provides an overview of the mentioned information.

5.6.3 Cervical Instability

A lack of motor control of the deep stabilizing muscles of the cervical spine is rarely formulated as a medical diagnosis. When such changes become symptomatic in the form of pain, this is often diagnosed as neck pain. In addition to the information already presented in 5.6.2, this chapter aims to contribute to a better identification of cervical instabilities in clinical practice.

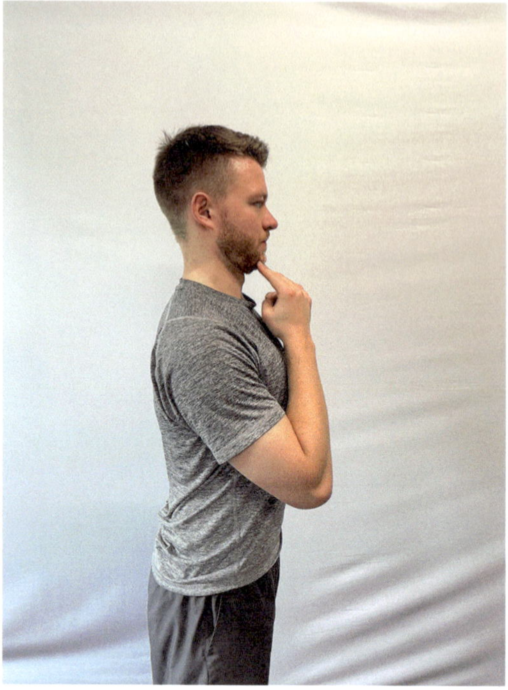

Fig. 5.174 MTT for neck pain—Chin-in exercise

Categories	Evidence-based training recommendation
Units	4-6 weeks, 5 times a week, 40-60 minutes per session is recommended
Exercises	Chin-in exercises / rowing in various starting positions (long sit, bent forward stand, upright stand, standing) / retraction of the shoulder blades against resistance using Theraband / lat pulldown / standing chest press / posture training by optimizing joint alignment / posture exercises in supine and standing position / strengthening of the deep neck extensors / biofeedback-associated strengthening of the deep neck flexors / sensorimotor exercises with the visual feedback rehab laser / motor control training / Pilates / traditional Chinese exercise programmes / yoga

Fig. 5.173 Summary of MTT for neck pain

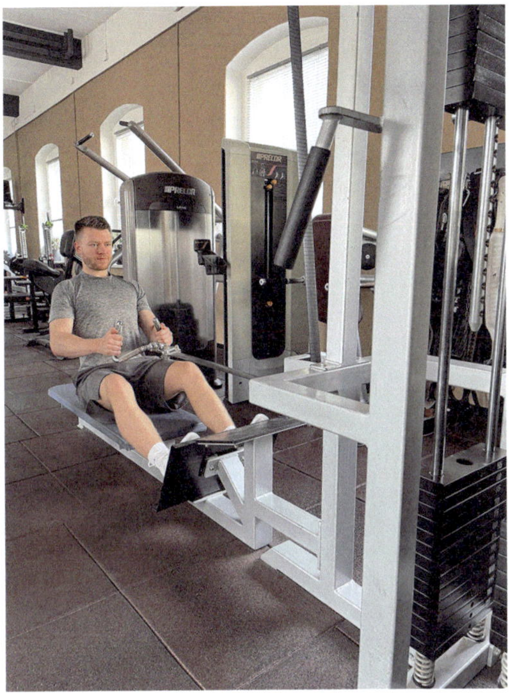

Fig. 5.175 MTT for neck pain—Rowing in different starting positions (long sitting, bent over standing, upright standing, sitting)

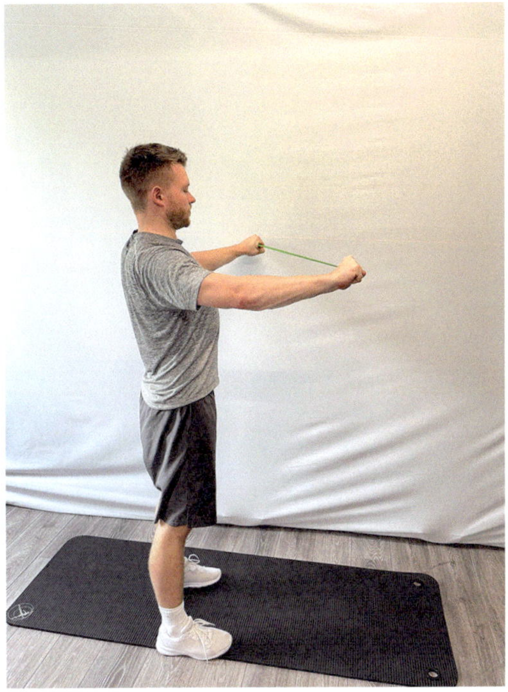

Fig. 5.176 MTT for neck pain—Retraction of the shoulder blades against resistance through Theraband

Subjectively, prolonged static activities or physical passivity can provoke symptoms. Also, stresses that require recurring muscular stabilization of the cervical spine can trigger pain or a feeling of instability.

From an objective perspective, the biofeedback-associated craniocervical flexion test can provide information about the recruitment ability of the deep cervical spine flexors (see Jull et al. 2008; Koning et al. 2008). In addition, the endurance test for the cervical spine flexors can be used (see Domenech et al. 2011; Childs et al. 2008). Furthermore, the endurance performance of the cervical spine extensors can also be checked (see Sebastian et al. 2015).

In particular, the biofeedback-associated craniocervical flexion test can be used not only as an assessment but also as a training method for the deep cervical spine flexors. For training the recruitment ability of the deep neck extensors, Schomacher and Falla (2013) propose a

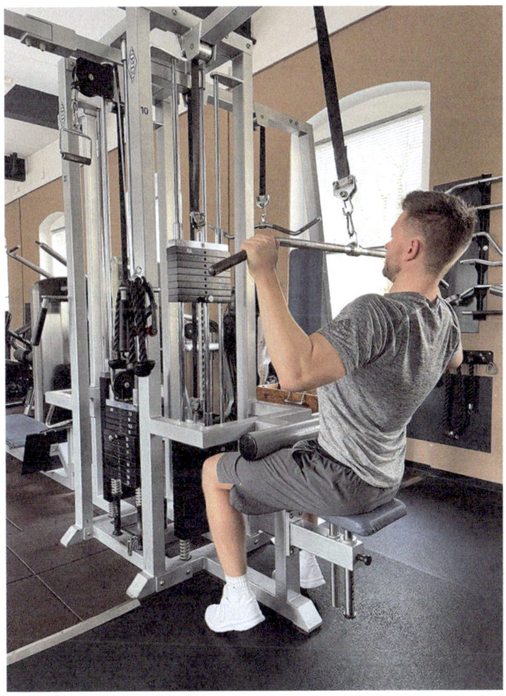

Fig. 5.177 MTT for neck pain—Lat pull

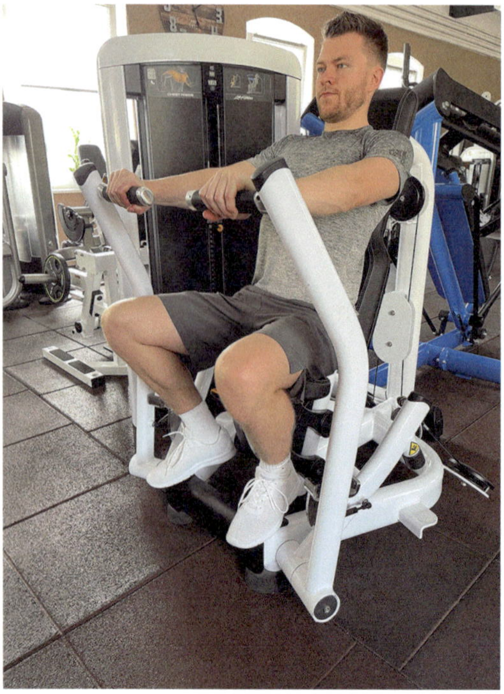

Fig. 5.178 MTT for neck pain—Chest press

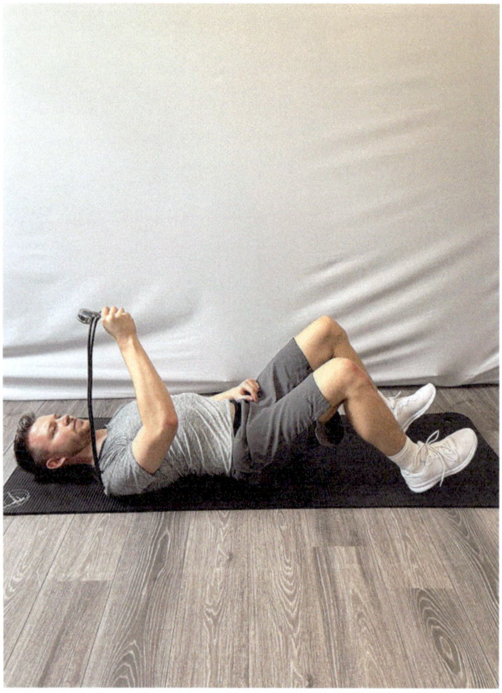

Fig. 5.179 MTT for neck pain—Strengthening of the deep neck extensors and neck flexors (Bio-feedback)

dorsal facilitation or resistance at the cervical spine with an active dorsal thrust by the trainee. More detailed information on the individual assessments can be found in the assessment list in the appendix of this book.

Useful visualizations can be found in Fig. 5.181 and 5.182.

> **Summary for Practice**
> This chapter complements Sect. 5.6.2 and emphasizes that in the case of cervical instability, the focus should be on the deep cervical spine flexors and the deep neck extensors.
>
> Positive effects can be achieved with the help of biofeedback mechanisms and targeted facilitation.
>
> Fig. 5.180 provides an overview of the information mentioned.

5.7 Shoulder Girdle/Shoulder Joint Area

5.7.1 Glenohumeral Instability

Both Warby et al. (2014) and Warby et al. (2016) lament the lack of homogeneity in existing studies. In addition, there is a high risk of bias in the included studies. These circumstances make it difficult to make statements about the effect of medical training therapy or to strive for a comparison with operations.

A meta-analysis from 2021 dealt with the effectiveness of conservative therapy in multidirectional instability of the shoulder joint. Medical training therapy was recognized as an important component of therapy. Training therapy is highly valued in instabilities that have not arisen from an injury. The practice of the Watson training program is currently considered the best instrument for the therapy of multidirectional instability (see Kłaptocz et al. 2021).

The research team led by Cools et al. (2016) recommends adapting medical training therapy to the type of existing glenohumeral instability.

Categories	Evidence-based training recommendation
Units	4-6 weeks, 5 times a week, 40-60 minutes per session is recommended
Exercises	Biofeedback-associated craniocervical flexion / dorsal facilitation and Resistance to the cervical spine with active dorsal thrust / Chin-in exercises / Rowing in various starting positions (long sit, bent forward stand, upright stand, sitting) / retraction of the shoulder blades against resistance with Theraband / lat pulldown / standing chest press / posture training by optimizing joint alignment / posture exercises in supine and standing position / strengthening of the deep neck extensors / biofeedback-associated strengthening of the deep neck flexors / sensorimotor exercises with the visual feedback rehab laser / motor control training / Pilates / traditional Chinese exercise programmes / yoga

Fig. 5.180 Summary MTT in cervical instability

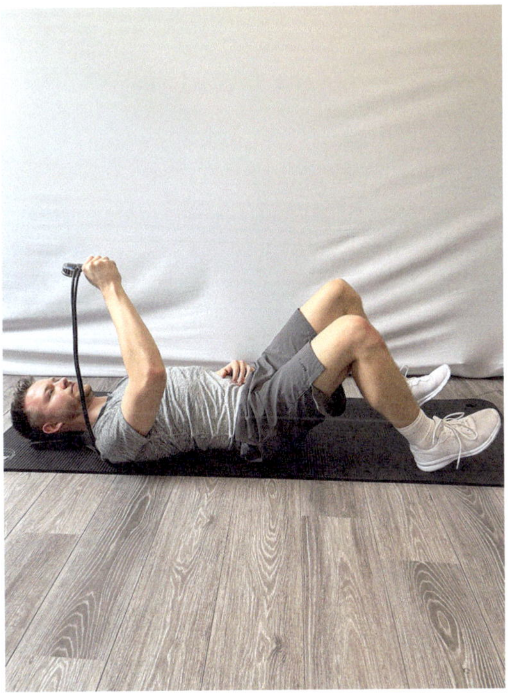

Fig. 5.181 MTT in cervical instability—Biofeedback-associated craniocervical flexion

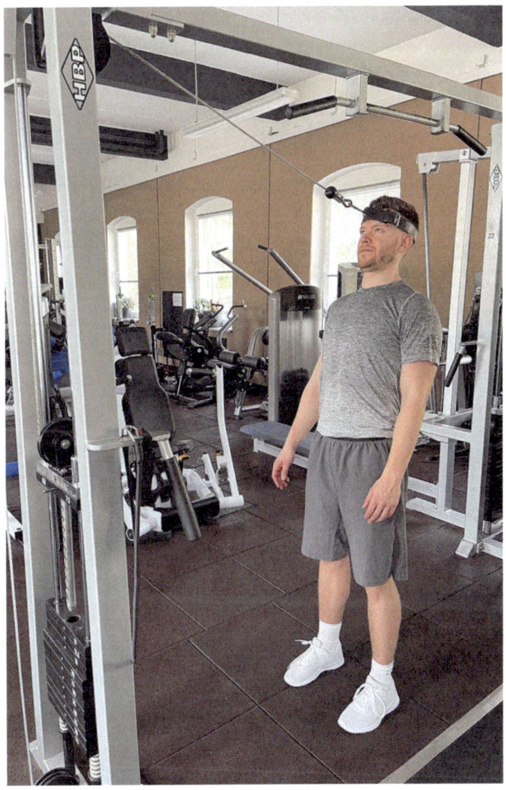

Fig. 5.182 MTT in cervical instability—Resistance at C-spine with active dorsal thrust

In general, strengthening of the rotator cuff with a focus on intermuscular balance is considered beneficial. In addition, the external rotators of the glenohumeral joint should be specifically trained eccentrically. The flexibility and strength of the muscles, which have an anatomical connection to the scapula, also play an important role in training therapy (see Cools et al. 2016).

In a randomized controlled study by Warby et al. (2018), the effect of training programs on a sample with multidirectional instability of the shoulder joint was examined. The Watson training program emerged as the most effective approach (see Watson et al. 2016, 2017). This training program is progressively structured and initially focuses on the individually adapted production of optimal glenohumeral alignment. While maintaining this alignment, the motor control of the scapula is trained. A rowing motion is performed from a 45° flexion angle to the neutral-zero position. In terms of the movement directions of the external and internal rotation of the shoulder joint, training is carried out with slight resistance from the neutral-zero position to 45°. The exercises of this phase are performed in an upright position. The following phase focuses on muscular build-up in the posterior shoulder area. For this purpose, rowing exercises are performed with a bent and upright upper body. In addition, the external rotators are practiced in a lateral position. Subsequently, the training program focuses on improving motor control in the sagittal plane. For this purpose, training is carried out into anteversion under resistance. In the next phase, the movement directions of external rotation, internal rotation, and flexion are trained under resistance to an extent of 45°–90°. Following this, the focus is on strengthening the deltoid muscle and its parts. Finally, integration into everyday activities or sport-specific load patterns takes place. Correct exercise execution with simultaneous freedom from pain is a prerequisite for progressing through the successive training phases. With this approach, both instability and pain intensity can be significantly reduced in a training period of twelve weeks (see Warby et al. 2018).

Jeon and Chon (2018) also point out the relevance of glenohumeral stabilization exercises and their centralizing effect on the humeral head.

The Melbourne Instability Shoulder Score and the Western Ontario Shoulder Index serve as assessments (see Warby et al. 2018). More detailed information on the individual assessments can be taken from the assessment list in the appendix of this book.

Useful visualizations can be taken from Fig. 5.184, 5.185, 5.186, 5.187, 5.188, 5.189 and 5.190.

Summary for Practice

Despite an increased risk of bias in numerous included studies, it can be concluded that medical training therapy, and in particular the Watson training program, can positively influence both pain intensity and instability in the shoulder joint. Important here are correct exercise execution with simultaneous freedom from pain.

The basis is the establishment of optimal glenohumeral alignment with simultaneous motor control of the scapula and strengthening of the rotator cuff.

Fig. 5.183 provides an overview of the mentioned information.

5.7.2 Frozen Shoulder

A meta-analysis from 2022 recognizes that both the sole application of medical training therapy and the combination of medical training therapy and other interventions are capable of positively influencing the mobility of the shoulder joint and the intensity of pain. The application of Muscle-Energy-Techniques is recommended with the aim of improving function (cf. Mertens et al. 2022).

Challoumas et al. (2020) present intra-articular corticosteroid supply in combination with home exercise programs as the most effective therapy method for frozen shoulder.

Categories	Evidence-based training recommendation
Exercises	12 weeks / establishing optimal glenohumeral alignment while standing / motor control of the scapula while maintaining alignment while standing / rowing movement from a flexion position of 45° to neutral zero position while maintaining alignment while standing / movement in 45° external and internal rotation from zero position against resistance while maintaining alignment while standing / rowing exercise with bent forward and upright body / training of the external rotators in lateral position / training of anteversion against resistance / training of external rotation, internal rotation, flexion against resistance at 45-90° / Strengthening the m. deltoid muscle with all parts / integration into everyday movements/sport-specific load patterns

Fig. 5.183 Summary of MTT in glenohumeral instability

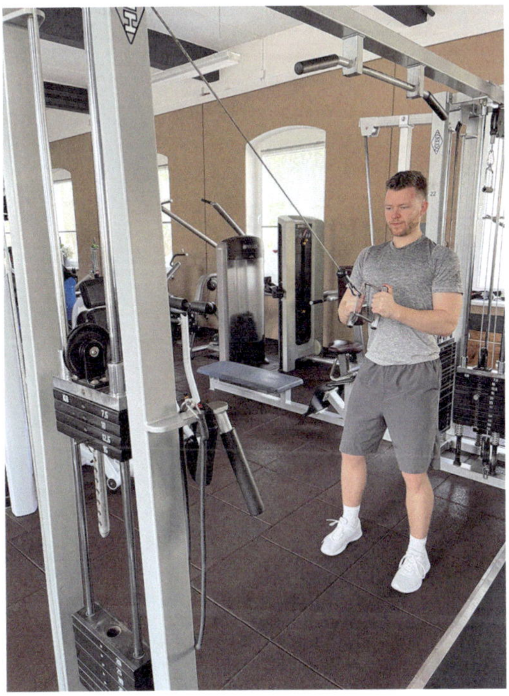

Fig. 5.184 MTT in glenohumeral instability—Rowing motion from a flexion position of 45° to neutral-zero position while maintaining alignment in standing

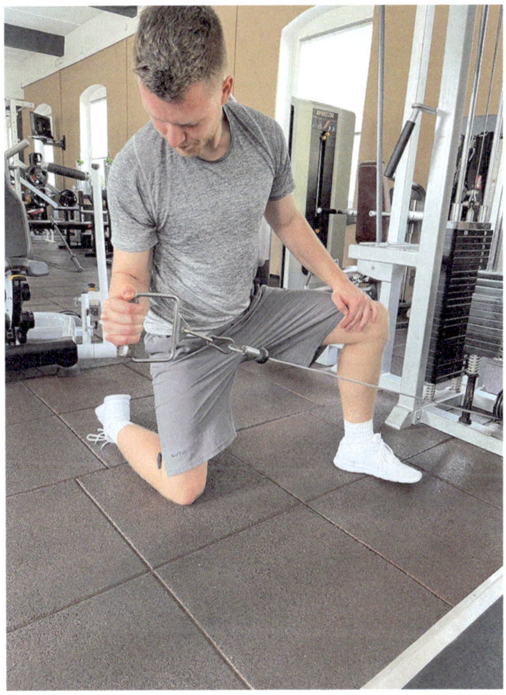

Fig. 5.185 MTT in glenohumeral instability—Movement in 45° external and internal rotation from zero position against resistance while maintaining alignment in standing

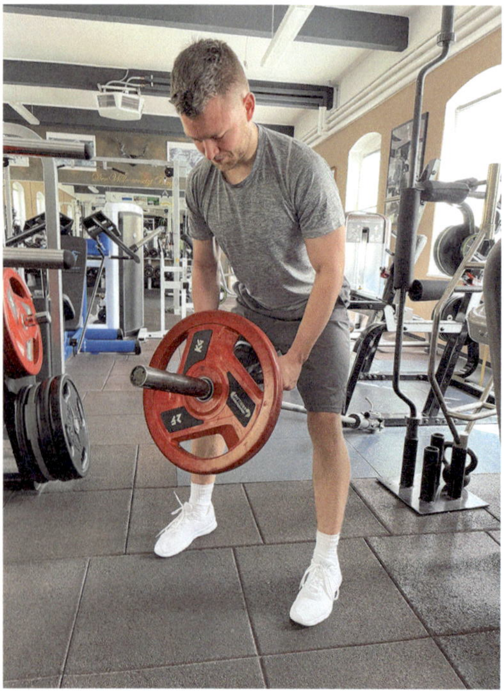

Fig. 5.186 MTT in glenohumeral instability—Rowing exercise with bent and upright body

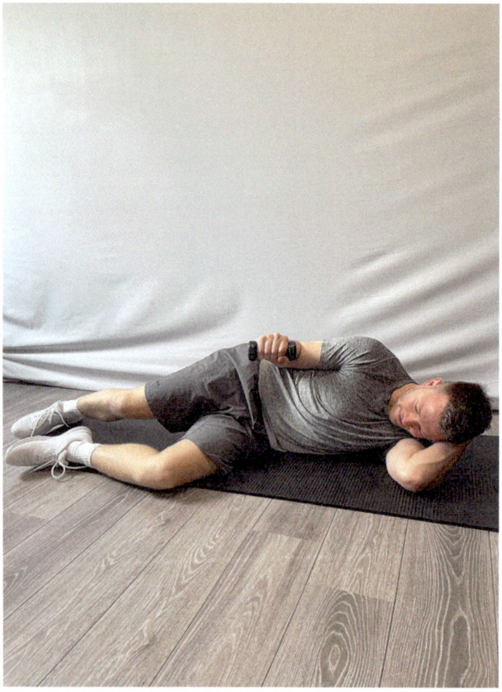

Fig. 5.187 MTT in glenohumeral instability—Training of the external rotators in lateral position

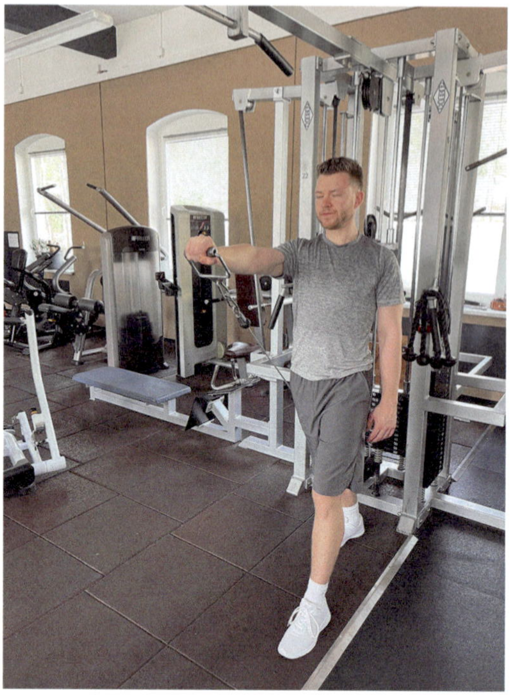

Fig. 5.188 MTT in glenohumeral instability—Training of anteversion against resistance

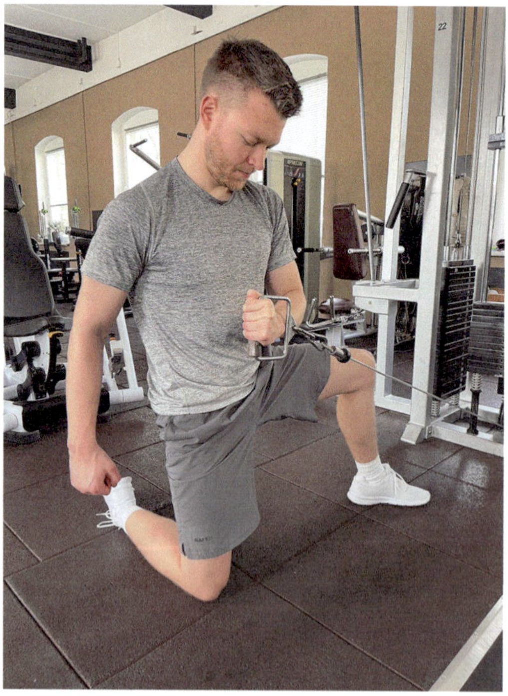

Fig. 5.189 MTT in glenohumeral instability—Training external rotation, internal rotation, flexion against resistance in the range 45–90°

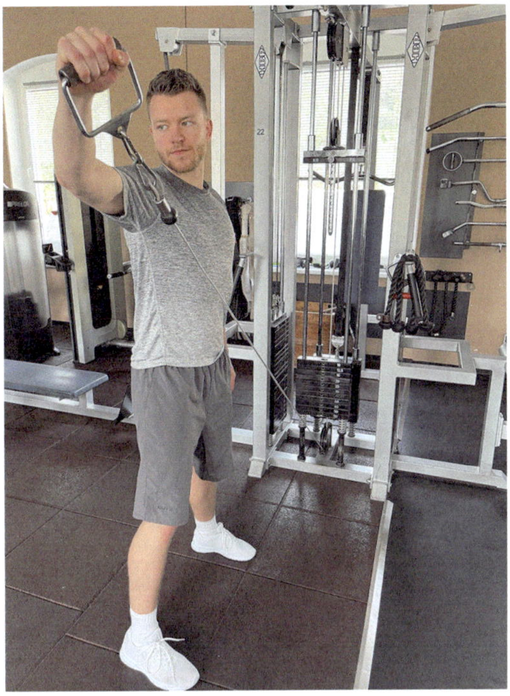

Fig. 5.190 MTT in glenohumeral instability—Strengthening of the M. deltoideus

The meta-analytical information from Lee et al. (2023) suggest that the training program used should be individually adapted to the needs, symptoms, and range of motion of those affected.

A recently conducted randomized controlled study by Wang et al. (2023) dealt with the influence of neuromuscular training and the combination of other therapeutic measures. The neuromuscular training was practiced on a device that allows strength, coordination, balance, and proprioceptive training (cf. Eshoj et al. 2020). In addition, the device enables a visual representation of the body's center of gravity. The sample with the diagnosis of frozen shoulder performed a total of six isometric tension exercises in various joint positions of the shoulder joint. Each joint position was held isometrically for 10 seconds using a Theraband. A rest period of 10 seconds was maintained between the eight sets per exercise. The starting positions included external and internal rotation in neutral position, external and internal rotation in 90° abduction, and external and internal rotation in 90° anteversion. The intensity was progressively increased in five stages by increasing the speed, acceleration, and amplitude of the device. The training was carried out five times a week over a period of two months. In addition, passive and active mobilization techniques and stretching exercises were practiced. This approach significantly reduced pain intensity and at the same time significantly increased the active anteversion, external and internal rotation in mobility (cf. Wang et al. 2023).

A randomized controlled study, which also used biofeedback, was conducted in 2020 by Mohamed et al. A motion sensor was attached to the skin in the area of the scapula spine. This sensor was able to detect the rotation of the scapula during abduction. The subjects were asked to actively move into shoulder joint abduction with maximum possible scapular rotation over a period of 15 minutes. As the scapular rotation increased, which was measured by the sensor, a louder auditory feedback occurred. In addition, a hot pack and passive scapula mobilization were practiced. Over a period of two weeks, three therapy sessions of 40 minutes each were conducted weekly. This approach significantly improved the external rotation of the scapula as well as the range of motion in anteversion, abduction, and external rotation of the shoulder joint and also the degree of pain and disability. These effects lasted six months after the end of the intervention period (cf. Mohamed et al. 2020).

Lin et al. (2022) were able to show that the implementation of techniques from the concept of proprioceptive-neuromuscular-facilitation in the area of the shoulder girdle or in the area of the shoulder girdle is a suitable means for the therapy of subjects with frozen shoulder.

The Shoulder-Pain-and-Disability-Index can be used as an assessment (cf. Mohamed et al. 2020). More detailed information on the individual assessments can be taken from the assessment list in the appendix of this book.

Useful visualizations can be taken from Fig. 5.192, 5.193 and 5.194.

Summary for Practice

The combination of medical training therapy and other interventions can positively influence both mobility and pain in patients with frozen shoulder. These include, among others, muscle-energy techniques, neuromuscular training, training with biofeedback, strength, coordination, and balance training, and proprioceptive-neuromuscular-facilitation in the area of the shoulder girdle. Hot packs and passive scapula mobilizers can also positively influence the result. The exercises should always be adapted to the needs, symptoms, and range of motion and be continuously completed as home exercises. An intra-articular corticosteroid supply in combination with a home exercise program can also have a positive effect.

Fig. 5.191 provides an overview of the mentioned information.

5.7.3 Impingement Syndrome

In their meta-analysis, Dong et al. (2015) recognized that the application of medical training therapy in impingement syndrome of the shoulder gains effectiveness when coupled with other measures. These combinable therapeutic measures include, for example, kinesiotape or acupuncture. It is also mentioned that surgical procedures should be implemented with caution, as medical training therapy can produce

Categories	Evidence-based training recommendation
Units	2-8 weeks, recommended 3-5 times per week, recommended 40-60 minutes per session
Exercises	Muscle energy techniques for the shoulder girdle and shoulder joint / neuromuscular training on the device (strength, coordination, balance, proprioceptive training) / isometric tension exercises with Theraband in various joint positions for 10 seconds, tension in external rotation, internal rotation in 0 position, tension in external rotation, internal rotation in 90° abduction, tension in external rotation, internal rotation in 90° anteversion / adjust intensity by increasing the speed and amplitude of the device, the acceleration and amplitude of the device / passive mobilization techniques of the scapula in all directions / biofeedback using a movement sensor on the skin in the area of the scapular spine) which detects the abduction and becomes louder the more scapular rotation occurs during an active shoulder joint abduction, exercise period 15 minutes / hot pack / PNF in the area of the shoulder girdle
Exercise parameters	Tension exercises: 8 sets of 10 Hold for seconds, pause time 10 Seconds / All other exercises: recommended 3-5 sets of 10-15 repetitions each

Fig. 5.191 Summary of MTT in Frozen Shoulder

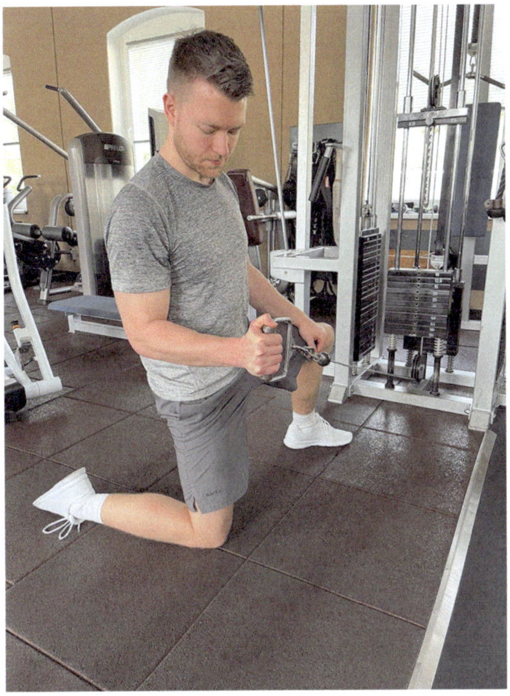

Fig. 5.192 MTT in Frozen Shoulder—Tension in External, Internal Rotation in 0 Position

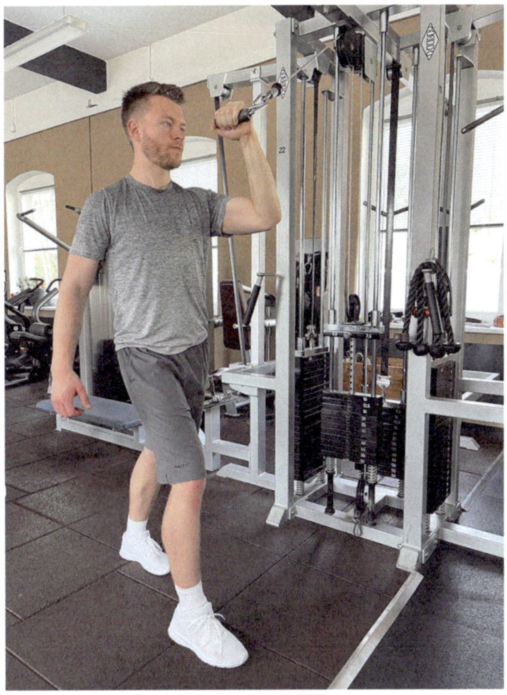

Fig. 5.194 MTT in Frozen Shoulder—Tension in External, Internal Rotation in 90° Anteversion

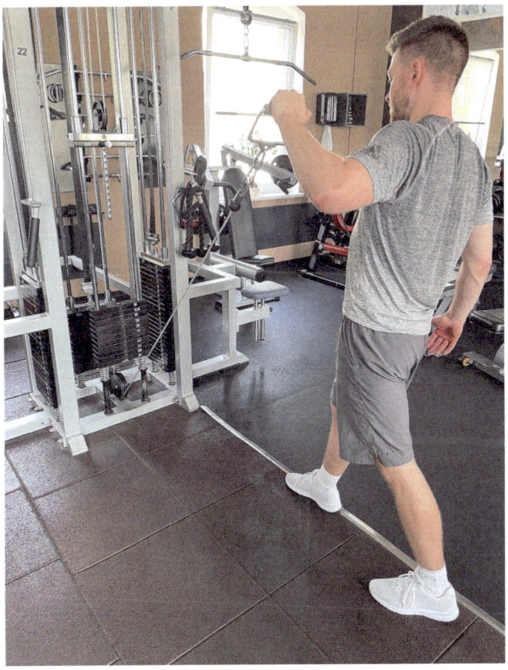

Fig. 5.193 MTT in Frozen Shoulder—Tension in External, Internal Rotation in 90° Abduction

simultaneous results in many cases (see Dong et al. 2015).

When comparing specific and global training approaches regarding impingement syndrome, no significant differences were found in the six included randomized controlled studies (see Shire et al. 2017).

Park et al. (2020) recognized that the size of the subacromial space does not represent a relationship to subacromial pain. Neither surgical nor training therapeutic care should therefore focus on enlarging the subacromial space. Rather, the inclusion of psychosocial factors should be pursued (see Park et al. 2020).

A randomized controlled study by Al Anazi et al. (2022) investigated the influence of an increase in grip strength on subacromial impingement syndrome. 58 subjects aged between 18-50 years underwent two training sessions per week over a period of two months. The control group practiced ultrasound, stretches of the external rotators of the shoulder joint, the pectoralis major muscle, and the

Categories	Evidence-based training recommendation
Units	8 weeks á 2 units per week
Exercises	Strength training of grip strength with equipment in the following positions (in 30°, 60°, 90° abduction of the shoulder joint with extended elbow, in 90° abduction with 90° elbow flexion) / general strengthening of the rotator cuff in external and internal rotation as well as under external rotation in abduction / strengthening of the shoulder girdle muscles / PNF
Exercise parameters	3 sets of 10 repetitions each, adjusting the resistance every two weeks
Elongation	Stretching the external rotators of the shoulder joint, pectoralis major muscle, posterior shoulder muscles, pectoralis minor muscle, levator scapulae muscle, latissimus dorsi muscle, trapezius pars descendens muscle, posterior shoulder joint capsule / Positioning the thoracic spine in extension / For all stretches, 10 sets of 10 seconds holding time each

Fig. 5.195 Summary of MTT in Impingement Syndrome

posterior shoulder musculature, and received ice application. Each stretch was practiced for 10 sets with a hold time of 10 seconds. In addition, the thoracic spine was positioned in extension for 10 sets of 10 seconds while sitting. The intervention group additionally performed grip strength training in various starting positions of the shoulder joint. The starting positions included 30°, 60°, and 90° shoulder abduction with extended elbow joint. In addition, grip strength was trained in 90° abduction with simultaneous 90° elbow flexion. Three sets of 10 repetitions were performed for each starting position. The resistance of the grip strength training device was adapted to the current performance level every two weeks. The application of the combined training variant of the intervention group resulted in a significant reduction in pain with simultaneous functional improvement. In addition, the strength of the rotator cuff could be significantly increased. The pain-free range of motion of the movement directions anteversion, abduction, and external rotation could also be significantly expanded. Therefore, the addition of grip strength training to conventional therapeutic measures is recommended (see AlAnazi et al. 2022).

Tahran and Yeşilyaprak (2020) also advocate the application of stretching exercises for the posterior shoulder musculature.

There is evidence that the combination of conventional physiotherapy or myofascial release techniques and interventions from the concept of proprioceptive neuromuscular facilitation can make a positive contribution to the therapy of subacromial impingement syndrome (see İğrek and Çolak 2022; Çelik et al. 2022).

Turgut et al. (2017) conclude that progressive strengthening of the rotator cuff in combination with stretching exercises of the shoulder girdle or shoulder joint muscles represents a sensible training therapeutic strategy for reducing pain intensity or alleviating the degree of disability. The muscles examined in relation to stretching exercises include the pectoralis minor muscle, the levator scapulae muscle, the latissimus dorsi muscle as well as the posterior shoulder muscles or posterior shoulder capsule. In the strengthening exercises, training should be done under progressive resistance into external rotation, internal rotation, and external rotation into abduction. Three sets of 10 repetitions each are recommended (see Turgut et al. 2017).

Eliason et al. (2021) were able to improve both the functional and pain situation in people with subacromial impingement through the combination of training therapy and passive translational humeral head mobilization. In addition to training the rotator cuff and stretching the pectoralis major muscle or the trapezius pars descendens muscle, the training execution focused on strengthening the shoulder girdle muscles (see Eliason et al. 2021).

Among other things, the Constant-Murley score and the Disabilities-of-the-Arm-Shoulder-and-Hand score serve as assessments (see İğrek and Çolak 2022). In addition, the Shoulder-Rating-Questionnaire can be used (see Schydlowsky et al. 2022). More detailed information on the individual assessments can be taken from the assessment list in the appendix of this book.

Useful visualizations can be taken from Fig. 5.196, 5.197, 5.198, 5.199 and 5.200.

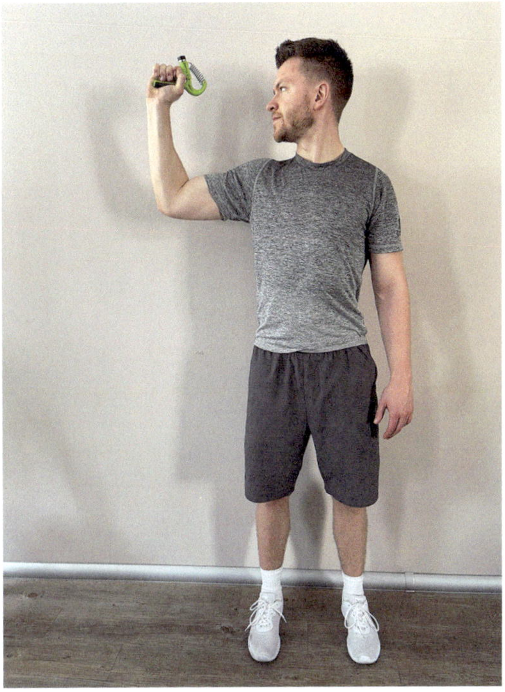

Fig. 5.197 MTT in Impingement Syndrome—Grip strength training with device at 90° abduction with 90° flexion in the elbow

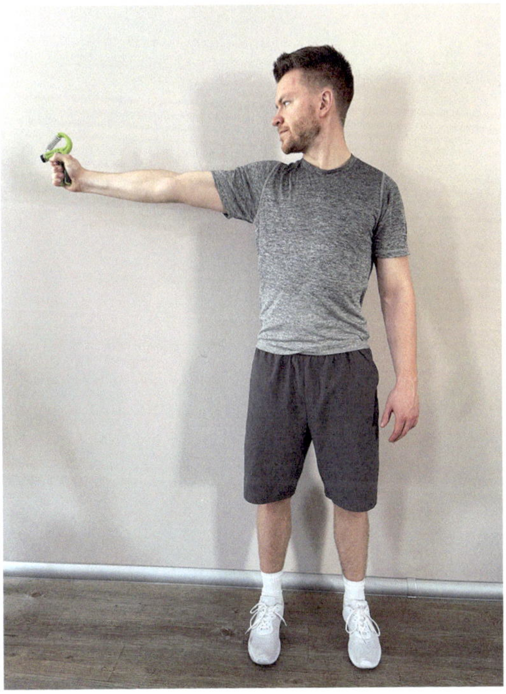

Fig. 5.196 MTT in Impingement Syndrome—Grip strength training with device at 30°, 60°, 90° abduction of the shoulder joint with extended elbow

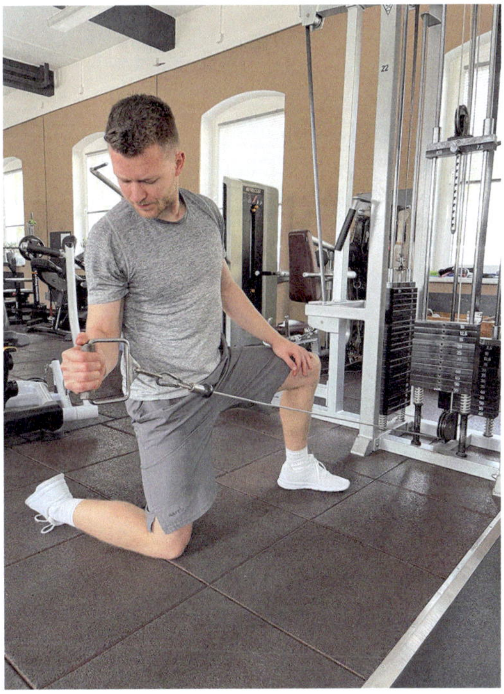

Fig. 5.198 MTT in Impingement Syndrome—General strengthening of the rotator cuff in external rotation

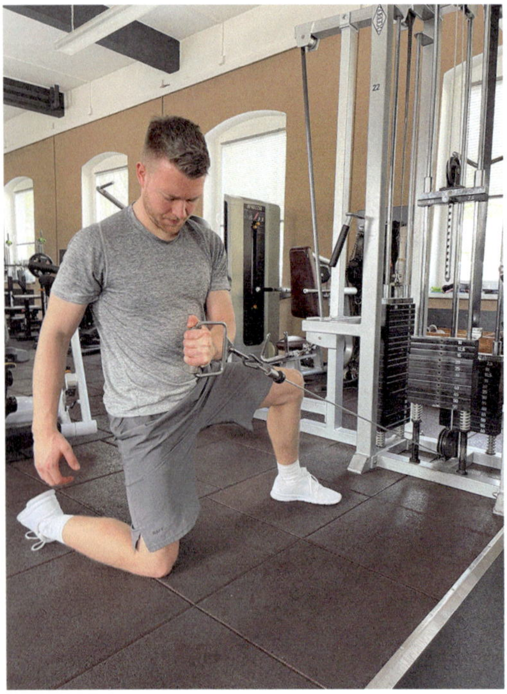

Fig. 5.199 MTT in Impingement Syndrome—General strengthening of the rotator cuff in internal rotation

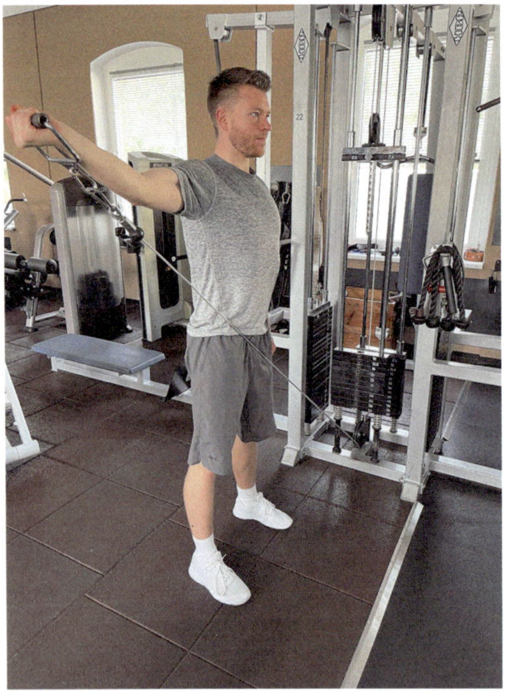

Fig. 5.200 MTT in Impingement Syndrome—General strengthening in abduction under maintained external rotation position

Summary for Practice

The study situation regarding medical training therapy for impingement syndrome in the area of the shoulder joint is very diverse and can overall lead to a reduction in pain and an improvement in function. All are united by targeted training in the area of strengthening the rotator cuff and grip strength as well as stretching the muscles in the area of the shoulder girdle and shoulder joint (shoulder joint external rotators, pectoralis major, posterior shoulder muscles, pectoralis minor, levator scapulae, latissimus dorsi, trapezius pars descendens) and the posterior shoulder joint capsule. Passive translational humeral head mobilization, proprioceptive-neuromuscular-facilitation, ultrasound, acupuncture and kinesiotaping as well as myofascial release techniques can also have a positive effect on pain intensity and the degree of disability.

It is advisable to initially prefer the conservative path to the surgical path, as medical training therapy can produce simultaneous results in many cases.

Fig. 5.195 provides an overview of the information mentioned.

5.7.4 Scapular Dyskinesis

The medical training therapy for scapular dyskinesis can be individually adapted to the dysfunction of the affected person. For this, the position of the scapula should be assessed by inspection in statics. In addition, an assessment of the dynamics should be made through movements of the shoulder girdle and shoulder joint (see Dexel et al. 2014).

Nowotny et al. (2018) recognized that a specific alignment of medical training therapy to the scapula-controlling musculature in the presence of scapular dyskinesis is capable of significantly reducing pain intensity. Kamonseki et al. (2023) advocate for the application of both specific and general training of the scapula-surrounding musculature in scapular dyskinesis.

Targeted posture training in those affected by scapular dyskinesis is capable of significantly reducing pain and improving quality of life (see Amorim et al. 2014).

Among other things, the SICK-scapula-rating-scale serves as an assessment (see Nowotny et al. 2018). In addition, the Disabilities-of-the-Arm-Shoulder-and-Hand-questionnaire can be used (see Amorim et al. 2014). More detailed information on the individual assessments can be taken from the assessment list in the appendix of this book.

Summary for Practice

Medical training therapy can have a positive influence on pain intensity and quality of life in patients with scapular dyskinesis. For this, it is important to analyze the statics and dynamics in advance in order to specifically train the scapula-controlling or scapula-surrounding musculature.

Fig. 5.201 provides an overview of the mentioned information.

5.8 Elbow Joint Area

5.8.1 Lateral Epicondylopathy of the Humerus

The results of Hoogvliet et al. (2013) suggest that medical training therapy in the form of strength training and stretching exercises can contribute to symptom reduction in existing lateral epicondylopathy of the humerus.

In terms of strength training, the application of eccentric exercise execution is recommended (see Landesa-Piñeiro and Leirós-Rodríguez 2022; Tyler et al. 2010). Cullinane et al. (2014) were able to determine an effect of eccentric training in a systematic review. In addition to an analgesic effect, an improvement in function and grip strength was induced. Giray et al. (2019) achieved the best results in their study with a combination of progressive eccentric hypertrophy training of the wrist flexors and wrist extensors, stretching of the forearm muscles, and a Kinesio tape application of the wrist extensors. When comparing different forms of training, it was shown that the eccentric-concentric exercise execution in combination with isometric contractions is the most effective form of training to reduce pain in tennis elbow (see Stasinopoulos D. and Stasinopoulos I. 2017). Viswas et al. (2012) recommend, in addition to eccentric strengthening of the wrist extensors with extended and pronated elbow joint, the stretching of the extensor carpi radialis brevis muscle.

Yilmaz et al. (2022) provide evidence for the application of neurodynamic mobilization of the radial nerve in relation to pain relief in lateral epicondylopathy of the humerus. For this, a home exercise program was carried out daily over a period of six weeks.

In a randomized controlled study, Schiffke-Juhász et al. (2021) demonstrated the effectiveness of training with the Flexibar®. The study included a sample of 71 people who had suffered from tennis elbow for more than three months. Over a period of twelve weeks, the intervention group trained daily for nine minutes with the Flexibar®. The exercises were performed in front of the body, to the side of the body, and overhead. The grip position varied depending on the starting position between

Categories	Evidence-based training recommendation
Exercises	As an initial assessment of the statics and dynamics of the scapula / Targeted strength training of the scapula muscles based on the findings

Fig. 5.201 Summary of MTT in Scapular Dyskinesis

a neutral, a pronated, and a supinated position. After the intervention period, the pain situation, grip strength, and quality of life improved significantly (see Schiffke-Juhász et al. 2021).

Assessments include, among others, the patient-rated tennis-elbow-evaluation, the Pain-visual-analogue-scale, the assessment of grip strength, and the disabilities-of-the-arm-shoulder-and-hand-scales (see Giray et al. 2019). More detailed information on the individual assessments can be found in the assessment list in the appendix of this book.

Useful visualizations can be found in Fig. 5.203, 5.204, 5.205 and 5.206.

Summary for Practice

A targeted medical training therapy can positively influence the pain intensity, function, grip strength, and quality of life in patients with tennis elbow. The focus is on strength training in the sense of eccentric hypertrophy training of the wrist extensors and flexors, as well as the stretching of the M. extensor carpi radialis brevis. A Kinesiotape application to the wrist extensors can positively influence the process and should therefore be applied additionally. Furthermore, a daily neurodynamic self-mobilization of the N. radialis over six weeks can alleviate symptoms.

Also, a daily 9-minute training with the Flexibar® in various starting positions has a positive effect on the symptoms.

Fig. 5.202 provides an overview of the mentioned information.

5.9 Wrist Area

5.9.1 Carpal Tunnel Syndrome

In a randomized controlled study, the intervention of neurodynamic mobilization was compared to a training program for the therapy of carpal tunnel syndrome using the data sets of 41 individuals. The neurodynamic group received a weekly therapy session of 60 minutes over a period of one month. During this, neurodynamic mobilizations of the median nerve were performed under supervision. Subsequently, the subjects were asked to perform two neurodynamic auto-mobilization units at home daily. The training group also received a supervised

Categories	Evidence-based training recommendation
Units	Neurodynamic mobilization of the radial nerve 6 weeks, 15 minutes daily recommended /Training with the Flexibar® 12 weeks, 9 minutes daily
Exercises	Eccentric hypertrophy training of wrist flexors and extensors / eccentric-concentric exercise execution with isometric contractions of wrist flexors and extensors / execution with extended and pronated elbow joint / neurodynamic mobilization of radial nerve as self-mobilization / training with flexibar in front of the body, sideways to the body, overhead, each with grip in neutral, pronated, supinated position
Elongation	Stretching the forearm muscles and explicitly the extensor carpi radialis brevis muscle

Fig. 5.202 Summary MTT for Epicondylopathia lateralis humeri

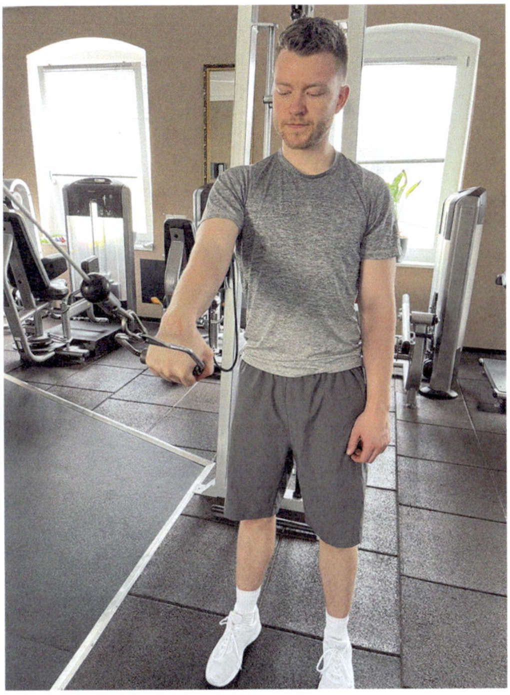

Fig. 5.203 MTT for Epicondylopathia lateralis humeri—Eccentric hypertrophy training of wrist flexors with extended and pronated elbow joint

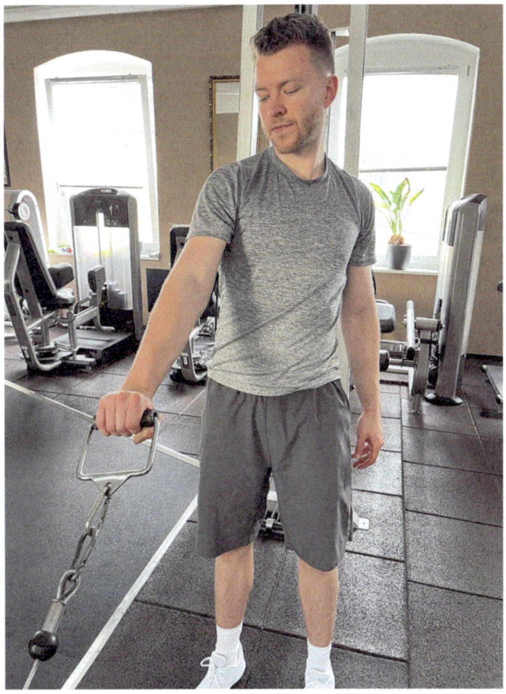

Fig. 5.204 MTT for Epicondylopathia lateralis humeri—Eccentric hypertrophy training of wrist extensors with extended and pronated elbow joint

therapy session weekly over a period of one month. In addition, the exercises were practiced twice daily at home. In addition to tendon gliding exercises, strengthening exercises for the forearm and hand muscles, stretching exercises, and active mobility exercises were used. After evaluating the collected data, it became apparent that both interventions contribute to a positive development. However, the neurodynamic intervention was superior to the training program in terms of pain reduction, improvement of strength, and functional improvement (see Hamzeh et al. 2021).

The implementation of nerve and tendon glide mobilization can also be used in pregnant women with the aim of symptom reduction and simultaneous improved function (see Keskin et al. 2020). Ijaz et al. (2022) also recommend the addition of neurodynamic mobilization to classical care based on a sample suffering from carpal tunnel syndrome for less than three months.

In a review, Page et al. (2012) point to the limited to very poor evidence of the effectiveness of medical training therapy or mobilization techniques. At the same time, the need for high-quality literature is described. In a meta-analysis, which checked the effectiveness of neurodynamic mobilization, no clinical relevance of the measure could be determined for mild to moderate carpal tunnel syndrome (see Paraskevopoulos et al. 2023). In contrast to this are the results of Arenas-Arroyo et al. (2021). Despite great uncertainty, they were able to demonstrate a positive effect of neurodynamic mobilization in terms of pain and function (see Arenas-Arroyo et al. 2021).

Assessments include the Symptom-Severity-Scale, the Functional-Status-Scale, and the Shortened-version-of-the-Disabilities-of-the-Arm-Shoulder-and-Hand. In addition, grip strength and the Numerical-Pain-Rating-Scale can be assessed (see Hamzeh et al. 2021; Ijaz et al. 2022). More detailed information on the

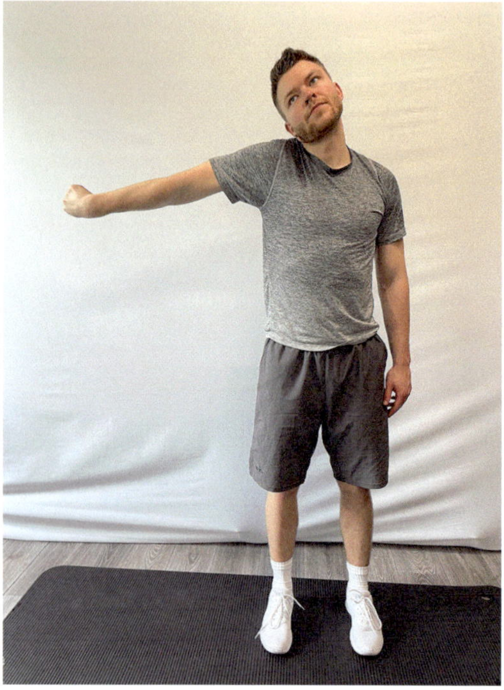

Fig. 5.205 MTT for Epicondylopathia lateralis humeri—Neurodynamic self-mobilization N. radialis as self-mobilization

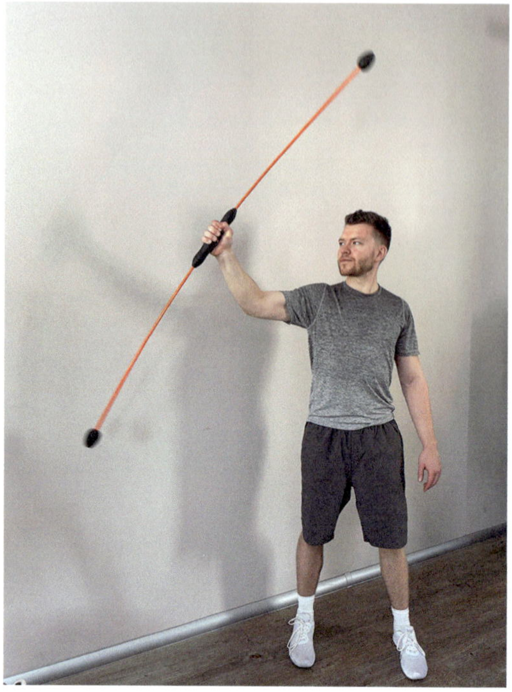

Fig. 5.206 MTT for Epicondylopathia lateralis humeri—Training with Flexibar in front of the body, to the side of the body, overhead each with grip in neutral, pronated, supinated position

individual assessments can be taken from the assessment list in the appendix of this book.

Useful visualizations can be found in Fig. 5.208 and 5.209.

Summary for Practice

In patients suffering from carpal tunnel syndrome, the focus should be on the neurodynamic mobilization of the median nerve as well as on the strengthening and stretching of the forearm and hand muscles. Active mobility exercises can also contribute to a positive development.

Fig. 5.207 provides an overview of the mentioned information.

Categories	Evidence-based training recommendation
Units	4 weeks, 2x daily 2 exercises plus once a week for 60 minutes under supervision
Exercises	Neurodynamic mobilization of the median nerve / tendon gliding exercises / strengthening exercises for forearm and hand muscles / active mobility exercises
Elongation	Stretching the forearm and hand muscles

Fig. 5.207 Summary of MTT in Carpal Tunnel Syndrome

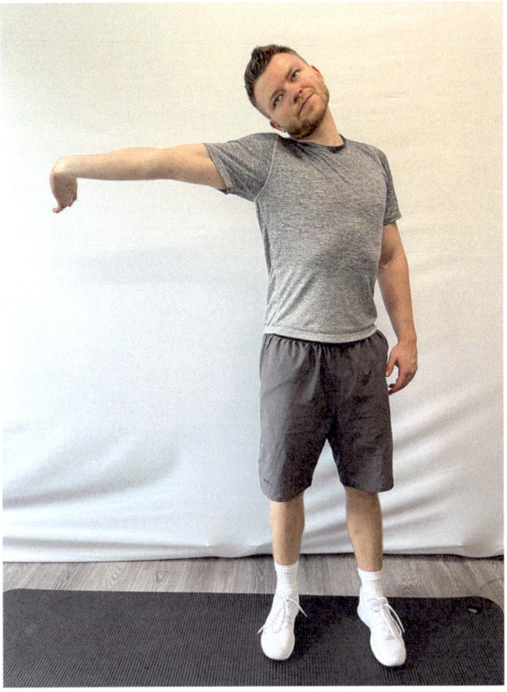

Fig. 5.208 MTT in Carpal Tunnel Syndrome—Neurodynamic Mobilization of the Median Nerve

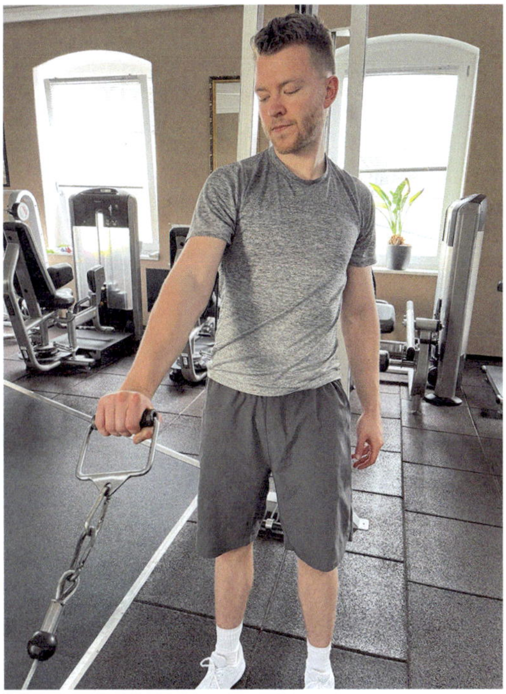

Fig. 5.209 MTT in Carpal Tunnel Syndrome—Strengthening Exercises for Forearm and Hand Muscles

Appendix

	Assessmentlise
6m-timed-up-and-hop-Test	The 6m-timed-up-and-go-Test is a simple assessment aimed at evaluating the functional mobility and balance of individuals, particularly older adults or individuals post-surgery. The test involves getting up from a chair, quickly walking a distance of six meters, turning around, returning to the chair, and sitting down again, with the time taken being measured to draw conclusions about the person's mobility.
6-Point-Likert-Scale	The 6-Point-Likert-Scale is a quantitative research tool used to capture individuals' attitudes, opinions, or perceptions towards specific statements or questions by offering six response options ranging from strong agreement to strong disagreement. This scale is frequently used in surveys and questionnaires in various fields such as market research, psychology, and social sciences to capture nuances in responses and enable a differentiated analysis of opinion trends or changes in attitudes.
ACL-return-to-sports-after-injury-scale	The ACL-return-to-sports-after-injury-scale is a specific assessment tool that was developed to determine when athletes can safely return to sports after an injury to the anterior cruciate ligament (ACL). It evaluates various factors such as physical performance, psychological well-being, and the specific sports ability of the athlete to make an informed decision about returning to competitive sports.
active-reproduction-of-a-passive-position-test	The Active Reproduction of a Passive Position Test is an assessment that measures an individual's proprioceptive accuracy by evaluating the ability to actively reproduce a previously passively assumed limb position. This test is often used in rehabilitation and sports medicine to assess the sensitivity and awareness of limb positioning following injuries or as part of recovery programs.

	Assessmentlise
Activity-Specific-Balance-Confidence-scale	The Activity-Specific Balance Confidence (ABC) Scale is a subjective assessment tool that measures a person's confidence in their ability to perform various daily activities without falling. It is primarily used in older adults or individuals affected by balance disorders to assess the risk of falls and identify specific intervention areas to improve balance and mobility.
Adam's test	The Adam's test is a clinical examination procedure used to assess spinal curvature, particularly for the identification of scoliosis. During the procedure, the test subject bends forward, with the arms hanging loosely, and the feet together, to reveal any asymmetries or abnormal curvatures of the spine that could indicate scoliosis or other spinal deformities.
ankylosing-spondylitis-quality-of-life-questionnaire	The Ankylosing Spondylitis Quality of Life (ASQoL) Questionnaire is a specific self-assessment tool that was developed to measure the quality of life of individuals with ankylosing spondylitis, a form of inflammatory arthritis that primarily affects the spine. The questionnaire includes questions that focus on various aspects of daily life and the well-being of those affected, in order to assess the impact of the disease on their quality of life and adjust the treatment accordingly.
anterior-posterior stability index of the Biodex Balance System	The Anterior-Posterior Stability Index of the Biodex Balance System is a quantitative measure of a person's balance and stability, specifically analyzing forward and backward movements. This assessment is typically used in rehabilitation centers and clinical settings to evaluate balance and postural stability after injuries or in certain diseases, and serves as a basis for the development of individually tailored rehabilitation programs.
Ashworth Scale	The Ashworth Scale is a clinically established instrument for assessing spasticity, that is, the resistance of muscles to passive movements, which occurs in various neurological disorders such as stroke, multiple sclerosis, or after severe traumatic brain injuries. It is applied by a doctor or therapist performing a passive movement in a specific joint and evaluating the resistance to quantify the extent of spasticity, which is of great importance for the planning of treatment and monitoring of progress.
bath-ankylosing-spondylitis-disease-activity-index	The Bath Ankylosing Spondylitis Disease Activity Index (BASDAI) is a patient-completed questionnaire specifically designed to measure disease activity in individuals with ankylosing spondylitis (AS). The index evaluates the intensity of symptoms such as fatigue, back and joint pain, stiffness, and inflammation using a scale, allowing doctors to assess the effectiveness of treatments and make adjustments as needed.
Beck-Depression-Inventory-II	The Beck Depression Inventory-II (BDI-II) is a widely used self-assessment tool used to measure the severity of depression symptoms in adolescents and adults aged 13 and over. It consists of 21 questions, which are rated on a 4-point scale, to capture aspects such as sadness, pessimism, sleep disturbances, and loss of interest in activities, thereby providing professionals with a comprehensive insight into the emotional state of the respondent and enabling them to develop appropriate treatment plans.
Berg Balance Scale	The Berg Balance Scale (BBS) is an objective, clinical assessment tool that was developed to evaluate the static and dynamic balance abilities in older adults. It consists of 14 tasks that include everyday activities such as getting up from a chair, standing on one leg, and walking backwards to assess the risk of falling and plan appropriate preventive measures.
Box-and-Block-Test	The Box-and-Block-Test is a standardized assessment for measuring manual dexterity and hand motor skills, in which a person's ability to move as many small blocks as possible from one area of the box to another within a minute is evaluated. This test is often used in occupational therapy and in the rehabilitation of patients with neurological damage, such as after a stroke, to measure and document progress in hand function and fine motor skills.

	Assessmentlise
British-Medical-Research-Council-questionnaire	The British Medical Research Council (BMRC) questionnaire is a standardized instrument used to assess respiratory function and the impact of respiratory diseases on patients' quality of life. It includes questions about symptoms such as coughing, sputum, shortness of breath, and their influence on everyday activities, thereby providing doctors with a comprehensive overview of the patient's condition and the effectiveness of treatments.
Chronic-Respiratory-Questionnaire-dyspnea-score	The Chronic Respiratory Questionnaire Dyspnea Score is a specialized assessment tool that focuses on measuring dyspnea (shortness of breath) in patients with chronic respiratory diseases. It evaluates how shortness of breath affects the patients' ability to perform everyday activities such as walking, climbing stairs, or carrying loads, and plays a crucial role in planning individual treatment strategies and monitoring disease progression.
Cobb Angle	The Cobb angle is a radiological measurement method used to determine the degree of spinal curvature, particularly in scoliosis. By drawing lines parallel to the endplates of the most tilted vertebral bodies above and below the curvature and then measuring the angle of intersection of these lines, the Cobb angle allows a precise assessment of the severity of scoliosis, which is crucial for treatment planning and monitoring progress.
Constant-Murley Score	The Constant-Murley Score is a comprehensive evaluation system specifically developed for assessing the function and pain of the shoulder. It combines patient self-assessments and clinical tests for pain, daily activities (such as sleeping, working, and leisure activities), range of motion, and muscle strength to provide detailed insight into the condition of the shoulder and monitor the success of treatment measures.
Corbin postural assessment scale	The Corbin Postural Assessment Scale is an instrument for evaluating body posture, which serves to identify postural deviations and asymmetries in children and adults. It is based on a visual assessment of body posture from the side and from the front, with special attention paid to the alignment of the head, shoulders, spine, pelvis, and knees in order to identify potential problem areas and develop targeted intervention strategies.
Cranio-cervical flexion test	The cranio-cervical flexion test is a clinical assessment used to evaluate the function and strength of the deep neck flexor muscles, particularly the longus colli muscle. In this test, the patient performs a series of five graded cranio-cervical flexion movements in a supine position, while an inflatable pressure measurement device is placed under the neck to measure the activation and endurance of the muscles, which is crucial for the diagnosis and treatment of neck pain and dysfunction.
Cumberland-ankle-instability-tool	The Cumberland Ankle Instability Tool (CAIT) is a self-administered questionnaire designed to assess the presence and severity of chronic ankle instability. It includes questions about past injuries, perceived instabilities during daily and athletic activities, as well as pain and functional limitations, making it a valuable tool for diagnosing and planning the treatment of ankle problems.
Disabilities-of-the-Arm-Shoulder-and-Hand-questionnaire	The Disabilities of the Arm, Shoulder, and Hand (DASH) questionnaire is a self-administered instrument that was developed to assess the functional limitations and symptoms of individuals with musculoskeletal disorders of the upper extremities. The questionnaire includes 30 items that relate to physical function, symptoms, and social function, and allows practitioners to assess the impact of the disease on the patients' everyday activities and quality of life, and to monitor the effectiveness of treatments.
Dynamic Gait Index	The Dynamic Gait Index (DGI) is a clinical assessment scale used to evaluate gait safety and balance during walking under various conditions. In this assessment, the patient performs eight specific tasks that mimic everyday challenges, such as walking at altered speeds, overcoming obstacles, and turning around to measure the ability to adapt the gait.

	Assessmentlise
Fear–Avoidance-Beliefs-Questionnaire	The Fear-Avoidance Beliefs Questionnaire (FABQ) is a psychometric tool aimed at assessing patients' beliefs about the relationship between their physical activities or their work and pain, particularly in the context of back pain. The questionnaire helps to gauge the extent to which a person believes that physical activities and work situations could exacerbate their pain, which is essential for planning treatment strategies in pain management and rehabilitation to address and modify maladaptive beliefs.
figure-8-hop-test-for-time	The Figure-8 Hop Test for Time is a functional assessment used to evaluate agility, coordination, and lower extremity function, particularly after injuries such as an anterior cruciate ligament tear. During the test, the person being tested is expected to hop as quickly as possible in a figure-eight around two markers, with the time being measured to assess performance and progress in rehabilitation.
Figure-8-Walk-Tests	The Figure-8-Walk-Test is a functional assessment for evaluating gait agility and control, in which the patient is asked to walk in the shape of an eight to test their ability to change direction and control speed. This test measures the patient's coordination and balance ability and is often used to assess motor skills in individuals with neurological diseases or after injuries.
foot-and-ankle-ability-measure	The Foot and Ankle Ability Measure (FAAM) is a self-reported questionnaire that was developed to assess the functional performance of individuals with various foot and ankle disorders. It consists of two parts: the Activities of Daily Living (ADL) subscale and the Sports subscale, each aiming to capture limitations in everyday activities and sporting endeavors in order to assess the impact of foot and ankle problems on quality of life and monitor the effectiveness of treatments.
foot-lift-test	The Foot Lift Test is a simple, clinical examination that serves to evaluate the strength and stability of the foot and ankle by assessing a person's ability to balance the weight of the body on one foot and lift the other foot off the ground. This test is often used to evaluate functional restoration and balance after injuries to the lower extremity area or in diseases that impair foot function, such as plantar fasciitis or after ankle sprains.
Fugl-Meyer-Assessment-Upper Extremity	The Fugl-Meyer Assessment for the upper extremity is a standardized test procedure specifically developed to assess the degree of motor recovery after a stroke. It includes various tasks that evaluate mobility, motor function, joint function, and sensitivity of the arms and hands, and serves as an important tool in rehabilitation to measure progress and set specific therapy goals for the restoration of upper extremity function.
Functional-Independence-Measure	The Functional Independence Measure (FIM) is a comprehensive assessment tool that was developed to evaluate a person's degree of independence in performing daily activities before and after rehabilitation. It covers 18 items that extend to six areas of physical and cognitive function, including self-care, elimination, mobility, locomotion, communication, and social cognition, and is a crucial tool for planning rehabilitation goals and measuring rehabilitation progress.
Functional Status Scale	The Functional Status Scale (FSS) is an assessment tool used to evaluate the functional status and everyday skills of patients, particularly children with chronic diseases or following acute medical events. It measures the degree of independence and the ability to participate in age-appropriate activities in various areas such as mobility, self-care, communication, and social interaction, which is crucial for the development of individual treatment plans and the monitoring of progress in rehabilitation or long-term care.
Harris-Hip-Score	The Harris Hip Score is a clinically established evaluation system specifically developed for patients after hip surgeries, such as hip joint arthroplasty, to assess pain, function, range of motion, and the ability to perform everyday activities. This instrument helps doctors and therapists evaluate the success of treatment by providing a quantitative measurement of hip function based on the patient's responses to standardized questions, and is crucial for planning postoperative rehabilitation and long-term monitoring of the patient.

	Assessmentlise
HeartQoL	HeartQoL is a specific quality of life questionnaire developed for patients with heart diseases to assess the impact of cardiovascular diseases and treatments on quality of life. It includes questions about physical and emotional aspects associated with heart diseases, including symptoms such as chest pain, shortness of breath, emotional stress, and their influence on everyday activities, and serves as a valuable tool in clinical practice and research to optimize treatment plans and improve patient well-being.
heel-to-buttock test	The heel-to-buttock test is a simple physical examination used to assess the flexibility and range of motion of the quadriceps and the knee joint. In this test, the patient or subject is asked to pull the heel as close as possible to the buttock to identify possible limitations or pain in the front area of the thigh or in the knee joint, which is particularly useful in diagnosing injuries or diseases such as quadriceps shortening or patellofemoral pain syndrome.
Hip-and-Groin-Outcome-Score	The Hip-and-Groin-Outcome-Score (HAGOS) is a patient-specific questionnaire tool that was developed to assess pain, symptoms, physical function in everyday life, sporting activities, participation in sporting activities, and quality of life in young individuals with hip and groin complaints. This assessment is frequently used in clinical practice and research to evaluate the impact of hip and groin diseases and to monitor the effectiveness of treatments, being tailored to the specific needs and challenges of this patient group.
Hop-for-Distance Test	The Hop-for-Distance Test is a functional performance evaluation that aims to measure the strength and stability of the lower extremities, particularly after injuries or surgeries to the knee joint. In this test, the participant is asked to jump off one leg and land as far as possible on the same foot, with the jump distance being measured to assess recovery and the ability to return to athletic activities.
Interactive-Functional-Reach-Test	The Interactive-Functional-Reach-Test is a modern variant of the traditional Functional Reach Test, which measures a person's reach while they lean forward to assess the balance and stability of the trunk muscles. This assessment is often conducted interactively, using technologies such as motion sensors or virtual reality to capture more precise data about the movement dynamics and the patient's responsiveness in real time.
Jebsen-Hand-Function-Test	The Jebsen-Hand-Function-Test is a standardized procedure for assessing fine motor skills and hand dexterity, often used in occupational therapy and rehabilitation. It measures the time a person needs to perform various everyday hand tasks, thereby evaluating the functional performance of the hands.
KOOS- questionnaire-of-pain-and-quality-of-life	The KOOS questionnaire for pain and quality of life is an instrumental assessment used to evaluate the degree of impairment caused by knee injuries or diseases. It is frequently used in clinical trials, orthopedic practices, and rehabilitation facilities to capture the pain, functional limitations, and quality of life of patients with knee problems.
Korean-version-of-fear-avoidance-beliefs- questionnaire	The Korean Fear Avoidance Beliefs Questionnaire is a tool for assessing beliefs and attitudes regarding the avoidance of activities due to pain. It is used in clinical settings as well as in research to capture the extent of fear of pain and the associated avoidance behavior in Korean-speaking patients.
KT-1000-arthrometer	The KT-1000 Arthrometer is a diagnostic instrument used to measure the stability of the anterior cruciate ligament in the knee. It is typically used in orthopedic clinics and rehabilitation facilities to assess injuries to the anterior cruciate ligament and monitor the progress of rehabilitation.
Lumbar-spine-instability-questionnaire	The Lumbar Spine Instability Questionnaire is a tool for assessing symptoms and functional limitations associated with instability of the lumbar spine. It is frequently used in clinical settings, particularly in orthopedics and neurosurgery, to evaluate the impact of lumbar spine instability on the quality of life and functionality of patients.

	Assessmentlise
Lysholm-knee-score	The Lysholm Knee Score is an assessment tool used to evaluate the function and stability of the knee following injuries or surgeries. This questionnaire is frequently used in clinical settings and in orthopedic rehabilitation to measure the condition of the knee as well as the success of the treatment.
Manual-Function-Test	The Manual Function Test is a standardized procedure for assessing hand function and grip ability, used in occupational therapy and rehabilitation. It allows therapists and doctors to evaluate fine motor skills and the strength of the hands, as well as to track progress in the rehabilitation of hand injuries or diseases.
Melbourne Instability Shoulder Score	The Melbourne Instability Shoulder Score is an assessment tool used to measure the functional instability of the shoulder, particularly after injuries or surgeries. It is used in clinical settings such as orthopedic practices and rehabilitation centers to assess the condition of the shoulder, track treatment outcomes, and evaluate rehabilitation progress.
modified-Ashworth-Scale	The modified Ashworth Scale is an instrument for assessing muscle tone and spasticity in patients with neurological disorders such as cerebral palsy or stroke. It is used by doctors and therapists in clinical settings to quantify the severity of spasticity, monitor the course of treatment, and assess the effectiveness of therapeutic interventions.
modified-Biering-Sorensen -test	The modified Biering-Sorensen test is a method for assessing trunk stability and back muscle function by measuring a person's ability to maintain an isometric trunk extension. It is often used in clinical settings such as physiotherapy practices and sports medicine centers to assess the back muscles, especially in patients with back pain or to evaluate the performance of athletes.
modified-Borg-score-during-exercise	The modified Borg score during training is a subjective measure for the perceived exertion or strain during physical activity. It is often used during training and physical rehabilitation to monitor and adjust the intensity of the exercise by asking participants to rate their perceived exertion on a scale.
modified-Rankin-Scale	The modified Rankin Scale is an assessment tool for evaluating functional outcomes after a stroke or other neurological diseases. It is used by doctors and therapists in clinical settings to capture the degree of disability and impairment of daily activities, as well as to assess rehabilitation progress.
Neck Disability Index	The Neck Disability Index is a questionnaire used to assess functional impairment and the impact of neck pain on daily life. It is frequently used in clinical practices, particularly in orthopedics and physiotherapy, to measure the severity of neck complaints, monitor the effectiveness of treatments, and track rehabilitation progress.
Neck-flexors-endurance-test	The Neck-Flexors-Endurance-Test is a specific assessment method that aims to measure the endurance capacity of the neck flexor muscles by recording the duration a person can maintain a certain head position against gravity. This test is often used in clinical and athletic settings to assess muscle strength and endurance in the neck area and is relevant for the development of rehabilitation or training programs, especially after injuries or for the prevention of neck complaints.
Neck-Pain-and-Disability-Scale	The Neck Pain and Disability Scale (NPAD) is a questionnaire that was developed to measure the extent of pain and impairments experienced by individuals with neck complaints. It is typically used in clinical settings to assess the impact of neck pain on daily activities and the quality of life of those affected, and serves as a basis for planning treatment strategies as well as monitoring therapy progress.
Numerical-Pain-Rating-Scale	The Numerical Pain Rating Scale (NPRS) is a simple and widely used method for self-assessment of pain, in which individuals are asked to quantify their pain on a scale from 0 (no pain) to 10 (worst possible pain). This assessment is used in a variety of clinical contexts as well as in research to quickly and effectively measure pain intensity and capture changes over time or in response to treatments. In German, this assessment is known as Numerische Analogskala (NAS) or Numerische Ratingskala (NRS).

	Assessmentlise
one-leg-hop-for-distance-Test	The One-Leg-Hop-for-Distance-Test is a functional performance evaluation that aims to measure leg strength, stability, and balance by assessing the maximum distance a person can cover hopping on one leg. This test is often used in rehabilitation, particularly after injuries to the lower extremity area such as ACL tears, as well as in sports medicine performance diagnostics to evaluate progress in healing and support the decision for a safe return to sports.
Oswestry Disability Index	The Oswestry Disability Index (ODI) is a specific questionnaire used to assess the degree of disability and limitations in daily life due to back pain in patients. It is primarily used in clinical settings to measure the impact of lower back pain on various aspects of everyday life and is an important tool for planning treatment strategies and monitoring therapy success.
Pain-Catastrophizing-Scale	The Pain Catastrophizing Scale (PCS) is a psychological assessment tool used to measure a person's tendency towards catastrophizing thoughts and feelings about pain. It is primarily used in clinical and research-oriented settings to understand how catastrophizing attitudes towards pain influence pain perception, coping, and treatment outcomes, and to develop targeted psychological interventions or therapy approaches.
pain-on-palpation-test	The Pain-on-Palpation Test is a clinical examination method in which pressure is applied to certain body areas or structures to identify pain sensitivity or trigger points. This test is often used by doctors, physiotherapists, and other health professionals to diagnose the cause of pain and to detect inflammation, injuries, or other pathological conditions in muscles, joints, and other tissues.
Pain-Self-Efficacy-Questionnaire	The Pain Self-Efficacy Questionnaire (PSEQ) is a psychometric tool designed to assess the extent of a person's belief in their ability to perform certain activities or behaviors despite pain. It is primarily used in clinical settings to measure the self-efficacy expectations of patients with chronic pain, which is crucial for planning individual treatment strategies and promoting coping mechanisms.
Pain-visual-analogue-scale	The Pain Visual Analogue Scale (VAS) is a measurement tool used to assess pain intensity by asking patients to place their pain on a line without scale divisions, which typically ranges from "no pain" to "worst possible pain". This simple and effective assessment is widely used in clinical and research-related contexts to quickly capture a person's subjective perception of pain and track changes over time or in response to treatments.
passive-reproduction-of-a-passive-position-test	The Passive Reproduction of a Passive Position Test is a neuromuscular assessment method that aims to measure a person's proprioceptive accuracy by checking their ability to reproduce a previously assumed limb position without visual aids. This test is often used in rehabilitation and in sports medicine assessment to evaluate proprioceptive function after injuries and to monitor the effectiveness of rehabilitation programs, especially in injuries that affect the joints.
patient-rated tennis-elbow-evaluation	The Patient-Rated Tennis Elbow Evaluation (PRTEE) is a specific questionnaire developed to assess pain intensity and functional impairments in patients with tennis elbow (lateral epicondylitis). It is used in clinical settings to determine the extent of symptoms and the impact on daily activities and quality of life of those affected, which is essential for planning treatment strategies and monitoring therapy success.
quality of life (QoL)	Quality of Life (QoL) Assessments encompass a range of questionnaires and scales aimed at evaluating a person's overall well-being and quality of life from their own perspective. These assessments are applied in a variety of contexts, including clinical research, public health, and in direct patient care, to understand and monitor the impact of diseases, disabilities, and treatments on daily life and the subjective satisfaction of individuals.

	Assessmentlise
roland-morris-disability-questionnaire	The Roland-Morris Disability Questionnaire (RMDQ) is a specific assessment tool that was developed to measure the functional impairments experienced by individuals with back pain in their daily lives. It is primarily used in clinical and research environments to assess the degree of disability and changes in the patient's condition over time, which is crucial for planning treatment strategies and monitoring therapy progress in individuals with acute and chronic back pain.
Roland-Morris-low-back-pain-and-disability-questionnaire	The Roland-Morris Low Back Pain and Disability Questionnaire is an assessment tool specifically designed for individuals with low back pain to capture the extent of their functional impairments in daily life. This questionnaire is frequently used in clinical settings as well as in research to evaluate the impact of back pain on daily activities and to monitor the effectiveness of treatments, which is crucial for the development of individual therapy plans and the improvement of patient care.
Romberg Test	The Romberg Test is a neurological examination method used to assess a patient's balance and proprioceptive function. During the test, the patient stands with closed eyes and feet together to determine whether there are any fluctuations or impairments in balance, which could indicate disturbances in the sensorimotor system.
Scoliosis-Research-Society-22-questionnaire	The Scoliosis Research Society-22 questionnaire (SRS-22) is a specialized assessment tool designed to capture the quality of life of individuals with scoliosis in terms of pain, function, self-image, and mental health. It is primarily used in clinical and research contexts to evaluate the impact of scoliosis on the daily life of those affected and to monitor the outcomes of conservative or surgical treatments, which is crucial for individual treatment planning and adjustment.
self-paced walking test	The Self-Paced Walking Test is an evaluation method in which the test subject is asked to walk a certain distance at their own speed choice, based on their comfort and abilities, to measure their endurance and functional mobility. This test is often used in clinical settings as well as in rehabilitation medicine to assess the progress of patients with various health conditions, including cardiovascular diseases, respiratory diseases, and after orthopedic procedures, and to adjust individual training and rehabilitation programs.
Short-Form-36	The Short-Form-36 (SF-36) is a general health survey questionnaire designed to assess general health states and quality of life from the patient's perspective by covering eight essential health domains, including physical function, bodily pain, general health perception, vitality, social function, emotional role, mental well-being, and role function due to physical problems. It is used in a variety of medical and health-related research contexts as well as in clinical practice to measure treatment impacts, monitor health care, and assess the quality of life of patients with different medical conditions.
Shortened-version-of-the-Disabilities-of-the-Arm-Shoulder-and-Hand	The shortened version of the Disabilities of the Arm, Shoulder and Hand (DASH) questionnaire, known as QuickDASH, is an assessment tool that was developed to measure the degree of impairment and functional limitations in the arms, shoulders, and hands. It is frequently used in clinical settings as well as in research to quickly assess the impact of injuries, diseases, or treatments on the patient's ability to perform everyday tasks, and to monitor the progress and success of rehabilitation measures.
Shoulder-Pain-and-Disability-Index	The Shoulder Pain and Disability Index (SPADI) is a specific questionnaire that was developed to assess pain and functional limitations in the shoulder area. It is frequently used in clinical settings to measure the impact of shoulder complaints on daily activities and the overall quality of life of those affected, and is an important tool for planning treatment strategies as well as for monitoring therapy progress in patients with shoulder diseases or injuries.

	Assessmentlise
Shoulder-Rating-Questionnaire	The Shoulder Rating Questionnaire (SRQ) is a diagnostic tool used to assess the function and pain level of the shoulder in patients, in order to capture specific impairments and the overall performance of the shoulder. This questionnaire is widely used in orthopedics and sports medicine, both in clinical practice and in research, to evaluate the effects of injuries, diseases, or treatments on shoulder function and to monitor therapy success.
SICK-scapula-rating-scale	The SICK Scapula Rating Scale is a specialized assessment tool used for the diagnosis and evaluation of Scapular Dyskinesis, a dysfunction of the shoulder blade that often occurs in athletes and individuals with shoulder injuries. It assesses the visible signs of shoulder blade misalignments and movements during certain movements and activities, and is primarily used in sports medicine and orthopedic rehabilitation to determine the need for specific therapeutic interventions and to monitor the progress of treatment.
side-hop functional performance test	The Side-Hop Functional Performance Test is a functional assessment that was developed to measure the stability, strength, and endurance of the lower extremity area, particularly after injuries such as an anterior cruciate ligament tear. In this test, the person being tested performs a series of side jumps over a specified distance, which is used in clinical and sports settings to assess suitability for a return to sports activities and to monitor rehabilitation progress.
single-hop-for-distance-test	The Single-Hop-for-Distance Test is a simple but effective functional performance assessment that aims to measure explosive leg power and stability by determining the maximum distance a person can cover with a single hop on one leg. This test is often used in rehabilitation, particularly after injuries to the lower extremities, as well as in athletic performance diagnostics to assess progress in restoring functional mobility and to decide when a safe return to sport or daily life activities is possible.
single-leg-hops-for-time-test	The Single-Leg Hops for Time Test is a functional assessment aimed at measuring the endurance and stability of the lower extremity area by recording the time a person is able to continuously hop on one leg. It is primarily used in rehabilitation after injuries and in sports performance diagnostics to evaluate the restoration of leg function and to determine when a return to sports activities or daily activities is safely possible.
single-leg-landing-test	The Single-Leg Landing Test is a functional assessment tool used to evaluate a person's ability to land safely and effectively on one leg after a jump, indicating the stability, strength, and proprioceptive control of the lower extremities. This test is often used in rehabilitation and sports medicine to assess the risk of injuries, especially in athletes or individuals returning to normal physical activity after an injury, and to develop specific training programs to improve landing technique and strengthen the involved musculature.
single-leg-vertical-jump-test	The Single-Leg Vertical Jump Test measures an individual's vertical jumping performance and explosive power by determining the height of a jump performed with only one leg. It is primarily used in sports medicine and athletic performance evaluations to assess the strength and symmetry of the lower extremities, which is particularly useful for athletes undergoing rehabilitation after injuries, as well as for identifying performance asymmetries that could increase the risk of injury.
sit-to-stand test	The sit-to-stand test is a simple but effective functional assessment that serves to evaluate a person's lower body strength and functional mobility by measuring how often they can stand up from a chair within a certain period of time without using their arms. This test is often used in geriatric assessments, in rehabilitation, and in general physical fitness evaluation to assess the ability to perform everyday activities and to plan appropriate training or rehabilitation programs.

	Assessmentlise
six-min-walk-test	The Six-Minute Walk Test (6MWT) is a simple performance test that measures the maximum distance a person can walk in six minutes on a flat surface, and serves as an indicator of aerobic capacity and endurance. It is widely used in clinical settings, particularly in cardiopulmonary rehabilitation, for the evaluation of patients with heart or lung diseases, but also for assessing the functional mobility and general health status of older people or patients with chronic diseases.
St.-George's-Respiratory-Questionnaire	The St. George's Respiratory Questionnaire (SGRQ) is a specific self-assessment tool that was developed to measure the impact of respiratory diseases on quality of life by capturing symptoms, activity limitations, and perceptions of current health states. This questionnaire is primarily used in clinical and research contexts to assess and monitor the severity and treatment effects in patients with chronic obstructive pulmonary disease (COPD), asthma, and other respiratory conditions.
stability-index-scores	Stability Index Scores are quantitative measurements used in biomechanics and clinical assessments to evaluate a person's balance and postural stability. These scores are typically determined using force platforms or similar technologies that capture the body movements and fluctuations of a standing person under various conditions (such as eyes open/closed, standing on one or two legs), and are particularly important in rehabilitation, sports, and research for assessing injury risk and developing training programs to improve stability.
stair-climb-test	The Stair Climb Test is a functional assessment aimed at measuring a person's leg strength and cardiorespiratory fitness by recording how quickly they can climb a set number of stairs. This test is often used in physical therapy and rehabilitation, as well as in pre- and postoperative evaluation, to assess the functional mobility of patients, especially those with orthopedic or cardiopulmonary diseases, and to monitor progress within the treatment.
star-excursion-balance-test	The Star Excursion Balance Test (SEBT) is a comprehensive assessment method that aims to measure a person's dynamic balance, mobility, and proprioceptive control of the lower extremities by their ability to maintain balance while reaching out with their foot in various directions following a star pattern. This test is often used in rehabilitation, sports medicine, and performance diagnostics to assess injury risk, monitor rehabilitation progress, and to develop individual training programs to improve functional stability and mobility.
Stroke-Impact-Scale	The Stroke Impact Scale (SIS) is a specific assessment tool that was developed to measure the impact of a stroke on the physical function, mobility, hand function, daily activities, communication, emotions, memory, and social participation of the affected individuals. This questionnaire is used in stroke rehabilitation to assess individual impairments and progress, which is crucial for therapy planning, setting rehabilitation goals, and improving the quality of life of the affected individuals.
subjective-international-knee-documentation-committee-score	The Subjective International Knee Documentation Committee (IKDC) Score is a self-reported questionnaire designed to assess the subjective function of the knee, symptoms, and the ability to participate in sports activities from the patient's perspective, particularly in the context of knee injuries and diseases. It is frequently used in clinical settings and research to evaluate the impact of knee problems on daily life and athletic performance, and to monitor the effectiveness of treatments and rehabilitation measures.
Symptom-Severity-Scale	The Symptom Severity Scale (SSS) is an assessment tool used to capture the severity and frequency of specific symptoms, often in relation to mental disorders or other health conditions. It is used in clinical and research contexts to assess a patient's condition, monitor the effects of treatments, and determine the need for therapeutic interventions by providing a quantitative value to the patient's self-reported symptoms.

	Assessmentlise
Tampa-scale-of-kinesiophobia	The Tampa Scale of Kinesiophobia (TSK) is a psychological assessment tool designed to measure fear of movement and re-experiencing anxiety in individuals with chronic pain conditions. It is frequently used in physiotherapy practice, pain therapy, and research to assess the impact of kinesiophobia on rehabilitation and general well-being, and to develop specific therapeutic approaches to overcome these fears.
Tandem Stand	The tandem stand is a balance exercise often used to assess coordination and stability. In this exercise, the patient stands on a line by placing one foot directly in front of the other and tries to maintain this position for a certain period of time, which tests the ability to maintain postural control under challenging conditions.
Tandem gait	The tandem gait is an assessment for checking balance and motor coordination, in which the patient is asked to walk in a straight line, with each step taken so that the heel of one foot touches the tip of the other. This exercise simulates a situation with increased balance requirements and is often used to identify disorders in the areas of the proprioceptive or vestibular systems.
Tegner-level-of-activity-score	The Tegner Activity Level Score is a rating system used to quantify and compare the activity level of individuals before and after knee injuries, particularly cruciate ligament injuries. It is frequently used in orthopedics and sports medicine to evaluate the return to sports and professional activities, and to assess the impact of the injury and subsequent treatment on the patient's quality of life and physical performance.
time-in-balance-test	The Time-in-Balance-Test is an evaluation method for measuring a person's balance and stability by recording the time they can spend in a specific position, often standing on one leg or on an unstable surface, without support. This test is frequently used in physical therapy, in rehabilitation after injuries, and in geriatric assessment to monitor progress in balance ability and to develop individual exercise programs to improve stability and prevent falls.
time-to-boundary measurements	Time-to-Boundary (TTB) measurements are biomechanical analyses used to assess a person's postural stability and balance control by calculating the time it takes for the body's center of gravity to reach a theoretical stability limit. These measurements are primarily used in research and clinical settings to assess the balance abilities of individuals with balance disorders, older adults, and athletes, or to monitor rehabilitation after injuries, providing detailed insights into dynamic balance capabilities.
Timed-Up-and-Go-Test	The Timed-Up-and-Go-Test (TUG) is a simple, standardized assessment used to evaluate mobility, balance, and fall risk, particularly in older adults, by measuring the time it takes for a person to stand up from a chair, walk three meters, turn around, return, and sit down again. This test is frequently used in geriatric medicine, rehabilitation, and home care to assess functional mobility, monitor progress in physical therapy, and plan appropriate interventions to improve mobility or reduce fall risk.
transitional-dyspnea-index	The Transitional Dyspnea Index (TDI) is a clinical assessment tool specifically designed to measure changes in patients' breathlessness symptoms over time, particularly in response to treatment for chronic respiratory diseases such as COPD. The index is used in clinical trials and in everyday clinical practice to evaluate the effectiveness of therapies by capturing the deterioration or improvement of dyspnea (shortness of breath) from the patient's perspective, which can be crucial for adjusting treatment plans.
triple-crossover-hop-test-for-distance	The Triple Crossover Hop Test for Distance is a functional assessment that aims to measure the lateral stability, strength, and coordination of the lower extremities by evaluating the total distance a person can cover in three consecutive lateral hops on one leg. This test is often used in rehabilitation and in sports medicine evaluation to assess progress in recovery after injuries such as cruciate ligament tears and to determine readiness for a safe return to athletic activities.

	Assessmentlise
trunk-flexion-endurance-test	The Trunk Flexion Endurance Test is a physical fitness assessment that aims to measure the endurance capability of the abdominal muscles by recording the time a person can hold a specific trunk flexion position without support. This test is often used in physiotherapy, sports, and fitness assessment to evaluate core strength and stability, which is crucial for the development of training programs to improve posture, performance, and prevent back pain.
visual analogue scale	The Visual Analogue Scale (VAS) is a simple, yet effective tool for measuring the intensity of pain or other subjective sensations, in which patients are asked to mark their current state on a line between two endpoints, representing the minimum and maximum of the sensation. This assessment is widely used in clinical settings, pain research, and patient satisfaction studies to quickly and easily collect subjective data relevant for the evaluation of pain conditions, therapeutic interventions, and patient well-being.
Walter-Reed-Visual-Assessment-Scale	The Walter Reed Visual Assessment Scale is a specific evaluation tool used in orthopedic medicine and rehabilitation to assess the extent of visually perceptible deformities and functional limitations in patients with musculoskeletal diseases or injuries. This scale allows doctors and therapists to evaluate changes in physical appearance and functionality over time through visual observation and patient feedback, which is important for planning treatment strategies and monitoring the progress of rehabilitation measures.
Western Ontario Shoulder Index	The Western Ontario Shoulder Index (WOSI) is a specific questionnaire developed to assess individuals with shoulder complaints, to measure the impact of these complaints on quality of life, physical activity, and pain intensity. It is frequently used in orthopedic practice and research to evaluate the effectiveness of treatment measures, monitor the progress of rehabilitation, and develop individual therapy approaches for patients with shoulder diseases or injuries.
Wolf-Motor-Function-Test	The Wolf Motor Function Test (WMFT) is a functional assessment specifically designed to evaluate the motor skills of patients after a stroke by measuring performance and time to complete everyday motor tasks. It is often used in the rehabilitation of stroke patients to assess progress in restoring arm and hand functions and to develop individually tailored therapy plans to improve motor skills and functional independence.
Y-Balance Test	The Y-Balance Test is a dynamic balance assessment that was developed to measure the functional symmetry and stability of the lower extremities by evaluating a person's maximum reach in three directions (anterior, posteromedial, and posterolateral) from a central standing position. It is frequently used in sports medicine, rehabilitation, and injury prevention to assess the risk of injuries, monitor rehabilitation progress, and develop targeted exercise programs to improve balance and proprioceptive abilities.
Zurich-Claudication-Questionnaire	The Zurich Claudication Questionnaire, also known as the Swiss Spinal Stenosis Questionnaire, is a specifically developed self-assessment tool aimed at measuring the symptoms, functional impairments, and quality of life of patients with spinal stenosis. This questionnaire is used in clinical settings and research to evaluate the severity of symptoms such as pain, numbness, and weakness in the legs, and to assess the effectiveness of conservative or surgical treatments in patients with this condition.

References

Abdi A, Bagheri S, Shekarbeigi Z, Usefvand S, Alimohammadi E (January 2023) The effect of repeated flexion-based exercises versus extension-based exercises on the clinical outcomes of patients with lumbar disk herniation surgery: a randomized clinical trial. Neurol Res 45(1):28–40. https://doi.org/10.1080/01616412.2022.2116686

Acar Y, İlçin N, Gürpınar B, Can G (January 2023) The effects of clinical pilates training on disease-specific indices, core stability, and balance in patients with ankylosing spondylitis. J Bodyw Mov Ther 33:69–75. https://doi.org/10.1016/j.jbmt.2022.09.010

Akkan H, Gelecek N (2018) The effect of stabilization exercise training on pain and functional status in patients with cervical radiculopathy. J Back Musculoskelet Rehabil 31(2):247–252. https://doi.org/10.3233/BMR-169583

Alam F, Raza S, Moiz J, Bhati P, Anwer S, Alghadir A (September 2019) Effects of selective strengthening of tibialis posterior and stretching of iliopsoas on navicular drop, dynamic balance, and lower limb muscle activity in pronated feet: A randomized clinical trial. Phys Sportsmed 47(3):301–311. https://doi.org/10.1080/00913847.2018.1553466

Alammari A, Spence N, Narayan A, Karnad S, Ottayil Z (2023) Effect of hip abductors and lateral rotators' muscle strengthening on pain and functional outcome in adult patients with patellofemoral pain: A systematic review and meta-analysis. J Back Musculoskelet Rehabil 36(1):35–60. https://doi.org/10.3233/BMR-220017

AlAnazi A, Alghadir A, Gabr S (30. August 2022). Handgrip Strength Exercises Modulate Shoulder Pain, Function, and Strength of Rotator Cuff Muscles of Patients with Primary Subacromial Impingement Syndrome. Biomed Res Int 2022:9151831. https://doi.org/10.1155/2022/9151831

Ammendolia C, Hofkirchner C, Plener J, Bussières A, Schneider M, Young J, Ornelas J (19. January 2022) Non-operative treatment for lumbar spinal stenosis with neurogenic claudication: an updated systematic review. BMJ Open 12(1):e057724. https://doi.org/10.1136/bmjopen-2021-057724

Amorim C, Gracitelli M, Marques A, Alves V (July-August 2014) Effectiveness of global postural reeducation compared to segmental exercises on function, pain, and quality of life of patients with scapular dyskinesis associated with neck pain: a preliminary clinical trial. J Manipulative Physiol Ther 37(6):441–447. https://doi.org/10.1016/j.jmpt.2013.08.011

Anwer S, Alghadir A, Shaphe, M, Anwar D (2015) Effects of Exercise on Spinal Deformities and Quality of Life in Patients with Adolescent Idiopathic Scoliosis. Biomed Res Int 2015:123848. https://doi.org/10.1155/2015/123848

Aoyama M, Ohnishi Y, Utsunomiya H, Kanezaki S, Takeuchi H, Watanuki M, Uchida S (July2019) A Prospective, Randomized, Controlled Trial Comparing Conservative Treatment With Trunk Stabilization Exercise to Standard Hip Muscle Exercise for Treating Femoroacetabular Impingement: A Pilot Study. Clin J Sport Med 29(4):267–275. https://doi.org/10.1097/JSM.0000000000000516

Arenas-Arroyo S, Cavero-Redondo I, Torres-Costoso A, Reina-Gutiérrez S, Álvarez-Bueno C, Martínez-Vizcaíno V (December 2021) Short-term Effects of Neurodynamic Techniques for Treating Carpal Tunnel Syndrome: A Systematic Review With Meta-analysis. J Orthop Sports Phys Ther 51(12):566–580. https://doi.org/10.2519/jospt.2021.10533

Arundale A, Bizzini M, Giordano A, Hewett T, Logerstedt D, Mandelbaum B, Snyder-Mackler L (September 2018) Exercise-Based Knee and Anterior Cruciate Ligament Injury Prevention. J Orthop Sports Phys Ther 48(9):A1–A42. https://doi.org/10.2519/jospt.2018.0303

Attar W, Bakhsh J, Khaledi E, Ghulam H, Sanders R (October 2022) Injury prevention programs that include plyometric exercises reduce the incidence of anterior cruciate ligament injury: a systematic review of cluster randomised trials. J Physiother 68(4):255–261. https://doi.org/10.1016/j.jphys.2022.09.001

Bandak E, Christensen R, Overgaard A, Kristensen L, Ellegaard K, Guldberg-Møller J, Henriksen M (April 2022) Exercise and education versus saline injections for knee osteoarthritis: a randomised controlled equivalence trial. Ann Rheum Dis 81(4):537–543. https://doi.org/10.1136/annrheumdis-2021-221129

Bartels E, Juhl C, Christensen R, Hagen K, Danneskiold-Samsøe B, Dagfinrud H, Lund H (23. March 2016) Aquatic exercise for the treatment of knee and hip osteoarthritis. Cochrane Database Syst Rev 3(3):CD005523. https://doi.org/10.1002/14651858.CD005523.pub3

Basbug G, Gurses H, Zeren M, Elmadag N (June 2023) Effects of inspiratory muscle training on respiratory muscle strength, respiratory function and functional capacity in adolescents with idiopathic scoliosis : A randomized, controlled trial. Wien Klin Wochenschr 135(11–12):282–29 https://doi.org/10.1007/s00508-023-02197-1

Bauer R, Wolfram S (2022) Palpationsatlas. Springer-Verlag, Berlin, Heidelberg. https://doi.org/10.1007/978-3-662-64241-2

Bayraktar D, Guclu-Gunduz A, Lambeck J, Yazici G, Aykol S, Demirci H (2016) A comparison of water-based and land-based core stability exercises in patients with lumbar disc herniation: a pilot study. Disabil Rehabil 38(12):1163–1171. https://doi.org/10.3109/09638288.2015.1075608

Bennell K, Nelligan R, Kimp A, Schwartz S, Kasza J, Wrigley T, Hinman R (June 2020) What type of exercise is most effective for people with knee osteoarthritis and co-morbid obesity?: The TARGET randomized controlled trial. Osteoarthritis Cartilage 28(6):755–765. https://doi.org/10.1016/j.joca.2020.02.838

Berschin G, Sommer B, Behrens A, Sommer H-M, (1. (September 2014) Whole Body Vibration Exercise Protocol versus a Standard Exercise Protocol after ACL Reconstruction: A Clinical Randomized Controlled Trial with Short Term Follow-Up. J Sports Sci Med 13(3):580–589

Bieler T, Sobol N, Andersen L, Kiel P, Løfholm P, Aagaard P, Beyer N (2014) The effects of high-intensity versus low-intensity resistance training on leg extensor power and recovery of knee function after ACL-reconstruction. Biomed Res Int 2014:278512. https://doi.org/10.1155/2014/278512

Bitar A, Demange M, D'Elia C, Camanho G (January 2012) Traumatic patellar dislocation: nonoperative treatment compared with MPFL reconstruction using patellar tendon. Am J Sports Med 40(1):114–122. https://doi.org/10.1177/0363546511423742

Bleakley C, Taylor J, Dischiavi S, Doherty C, Delahunt E (July 2019) Rehabilitation Exercises Reduce Reinjury Post Ankle Sprain, But the Content and Parameters of an Optimal Exercise Program Have Yet to Be Established: A Systematic Review and Meta-analysis. Arch Phys Med Rehabil 100(7):1367–1375. https://doi.org/10.1016/j.apmr.2018.10.005

Boudjani R, Challal S, Semerano L, Sigaux J (December 2023) Impact of different types of exercise programs on ankylosing spondylitis: a systematic review and meta-analysis. Disabil Rehabil 45(24):3989–4000. https://doi.org/10.1080/09638288.2022.2140842

Brech G, Guarnieiro R (December 2006) Evaluation of physiotherapy in the treatment of Legg-Calvé-Perthes disease. Clinics (Sao Paulo) 61(6):521–528. https://doi.org/10.1590/s1807-59322006000600006

Bremander A, Dahl L, Roos E (April 2007) Validity and reliability of functional performance tests in meniscectomized patients with or without knee osteoarthritis. Scand J Med Sci Sports 17(2):120–127. https://doi.org/10.1111/j.1600-0838.2006.00544.x

Brijwasi T, Borkar P (January 2023) A comprehensive exercise program improves foot alignment in people with flexible flat foot: a randomised trial. J Physiother 69(1):42–46. https://doi.org/10.1016/j.jphys.2022.11.011

Buyukturan B, Guclu-Gunduz A, Buyukturan O, Dadali Y, Bilgin S, Kurt E (November 2017) Cervical stability training with and without core stability training for patients with cervical disc herniation: A randomized, single-blind study. Eur J Pain 21(10):1678–1687. https://doi.org/10.1002/ejp.1073

Cain M, Ban R, Chen Y-P, Geil M, Goerger B, Linens S, (1. (August 2020) Four-Week Ankle-Rehabilitation Programs in Adolescent Athletes With Chronic Ankle Instability. J Athl Train 55(8):801–810. https://doi.org/10.4085/1062-6050-41-19

Calik B, Kabul E, Taskın H, Atalay O, Aslan U, Tascı M, Yıldız A (September 2018) The efficiency of inspiratory muscle training in patients with ankylosing spondylitis. Rheumatol Int 38(9):1713–1720. https://doi.org/10.1007/s00296-018-4093-2

Campo M, Zadro J, Pappas E, Monticone M, Secci C, Scalzitti D, Graham P (April 2021) The effectiveness of biofeedback for improving pain, disability and work ability in adults with neck pain: A systematic review and meta-analysis. Musculoskelet Sci Pract 52:102317. https://doi.org/10.1016/j.msksp.2021.102317

Ceballos-Laita L, Carrasco-Uribarren A, Cabanillas-Barea S, Pérez-Guillén S, Pardos-Aguilella P, Barrio S (April 2023) The effectiveness of Schroth method in Cobb angle, quality of life and trunk rotation angle in adolescent idiopathic scoliosis: a systematic review and meta-analysis. Eur J Phys Rehabil Med 59(2):228–236. https://doi.org/10.23736/S1973-9087.23.07654-2

Ceballos-Laita L, Jiménez-Del-Barrio S, Marín-Zurdo J, Moreno-Calvo A, Marín-Boné J, Albarova-Corral M, Estébanez-de-Miguel E (November 2022) Comparison of dry needling and self-stretching in muscle extensibility, pain, stiffness, and physical function in hip osteoarthritis: A randomized controlled trial. Complement Ther Clin Pract 49:101667. https://doi.org/10.1016/j.ctcp.2022.101667

Challoumas D, Biddle M, McLean M, Millar N (1. December 2020) Comparison of Treatments for Frozen Shoulder: A Systematic Review and Meta-analysis. JAMA Netw Open 3(12):e2029581. https://doi.org/10.1001/jamanetworkopen.2020.29581

Chen Y, Zhang Z, Zhu Q (4. September 2023) The effect of an exercise intervention on adolescent idiopathic scoliosis: a network meta-analysis. J Orthop Surg Res 18(1):655. https://doi.org/10.1186/s13018-023-04137-1

Childs J, Cleland J, Elliott J, Teyhen D, Wainner R, Whitman J, Association APT (September 2008) Neck pain: Clinical practice guidelines linked to the International Classification of Functioning, Disability, and Health from the Orthopedic Section of the American Physical Therapy Association. J Orthop Sports Phys Ther 38(9):A1–A34. https://doi.org/10.2519/jospt.2008.0303

Cho W, Park C, Kim B (October 2023) Effects of exercise therapy on pain and disability in patients with non-specific neck pain: A systematic review and meta-analysis. J Bodyw Mov Ther 36:213–220. https://doi.org/10.1016/j.jbmt.2023.07.010

Choi G, Raiturker P, Kim M-J, Chung D, Chae Y-S, Lee S-H (October 2005) The effect of early isolated lumbar extension exercise program for patients with herniated disc undergoing lumbar discectomy. Neurosurgery 57(4):764–772. https://doi.org/10.1093/neurosurgery/57.4.764

Choo Y, Chang M (December 2023) The effect of exercise for stabilizing and strengthening core muscles for patients with symptomatic herniated lumbar disc: A systematic review and meta-analysis. Asian J Surg 23(02010–9):S1015-9584. https://doi.org/10.1016/j.asjsur.2023.12.045

Comer C, Williamson E, McIlroy S, Srikesavan C, Dalton S, Melendez-Torres G, Lamb S (16.

September 2023) Exercise treatments for lumbar spinal stenosis: A systematic review and intervention component analysis of randomised controlled trials. Clin Rehabil 2692155231201048. https://doi.org/10.1177/02692155231201048

Cools A, Borms D, Castelein B, Vanderstukken F, Johansson F (February 2016) Evidence-based rehabilitation of athletes with glenohumeral instability. Knee Surg Sports Traumatol Arthrosc 24(2):382–389. https://doi.org/10.1007/s00167-015-3940-x

Cullinane F, Boocock M, Trevelyan F (January 2014) Is eccentric exercise an effective treatment for lateral epicondylitis? A systematic review. Clin Rehabil 28(1):3–19. https://doi.org/10.1177/0269215513491974

Çelik M, Sönmezer E, Acar M (June-December 2022) Effectiveness of proprioceptive neuromuscular facilitation and myofascial release techniques in patients with subacromial impingement syndrome. Somatosens Mot Res 39(2–4):97–105. https://doi.org/10.1080/08990220.2021.2018293

de Jong S, van Caspel D, van Haeff M, Saris D (January 2007) Functional assessment and muscle strength before and after reconstruction of chronic anterior cruciate ligament lesions. Arthroscopy 23(1):21–28. https://doi.org/10.1016/j.arthro.2006.08.024

Dexel J, Kopkow C, Kasten P (March 2014) Scapulothoracic dysbalance in overhead athletes. Causes and therapy strategies. Orthopade 43(3):215–222. https://doi.org/10.1007/s00132-013-2143-8

Diasuke K, Akiraa M, Masatoshia N, Shigekib M, Ichiroa Y, Yoshinaria N, Takahikoa K, (20. (May2013) Dynamic hip stability, strength and pain before and after hip abductor strengthening exercises for patients with dysplastic hips. Isokinet Exerc Sci 21(2):95–100. https://doi.org/10.3233/IES-130480

Doherty C, Bleakley C, Delahunt E, Holden S (January 2017) Treatment and prevention of acute and recurrent ankle sprain: an overview of systematic reviews with meta-analysis. Br J Sports Med 51(2):113–125. https://doi.org/10.1136/bjsports-2016-096178

Dolak K, Silkman C, McKeon J, Hosey R, Lattermann C, Uhl T (August 2011) Hip strengthening prior to functional exercises reduces pain sooner than quadriceps strengthening in females with patellofemoral pain syndrome: a randomized clinical trial. J Orthop Sports Phys Ther 41(8):560–570. https://doi.org/10.2519/jospt.2011.3499

Domenech M, Sizer P, Dedrick G, McGalliard M, Brismee J-M (February 2011) The deep neck flexor endurance test: normative data scores in healthy adults. PM R 3(2):105–110. https://doi.org/10.1016/j.pmrj.2010.10.023

Dong W, Goost H, Lin X.-B, Burger C, Paul C, Wang Z.-L, Kabir K (March 2015) Treatments for shoulder impingement syndrome: a PRISMA systematic review and network meta-analysis. Medicine (Baltimore), 94(10):e510. https://doi.org/10.1097/MD.0000000000000510

Dydyk A, Sapra A (2023) Williams Back Exercises. (S. [Internet], Hrsg.) Treasure Island (FL): StatPearls Publishing

Eliason A, Harringe M, Engström B, Werner S (11. May 2021) Guided exercises with or without joint mobilization or no treatment in patients with subacromial pain syndrome: A clinical trial. J Rehabil Med 53(5):jrm00190. https://doi.org/10.2340/16501977-2806

Elsayed W, Alotaibi S, Shaheen A, Farouk M, Farrag A (June2023) The combined effect of short foot exercises and orthosis in symptomatic flexible flatfoot: a randomized controlled trial. Eur J Phys Rehabil Med 59(3):396–405. https://doi.org/10.23736/S1973-9087.23.07846-2

Emamvirdi M, Letafatkar A, Tazji M (May-June 2019) The Effect of Valgus Control Instruction Exercises on Pain, Strength, and Functionality in Active Females With Patellofemoral Pain Syndrome. Sports Health 11(3):223–237. https://doi.org/10.1177/1941738119837622

Eshoj H, Rasmussen S, Frich L, Hvass I, Christensen R, Boyle E, Juul-Kristensen B (30. January 2020) Neuromuscular Exercises Improve Shoulder Function More Than Standard Care Exercises in Patients With a Traumatic Anterior Shoulder Dislocation: A Randomized Controlled Trial. Orthop J Sports Med 8(1):2325967119896102. https://doi.org/10.1177/2325967119896102

Fernández-Matías R, García-Pérez F, Gavín-González C, Martínez-Martín J, Valencia-García H, Flórez-García M (May2023) Effectiveness of exercise versus arthroscopic partial meniscectomy plus exercise in the management of degenerative meniscal tears at 5-year follow-up: a systematic review and meta-analysis. Arch Orthop Trauma Surg 143(5):2609–2620. https://doi.org/10.1007/s00402-022-04579-y

Fernández-Rodríguez R, Álvarez-Bueno C, Cavero-Redondo I, Torres-Costoso A, Pozuelo-Carrascosa D, Reina-Gutiérrez S, Martínez-Vizcaíno V (August 2022) Best Exercise Options for Reducing Pain and Disability in Adults With Chronic Low Back Pain: Pilates, Strength, Core-Based, and Mind-Body. A Network Meta-analysis. J Orthop Sports Phys Ther 52(8):505–521. https://doi.org/10.2519/jospt.2022.10671

Fernandes T, Méndez-Sánchez R, Puente-González A, Martín-Vallejo F, Falla D, Vila-Chã C (February 2023) A randomized controlled trial on the effects of „Global Postural Re-education" versus neck specific exercise on pain, disability, postural control, and neuromuscular features in women with chronic non-specific neck pain. Eur J Phys Rehabil Med 59(1):42–53. https://doi.org/10.23736/S1973-9087.22.07554-2

Ferreira R, Torres R, Duarte J, Gonçalves R (29 July 2019) Non-Pharmacological and Non-Surgical Interventions for Knee Osteoarthritis: A Systematic Review and Meta-Analysis. Acta Reumatol Port 44(3):173–217

Ferri-Caruana A, Prades-Insa B, Serra-AÑÓ P (August 2020) Effects of pelvic and core strength training on biomechanical risk factors for anterior cruciate ligament injuries. J Sports Med Phys Fitness 60(8):1128–1136. https://doi.org/10.23736/S0022-4707.20.10552-8

Fitzgerald G, Piva S, Irrgang J (September 2003) A modified neuromuscular electrical stimulation protocol for quadriceps strength training following anterior cruciate ligament reconstruction. J Orthop Sports Phys Ther 33(9):492–501. https://doi.org/10.2519/jospt.2003.33.9.492

Flores G, de Oliveira D, Ramos A, Sanada L, Migliorini F, Maffulli N, Okubo R (30. May 2023) Conservative management following patellar dislocation: a level I systematic review. J Orthop Surg Res 18(1):393. https://doi.org/10.1186/s13018-023-03867-6

Freke M, Kemp J, Svege I, Risberg M, Semciw A, Crossley K (October 2016) Physical impairments in symptomatic femoroacetabular impingement: a systematic review of the evidence. Br J Sports Med 50(19):1180. https://doi.org/10.1136/bjsports-2016-096152

Fu C, Yung S, Law K, Leung K, Lui P, Siu H, Chan K (April 2013) The effect of early whole-body vibration therapy on neuromuscular control after anterior cruciate ligament reconstruction: a randomized controlled trial. Am J Sports Med 41(4):804–814. https://doi.org/10.1177/0363546513476473

Fukuda T, Rossetto F, Magalhães E, Bryk F, Lucareli P, Carvalho N (November 2010) Short-term effects of hip abductors and lateral rotators strengthening in females with patellofemoral pain syndrome: a randomized controlled clinical trial. J Orthop Sports Phys Ther 40(11):736–742. https://doi.org/10.2519/jospt.2010.3246

Fukumoto Y, Tateuchi H, Ikezoe T, Tsukagoshi R, Akiyama H, So K, Ichihashi N (January 2014) Effects of high-velocity resistance training on muscle function, muscle properties, and physical performance in individuals with hip osteoarthritis: a randomized controlled trial. Clin Rehabil 28(1):48–58. https://doi.org/10.1177/0269215513492161

Fukumoto Y, Tateuchi H, Tsukagoshi R, Okita Y, Akiyama H, So K, Ichihashi N (June 2017) Effects of High- and Low-Velocity Resistance Training on Gait Kinematics and Kinetics in Individuals with Hip Osteoarthritis: A Randomized Controlled Trial. Am J Phys Med Rehabil 96(6):417–423. https://doi.org/10.1097/PHM.0000000000000640

Gámiz-Bermúdez F, Obrero-Gaitán E, Zagalaz-Anula N, Lomas-Vega R (May 2022) Corrective exercise-based therapy for adolescent idiopathic scoliosis: Systematic review and meta-analysis. Clin Rehabil 36(5):597–608. https://doi.org/10.1177/02692155211070452

Gatz M, Betsch M, Dirrichs T, Schrading S, Tingart M, Michalik R, Quack V (July-August 2020) Eccentric and Isometric Exercises in Achilles Tendinopathy Evaluated by the VISA-A Score and Shear Wave Elastography. Sports Health 12(4):373–381. https://doi.org/10.1177/1941738119893996

Gerber J, Marcus R, Dibble L, Greis P, Burks R, LaStayo P (March 2007) Effects of early progressive eccentric exercise on muscle structure after anterior cruciate ligament reconstruction. J Bone Joint Surg Am 89(3):559–570. https://doi.org/10.2106/JBJS.F.00385

Ghanati H, Letafatkar A, Shojaedin, S, Hadadnezhad, M, Schöllhorn W (15. August 2022) Comparing the Effects of Differential Learning, Self-Controlled Feedback, and External Focus of Attention Training on Biomechanical Risk Factors of Anterior Cruciate Ligament (ACL) in Athletes: A Randomized Controlled Trial. Int J Environ Res Public Health 19(16):10052. https://doi.org/10.3390/ijerph191610052

Gibbs M, Morrison N, Raftry S, Jones M, Marshall P (September 2022) Does a powerlifting inspired exercise programme better compliment pain education compared to bodyweight exercise for people with chronic low back pain? A multicentre, single-blind, randomised controlled trial. Clin Rehabil 36(9):1199–1213. https://doi.org/10.1177/02692155221095484

Giray E, Karali-Bingul D, Akyuz G (July 2019) The Effectiveness of Kinesiotaping, Sham Taping or Exercises Only in Lateral Epicondylitis Treatment: A Randomized Controlled Study. PM R 11(7):681–693. https://doi.org/10.1002/pmrj.12067

Goh S-L, Persson M, Stocks J, Hou Y, Lin J, Hall M, Zhang W (September 2019) Efficacy and potential determinants of exercise therapy in knee and hip osteoarthritis: A systematic review and meta-analysis. Ann Phys Rehabil Med 62(5):356–365. https://doi.org/10.1016/j.rehab.2019.04.006

Goh S-L, Persson M, Stocks J, Hou Y, Welton N, Lin J, Zhang W (May 2019) Relative Efficacy of Different Exercises for Pain, Function, Performance and Quality of Life in Knee and Hip Osteoarthritis: Systematic Review and Network Meta-Analysis. Sports Med 49(5):743–761. https://doi.org/10.1007/s40279-019-01082-0

Gokeler A, Bisschop M, Benjaminse A, Myer G, Eppinga P, Otten E (May 2014) Quadriceps function following ACL reconstruction and rehabilitation: implications for optimisation of current practices. Knee Surg Sports Traumatol Arthrosc 22(5):1163–1174. https://doi.org/10.1007/s00167-013-2577-x

Habets B, van Cingel R, Backx F, van Elten H, Zuithoff P, Huisstede B. (27. October 2021) No Difference in Clinical Effects When Comparing Alfredson Eccentric and Silbernagel Combined Concentric-Eccentric Loading in Achilles Tendinopathy: A Randomized Controlled Trial. Orthop J Sports Med, 9(10):23259671211031254. https://doi.org/10.1177/23259671211031254

Hahne A, Ford J, McMeeken J (15. May 2010) Conservative management of lumbar disc herniation with associated radiculopathy: a systematic review.

Spine (Phila Pa 1976) 35(11):E488–504. https://doi.org/10.1097/BRS.0b013e3181cc3f56

Hall E, Chomistek A, Kingma J, Docherty C (June 2018) Balance- and Strength-Training Protocols to Improve Chronic Ankle Instability Deficits, Part I: Assessing Clinical Outcome Measures. J Athl Train 53(6):568–577. https://doi.org/10.4085/1062-6050-385-16

Hall E, Docherty C, Simon J, Kingma J, Klossner J (January 2015) Strength-training protocols to improve deficits in participants with chronic ankle instability: a randomized controlled trial. J Athl Train 50(1):36–44. https://doi.org/10.4085/1062-6050-49.3.71

Hall M, Allison K, Hinman R, Bennell K, Spiers L, Knox G, Dobson F (18. April 2022) Effects of adding aerobic physical activity to strengthening exercise on hip osteoarthritis symptoms: protocol for the PHOENIX randomised controlled trial. BMC Musculoskelet Disord 23(1):361. https://doi.org/10.1186/s12891-022-05282-0

Hammami N, Mechraoui A, Hattabi S, Forte P, Sampaio T, Sortwell A, Bouassida A (20. July 2023) Concentric Isokinetic Strengthening Program's Impact on Knee Biomechanical Parameters, Physical Performance and Quality of Life in Overweight/Obese Women with Chronic Meniscal Lesions. Healthcare (Basel) 11(14):2079. https://doi.org/10.3390/healthcare11142079

Hamzeh H, Madi M, Alghwiri A, Hawamdeh Z (October-December 2021) The long-term effect of neurodynamics vs exercise therapy on pain and function in people with carpal tunnel syndrome: A randomized parallel-group clinical trial. J Hand Ther 34(4):521–530. https://doi.org/10.1016/j.jht.2020.07.005

Han Y, Duan D, Zhao K, Wang X, Ouyang L, Liu G, (January-February 2017) Investigation of the Relationship Between Flatfoot and Patellar Subluxation in Adolescents. J Foot Ankle Surg 56(1):15–18. https://doi.org/10.1053/j.jfas.2016.10.001

Hansen S, Mikkelsen L, Overgaard S, Mechlenburg I (1. June2020) Effectiveness of supervised resistance training for patients with hip osteoarthritis—a systematic review. Dan Med J 67(6):A08190424

Harpham C, Harpham Q, Barker A (June2022) The effect of exercise training programs with aerobic components on C-reactive protein, erythrocyte sedimentation rate and self-assessed disease activity in people with ankylosing spondylitis: A systematic review and meta-analysis. Int J Rheum Dis 25(6):635–649. https://doi.org/10.1111/1756-185X.14315

Hayden J, Ellis J, Ogilvie R, Stewart S, Bagg M, Stanojevic S, Saragiotto B (October 2021) Some types of exercise are more effective than others in people with chronic low back pain: a network meta-analysis. J Physiother 67(4):252–262. https://doi.org/10.1016/j.jphys.2021.09.004

Hebert J, Fritz J, Thackeray A, Koppenhaver S, Teyhen D (January 2015) Early multimodal rehabilitation following lumbar disc surgery: a randomised clinical trial comparing the effects of two exercise programmes on clinical outcome and lumbar multifidus muscle function. Br J Sports Med 49(2):100–106. https://doi.org/10.1136/bjsports-2013-092402

Hefti F (2015) Kinderorthopädie in der Praxis. Springer, Berlin

Heijne A, Werner S (April 2007) Early versus late start of open kinetic chain quadriceps exercises after ACL reconstruction with patellar tendon or hamstring grafts: a prospective randomized outcome study. Knee Surg Sports Traumatol Arthrosc 15(4):402–414. https://doi.org/10.1007/s00167-006-0246-z

Hlaing S, Puntumetakul R, Khine, E, Boucaut R (30. November 2021) Effects of core stabilization exercise and strengthening exercise on proprioception, balance, muscle thickness and pain related outcomes in patients with subacute nonspecific low back pain: a randomized controlled trial. BMC Musculoskelet Disord 22(1):998. https://doi.org/10.1186/s12891-021-04858-6

Hoang N.-T.-T, Chen S, Chou L.-W (29. July 2021) The Impact of Foot Orthoses and Exercises on Pain and Navicular Drop for Adult Flatfoot: A Network Meta-Analysis. Int J Environ Res Public Health 18(5):8063. https://doi.org/10.3390/ijerph18158063

Hoeksma H, Dekker J, Ronday H, Heering A, van der Lubbe N, Vel C, van den Ende C (15. (October 2014) Comparison of manual therapy and exercise therapy in osteoarthritis of the hip: a randomized clinical trial. Arthritis Rheum 51(5):722–729. https://doi.org/10.1002/art.20685

Hoit G, Whelan D, Dwyer T, Ajrawat P, Chahal J (July 2020) Physiotherapy as an Initial Treatment Option for Femoroacetabular Impingement: A Systematic Review of the Literature and Meta-analysis of 5 Randomized Controlled Trials. Am J Sports Med 48(8):2042–2050. https://doi.org/10.1177/0363546519882668

Honkonen E, Sillanpää P, Reito A, Mäenpää H, Mattila V (June2022) A Randomized Controlled Trial Comparing a Patella-Stabilizing, Motion-Restricting Knee Brace Versus a Neoprene Nonhinged Knee Brace After a First-Time Traumatic Patellar Dislocation. Am J Sports Med 50(7):1867–1875. https://doi.org/10.1177/03635465221090644

Hoogvliet P, Randsdorp M, Dingemanse R, Koes B, Huisstede B (November 2013) Does effectiveness of exercise therapy and mobilisation techniques offer guidance for the treatment of lateral and medial epicondylitis? A systematic review. Br J Sports Med 47(17):1112–1119. https://doi.org/10.1136/bjsports-2012-091990

Hu X, Chen, J, Tang, W, Chen, W, Sang, Y, Jia L (December 2020) Effects of exercise programmes on pain, disease activity and function in ankylosing spondylitis: A meta-analysis of randomized controlled trials. Eur J Clin Invest 50(12):e13352. https://doi.org/10.1111/eci.13352

Hu, H, Zheng, Y, Liu, X, Gong D, Chen, C, Wang, Y, . . . Wang, X. (9. July 2019). Effects of neuromuscular training on pain intensity and self-reported functionality for patellofemoral pain syndrome in runners: study protocol for a randomized controlled clinical trial. Trials 20(1):409. https://doi.org/10.1186/s13063-019-3503-4

Hua J, Sun L, Teng Y (1. April 2023) Effects of High-Intensity Strength Training in Adults With Knee Osteoarthritis: A Systematic Review and Meta-analysis of Randomized Controlled Trials. Am J Phys Med Rehabil 102(4):292–299. https://doi.org/10.1097/PHM.0000000000002088

Huang C, Chen L.-Y, Liao Y.-H, Masodsai K, Lin Y.-Y (22. September 2022) Effects of the Short-Foot Exercise on Foot Alignment and Muscle Hypertrophy in Flatfoot Individuals: A Meta-Analysis. Int J Environ Res Public Health 19(19):11994. https://doi.org/10.3390/ijerph191911994

Huang Y-L, Jung J, Mulligan C, Oh J, Norcross M (May 2020) A Majority of Anterior Cruciate Ligament Injuries Can Be Prevented by Injury Prevention Programs: A Systematic Review of Randomized Controlled Trials and Cluster-Randomized Controlled Trials With Meta-analysis. Am J Sports Med 48(6):1505–1515. https://doi.org/10.1177/0363546519870175

Husby V, Helgerud J, Bjørgen S, Husby O, Benum P, Hoff J (April 2010) Early postoperative maximal strength training improves work efficiency 6–12 months after osteoarthritis-induced total hip arthroplasty in patients younger than 60 years. Am J Phys Med Rehabil 89(4):304–314. https://doi.org/10.1097/PHM.0b013e3181cf5623

Ijaz M, Karimi H, Gillani S, Ahmad A, Chaudhary M (2022) Effect of median nerve neuromobilization on functional status in patients with carpal tunnel syndrome: A double blinded randomized control trial. J Pak Med Assoc 72(4):605–609. https://doi.org/10.47391/JPMA.2212

Ismail M, Gamaleldein M, Hassa K (October 2013) Closed kinetic chain exercises with or without additional hip strengthening exercises in management of patellofemoral pain syndrome: a randomized controlled trial. Eur J Phys Rehabil Med 49(5):687–698

İğrek S, Çolak T (April 2022) Comparison of the effectiveness of proprioceptive neuromuscular facilitation exercises and shoulder mobilization patients with Subacromial Impingement Syndrome: A randomized clinical trial. J Bodyw Mov Ther 30:42–52. https://doi.org/10.1016/j.jbmt.2021.10.015

Jacobi S, Beynon A, Dombrowski S, Wedderkopp N, Witherspoon R, Hébert J (November 2021) Effectiveness of Conservative Nonpharmacologic Therapies for Pain, Disability, Physical Capacity, and Physical Activity Behavior in Patients With Degenerative Lumbar Spinal Stenosis: A Systematic Review and Meta-Analysis. Arch Phys Med Rehabil 102(11):2247–2260. https://doi.org/10.1016/j.apmr.2021.03.033

Jacobsen J, Thorborg K, Sørensen D, Jakobsen S, Nielsen R, Oestergaard L, Mechlenburg I (October 2022) Feasibility and acceptability of a six-month exercise and patient education intervention for patients with hip dysplasia: A mixed methods study. Musculoskeletal Science and Practice 61:102615. https://doi.org/10.1016/j.msksp.2022.102615

Javadian Y, Behtash H, Akbari M, Taghipour-Darzi M, Zekavat H (2012) The effects of stabilizing exercises on pain and disability of patients with lumbar segmental instability. J Back Musculoskelet Rehabil 25(3):149–155. https://doi.org/10.3233/BMR-2012-0321

Javdaneh N, Saeterbakken A, Shams A, Barati A (22. August 2021) Pain Neuroscience Education Combined with Therapeutic Exercises Provides Added Benefit in the Treatment of Chronic Neck Pain. Int J Environ Res Public Health 18(16):8848. https://doi.org/10.3390/ijerph18168848

Jeon N-Y, Chon S-C (2018) Effect of glenohumeral stabilization exercises combined with scapular stabilization on shoulder function in patients with shoulder pain: A randomized controlled experimenter-blinded study. J Back Musculoskelet Rehabil 31(2):259–265. https://doi.org/10.3233/BMR-169612

Jeong H, Lee S-C, Jee H, Song J, Chang H, Lee S (April 2019) Proprioceptive Training and Outcomes of Patients With Knee Osteoarthritis: A Meta-Analysis of Randomized Controlled Trials. J Athl Train 54(4):418–428. https://doi.org/10.4085/1062-6050-329-17

Jeong J, Choi D-H, Shin C (January 2021) Core Strength Training Can Alter Neuromuscular and Biomechanical Risk Factors for Anterior Cruciate Ligament Injury. Am J Sports Med 49(1):183–192. https://doi.org/10.1177/0363546520972990

Jull G, O'Leary S, Falla D (September 2008) Clinical assessment of the deep cervical flexor muscles: the craniocervical flexion test. J Manipulative Physiol Ther 31(7):525–533. https://doi.org/10.1016/j.jmpt.2008.08.003

Kłaptocz P, Solecki W, Grzegorzewski A, Błasiak A, Brzóska R. (29. August 2021) Effectiveness of conservative treatment of multidirectional instability of the shoulder joint. Literature review and meta-analysis. Pol Przegl Chir, 94(1):6–11. https://doi.org/10.5604/01.3001.0015.2415

Kalichman L, Hunter D (March 2008) Diagnosis and conservative management of degenerative lumbar spondylolisthesis. Eur Spine J 17(3):327–335. https://doi.org/10.1007/s00586-007-0543-3

Kamonseki D, Haik M, Ribeiro L, Almeida R, Camargo P (September 2023) Scapular movement training is not superior to standardized exercises in the treatment of individuals with chronic shoulder pain and scapular dyskinesis: randomized controlled trial. Disabil

Rehabil 45(18):2925–2935. https://doi.org/10.1080/09638288.2022.2114552

Kang T, Kim B (30. September 2022) Cervical and scapula-focused resistance exercise program versus trapezius massage in patients with chronic neck pain: A randomized controlled trial. Medicine (Baltimore) 101(39):e30887. https://doi.org/10.1097/MD.0000000000030887

Kastrinis A, Koumantakis G, Tsekoura M, Nomikou E, Katsoulaki M, Theodosopoulos E, Dimitriadis Z (2023) The Effect of Schroth Method on Postural Control and Balance in Patients with Adolescent Idiopathic Scoliosis: A Literature Review. Adv Exp Med Biol 1425:469–476. https://doi.org/10.1007/978-3-031-31986-0_45

Kemp J, Coburn S, Jones D, Crossley K (April 2018) The Physiotherapy for Femoroacetabular Impingement Rehabilitation STudy (physioFIRST): A Pilot Randomized Controlled Trial. J Orthop Sports Phys Ther 48(4):307–315. https://doi.org/10.2519/jospt.2018.7941

Kemp J, King M, Barton C, Schache A, Thorborg K, Roos E, Crossley K (October 2019) Is exercise therapy for femoroacetabular impingement in or out of FASHIoN? We need to talk about current best practice for the non-surgical management of FAI syndrome. Br J Sports Med 53(19):1204–1205. https://doi.org/10.1136/bjsports-2018-100173

Keskin Y, Kilic G, Taspinar O, Posul S, Halac G, Eren F, Aydin T (February 2020) Effectiveness of home exercise in pregnant women with carpal tunnel syndrome: Randomized Control Trial. J Pak Med Assoc 70(2):202–207. https://doi.org/10.5455/JPMA.1846

Kim B, Yim J (July 2020) Core Stability and Hip Exercises Improve Physical Function and Activity in Patients with Non-Specific Low Back Pain: A Randomized Controlled Trial. Tohoku J Exp Med 251(3):193–206. https://doi.org/10.1620/tjem.251.193

Kim J, Choi M, Kong D, Ha J, Chung K (June 2023) Does a Lower Limb Balance Test after Anterior Cruciate Ligament Reconstruction Have a Significant Correlation with Postoperative Clinical Score, Stability, and Functional Performance Test? Clin Orthop Surg 15(3):402–409. https://doi.org/10.4055/cios21218

Kim J, Hwang U, Choi M, Kong D, Chung K, Ha J, Kwon O (1. February 2022) Correlation Between Y-Balance Test and Balance, Functional Performance, and Outcome Measures in Patients Following ACL Reconstruction. Int J Sports Phys Ther 17(2):193–200. https://doi.org/10.26603/001c.31873

Kim J, Lee Y, Yang B, Oh S, Yang S (December 2013) Rehabilitation after posterior cruciate ligament reconstruction: a review of the literature and theoretical support. Arch Orthop Trauma Surg 133(12):1687–1695. https://doi.org/10.1007/s00402-013-1854-y

Kim Y, Kim N, Chang W, Lee S (1. (January 2018) Comparison of the Therapeutic Effects of a Sling Exercise and a Traditional Stabilizing Exercise for Clinical Lumbar Spinal Instability. J Sport Rehabil 27(1):47–54. https://doi.org/10.1123/jsr.2016-0083

Kise N, Risberg M, Stensrud S, Ranstam J, Engebretsen L, Roos E (20 July 2016) Exercise therapy versus arthroscopic partial meniscectomy for degenerative meniscal tear in middle aged patients: randomised controlled trial with two year follow-up. BMJ 354:i3740. https://doi.org/10.1136/bmj.i3740

Kocaman H, Bek, N, Kaya M, Büyükturan B, Yetiş M, Büyükturan Ö (15. April 2021) The effectiveness of two different exercise approaches in adolescent idiopathic scoliosis: A single-blind, randomized-controlled trial. PLoS One 16(4):e0249492. https://doi.org/10.1371/journal.pone.0249492

Koning C, Heuvel S, Staal J, Smits-Engelsman B, Hendriks E (19. October 2008) Clinimetric evaluation of methods to measure muscle functioning in patients with non-specific neck pain: a systematic review. BMC Musculoskelet Disord 9:142. https://doi.org/10.1186/1471-2474-9-142

Kostadinović S, Milovanović N, Jovanović J, Tomašević-Todorović S (2020) Efficacy of the lumbar stabilization and thoracic mobilization exercise program on pain intensity and functional disability reduction in chronic low back pain patients with lumbar radiculopathy: A randomized controlled trial. J Back Musculoskelet Rehabil 33(6):897–907. https://doi.org/10.3233/BMR-201843

Krieg A, Schell R, Neuhaus C (2018) Legg-Calvé-Perthes Disease and Its Physiotherapy—"If the Hip Melts Away". HSOA Journal of Orthopedic Research and Physiotherapy 3:037. https://doi.org/10.24966/ORP-2052/100037

Kruse L, Gray B, Wright R (3. October 2012) Rehabilitation after anterior cruciate ligament reconstruction: a systematic review. J Bone Joint Surg Am 94(19):1737–1748. https://doi.org/10.2106/JBJS.K.01246

la Fuente C, Silvestre R, Baechler P, Gemigniani A, Grunewaldt K, Vassiliu M, Carpes F (October 2020) Intrasession Real-time Ultrasonography Feedback Improves the Quality of Transverse Abdominis Contraction. J Manipulative Physiol Ther 43(8):816–823. https://doi.org/10.1016/j.jmpt.2019.10.017

Landesa-Piñeiro L, Leirós-Rodríguez R (2022) Physiotherapy treatment of lateral epicondylitis: A systematic review. J Back Musculoskelet Rehabil 35(3):463–477. https://doi.org/10.3233/BMR-210053

Lane B, McCullagh R, Cardoso J, McVeigh J (December 2022) The effectiveness of group and home-based exercise on psychological status in people with ankylosing spondylitis: A systematic review and meta-analysis. Musculoskeletal Care 20(4):758–771. https://doi.org/10.1002/msc.1641

Lazarou L, Kofotolis N, Pafis G, Kellis E (2018) Effects of two proprioceptive training programs on ankle range of motion, pain, functional and balance performance in individuals with ankle sprain. J Back Musculoskelet Rehabil 31(3):437–446. https://doi.org/10.3233/BMR-170836

Lee D, Yang S, Cho S, Lee J, Kim J (December 2018) Single-leg vertical jump test as a functional test after anterior cruciate ligament reconstruction. Knee 25(6):1016–1026. https://doi.org/10.1016/j.knee.2018.07.014

Lee J, Jang K-M, Kim E, Rhim H, Kim H-D (September-October 2021a) Static and Dynamic Quadriceps Stretching Exercises in Patients With Patellofemoral Pain: A Randomized Controlled Trial. Sports Health 13(5):482–489. https://doi.org/10.1177/1941738121993777

Lee J, Jang K-M, Kim E, Rhim H, Kim H-D (January-February 2021b) Effects of Static and Dynamic Stretching With Strengthening Exercises in Patients With Patellofemoral Pain Who Have Inflexible Hamstrings: A Randomized Controlled Trial. Sports Health 13(1):49–56. https://doi.org/10.1177/1941738120932911

Lee J, Jeon H, Yoon Y (22. May 2023) Effects of Exercise Intervention (with and without Joint Mobilization) in Patients with Adhesive Capsulitis: A Systematic Review and Meta-Analysis. Healthcare (Basel) 11(10):1504. https://doi.org/10.3390/healthcare11101504

Liang Z, Fu C, Zhang Q, Xiong F, Peng L, Chen L, Wei Q (April 2021) Effects of water therapy on disease activity, functional capacity, spinal mobility and severity of pain in patients with ankylosing spondylitis: a systematic review and meta-analysis. Disabil Rehabil 43(7):895–902. https://doi.org/10.1080/09638288.2019.1645218

Liang L, Feng M, Cui X, Zhou S, Yin X, Wang X, Wei X (November 2019) The effect of exercise on cervical radiculopathy: A systematic review and meta-analysis. Medicine (Baltimore), 98(45):e17733. https://doi.org/10.1097/MD.0000000000017733

Lin P, Yang M, Huang D, Lin H, Wang J, Zhong C, Guan L (20. April 2022) Effect of proprioceptive neuromuscular facilitation technique on the treatment of frozen shoulder: a pilot randomized controlled trial. BMC Musculoskelet Disord, 23(1):367. https://doi.org/10.1186/s12891-022-05327-4

Lu C.-C, Yao H.-I, Fan T.-Y, Lin Y.-C, Lin H.-T, Chou P.-H. (December 2021). Twelve Weeks of a Staged Balance and Strength Training Program Improves Muscle Strength, Proprioception, and Clinical Function in Patients with Isolated Posterior Cruciate Ligament Injuries. Int J Environ Res Public Health 18(23):12849. https://doi.org/10.3390/ijerph182312849

Luan L, Bousie J, Pranata A, Adams R, Han J (April 2021) Stationary cycling exercise for knee osteoarthritis: A systematic review and meta-analysis. Clin Rehabil 35(4):522–533. https://doi.org/10.1177/0269215520971795

Luan L, El-Ansary D, Adams R, Wu S, Han J (March 2022) Knee osteoarthritis pain and stretching exercises: a systematic review and meta-analysis. Physiotherapy 114:16–29. https://doi.org/10.1016/j.physio.2021.10.001

Luc-Harkey B, Safran-Norton C, Mandl L, Katz J, Losina E (27. July 2018) Associations among knee muscle strength, structural damage, and pain and mobility in individuals with osteoarthritis and symptomatic meniscal tear. BMC Musculoskelet Disord 19(1):258. https://doi.org/10.1186/s12891-018-2182-8

Ma J, Chen H, Liu A, Cui Y, Ma X (15. June 2020) Medical exercise therapy alone versus arthroscopic partial meniscectomy followed by medical exercise therapy for degenerative meniscal tear: a systematic review and meta-analysis of randomized controlled trials. J Orthop Surg Res 15(1):219. https://doi.org/10.1186/s13018-020-01741-3

Małecki K, Fabiś J, Flont P, Fabiś-Strobin A, Niedzielski K (28. August 2021) Assessment of knee flexor muscles strength in patients with patellar instability and its clinical implications for the non-surgical treatment of patients after first patellar dislocation—pilot study. BMC Musculoskelet Disord 22(1):740. https://doi.org/10.1186/s12891-021-04636-4

Macedo L, Kuspinar A, Roberts M, Maher C (July 2021) A Rasch analysis of the lumbar spine instability questionnaire. Physiother Theory Pract 37(7):844–851. https://doi.org/10.1080/09593985.2019.1642429

MacLean C, Taunton J, Clement D, Regan W, Stanish W (July 1999) Eccentric kinetic chain exercise as a conservative means of functionally rehabilitating chronic isolated insufficiency of the posterior cruciate ligament. Clin J Sport Med 9(3):142–150. https://doi.org/10.1097/00042752-199907000-00005

Mansell N, Rhon D, Meyer J, Slevin J, Marchant B (May 2018) Arthroscopic Surgery or Physical Therapy for Patients With Femoroacetabular Impingement Syndrome: A Randomized Controlled Trial With 2-Year Follow-up. Am J Sports Med 46(6):1306–1314. https://doi.org/10.1177/0363546517751912

Månsson O, Kartus J, Sernert N (February 2013) Pre-operative factors predicting good outcome in terms of health-related quality of life after ACL reconstruction. Scand J Med Sci Sports 23(1):15–22. https://doi.org/10.1111/j.1600-0838.2011.01426.x

Martins N, Furtado G, Campos M, Leitão J, Filaire E, Ferreira J (Ocotber-December 2014) Exercise and ankylosing spondylitis with New York modified criteria: a systematic review of controlled trials with meta-analysis. Acta Reumatol Port 39(4):298–308

McHugh M, Tyler T, Browne M, Gleim G, Nicholas S, (May-June 2002) Electromyographic predictors of residual quadriceps muscle weakness after anterior cruciate ligament reconstruction. Am J Sports Med 30(3):334–339. https://doi.org/10.1177/03635465020300030601

McKeon P, Ingersoll C, Kerrigan D, Saliba E, Bennett B, Hertel J (October 2008) Balance training improves function and postural control in those with chronic ankle instability. Med Sci Sports Exerc 40(10):1810–1819. https://doi.org/10.1249/MSS.0b013e31817e0f92

Melin L, Rendek Z, Hailer Y (16 August 2023) Recommendations for physiotherapy and physical activity for children with Legg-Calvé-Perthes disease: a survey of pediatric orthopedic surgeons and physiotherapists in Sweden. Acta Orthop 94:432–437. https://doi.org/10.2340/17453674.2023.18341

Mertens M, Meert L, Struyf F, Schwank A, Meeus M (May 2022) Exercise Therapy Is Effective for Improvement in Range of Motion, Function, and Pain in Patients With Frozen Shoulder: A Systematic Review and Meta-analysis. Arch Phys Med Rehabil 103(5):998–1012. https://doi.org/10.1016/j.apmr.2021.07.806

Minetama M, Kawakami M, Teraguchi M, Kagotani R, Mera Y, Sumiya T, Nakagawa Y (August 2019) Supervised physical therapy vs. home exercise for patients with lumbar spinal stenosis: a randomized controlled trial. Spine J, 19(8):1310–1318. https://doi.org/10.1016/j.spinee.2019.04.009

Mo Z, Zhang R, Chang M, Tang S (July-August 2018) Exercise therapy versus surgery for lumbar spinal stenosis: A systematic review and meta-analysis. Pak J Med Sci 34(4):879–885. https://doi.org/10.12669/pjms.344.14349

Mohamed A, Jan Y-K, Sayed W, Wanis M, Yamany A (July 2020) Dynamic scapular recognition exercise improves scapular upward rotation and shoulder pain and disability in patients with adhesive capsulitis: a randomized controlled trial. J Man Manip Ther 28(3):146–158. https://doi.org/10.1080/10669817.2019.1622896

Mohammadimajd E, Lotfinia I, Salahzadeh Z, Aghazadeh N, Noras P, Ghaderi, F, Choopani R (July 2020). Comparison of lumbar segmental stabilization and general exercises on clinical and radiologic criteria in grade-I spondylolisthesis patients: A double-blind randomized controlled trial. Physiother Res Int 25(3):e1843. https://doi.org/10.1002/pri.1843

Mortensen L, Schultz J, Elsner A, Jakobsen S, Søballe K, Jacobsen J, Mechlenburg I (22. August 2018) Progressive resistance training in patients with hip dysplasia: A feasibility study. J Rehabil Med 50(8):751–758. https://doi.org/10.2340/16501977-2371

Mueller J, Weinig J, Niederer D, Tenberg S, Mueller S (August 2023) Resistance, Motor Control, and Mindfulness-Based Exercises Are Effective for Treating Chronic Nonspecific Neck Pain: A Systematic Review With Meta-Analysis and Dose-Response Meta-Regression. J Orthop Sports Phys Ther 53(8):420–459. https://doi.org/10.2519/jospt.2023.11820

Nørregaard J, Larsen C, Bieler T, Langberg H (April 2007) Eccentric exercise in treatment of Achilles tendinopathy. Scand J Med Sci Sports 17(2):133–138. https://doi.org/10.1111/j.1600-0838.2006.00545.x

Namsawang J, Eungpinichpong W, Vichiansiri R, Rattanathongkom S (July 2019) Effects of the Short Foot Exercise With Neuromuscular Electrical Stimulation on Navicular Height in Flexible Flatfoot in Thailand: A Randomized Controlled Trial. J Prev Med Public Health 52(4):250–257. https://doi.org/10.3961/jpmph.19.072

Narouei S, Barati A, Akuzawa H, Talebian S, Ghiasi F, Akbari A, Alizadeh M (October 2020) Effects of core stabilization exercises on thickness and activity of trunk and hip muscles in subjects with nonspecific chronic low back pain. J Bodyw Mov Ther 24(4):138–146. https://doi.org/10.1016/j.jbmt.2020.06.026

Nava-Bringas T, Romero-Fierro L, Trani-Chagoya Y, Macías-Hernández S, García-Guerrero E, Hernández-López M, Roberto C.-Z (1. August 2021) Stabilization Exercises Versus Flexion Exercises in Degenerative Spondylolisthesis: A Randomized Controlled Trial. Phys Ther, 101(8):pzab108. https://doi.org/10.1093/ptj/pzab108

Nowotny J, Kasten P, Kopkow C, Biewener A, Mauch F (October 2018) Evaluation of a New Exercise Program in the Treatment of Scapular Dyskinesis. Int J Sports Med 39(10):782–790. https://doi.org/10.1055/a-0608-4584

Noyes F, Barber S, Mangine R (September-October 1991) Abnormal lower limb symmetry determined by function hop tests after anterior cruciate ligament rupture. Am J Sports Med 19(5):513–518. https://doi.org/10.1177/036354659101900518

Olivares-Jabalera J, Fílter-Ruger A, Dos'Santos T, Afonso J, Della Villa F, Morente-Sánchez J, Requena B (18. December 2021) Exercise-Based Training Strategies to Reduce the Incidence or Mitigate the Risk Factors of Anterior Cruciate Ligament Injury in Adult Football (Soccer) Players: A Systematic Review. Int J Environ Res Public Health 18(24):13351. https://doi.org/10.3390/ijerph182413351

O'Sullivan P, Phyty G, Twomey L, Allison, G. (15. December 1997). Evaluation of specific stabilizing exercise in the treatment of chronic low back pain with radiologic diagnosis of spondylolysis or spondylolisthesis. Spine (Phila Pa 1976) 22(24):2959–67. https://doi.org/10.1097/00007632-199712150-00020

Owen P, Miller C, Mundell N, Verswijveren S, Tagliaferri S, Brisby H, Belavy D (November 2020) Which specific modes of exercise training are most effective for treating low back pain? Network meta-analysis. Br J Sports Med 54(21):1279–1287. https://doi.org/10.1136/bjsports-2019-100886

Page M, O'Connor D, Pitt V, Massy-Westropp N. (13. June 2012) Exercise and mobilisation interventions for carpal tunnel syndrome. Cochrane Database Syst Rev 6:CD009899. https://doi.org/10.1002/14651858.CD009899

Paraskevopoulos E, Karanasios S, Gioftsos G, Tatsios P, Koumantakis G, Papandreou M, (3. (October 2023) The effectiveness of neuromobilization exercises in carpal tunnel syndrome: Systematic review and meta-analysis. Physiother Theory Pract 39(10):2037–2076. https://doi.org/10.1080/09593985.2022.2068097

Park J-H, Jeon H-S, Park H-W (June2018) Effects of the Schroth exercise on idiopathic scoliosis: a meta-analysis. Eur J Phys Rehabil Med 54(3):440–449. https://doi.org/10.23736/S1973-9087.17.04461-6

Park S, Chen Y, Thompson L, Kjoenoe A, Juul-Kristensen B, Cavalheri V, McKenna L (26. November 2020) No relationship between the acromiohumeral distance and pain in adults with subacromial pain syndrome: a systematic review and meta-analysis. Sci Rep 10(1): 20611. https://doi.org/10.1038/s41598-020-76704-z

Park S-H, Lee M-M, (7. (March 2019) Effects of a Progressive Stabilization Exercise Program Using Respiratory Resistance for Patients with Lumbar Instability: A Randomized Controlled Trial. Med Sci Monit 25:1740–1748. https://doi.org/10.12659/MSM.913036

Park S.-H, Oh Y.-J, Seo J.-H, Lee M.-M (18. November 2022) Effect of stabilization exercise combined with respiratory resistance and whole body vibration on patients with lumbar instability: A randomized controlled trial. Medicine (Baltimore) 101(46):e31843. https://doi.org/10.1097/MD.0000000000031843

Pécourneau V, Degboé Y, Barnetche T, Cantagrel A, Constantin A, Ruyssen-Witrand A (February 2018) Effectiveness of Exercise Programs in Ankylosing Spondylitis: A Meta-Analysis of Randomized Controlled Trials. Arch Phys Med Rehabil 99(2):383–389. https://doi.org/10.1016/j.apmr.2017.07.015

Pennock A, Bomar J, Johnson K, Randich K, Upasani V (December 2018) Nonoperative Management of Femoroacetabular Impingement: A Prospective Study. Am J Sports Med 46(14):3415–3422. https://doi.org/10.1177/0363546518804805

Petri M, Liodakis E, Hofmeister M, Despang F, Maier M, Balcarek P, Jagodzinski M (February 2013) Operative vs conservative treatment of traumatic patellar dislocation: results of a prospective randomized controlled clinical trial. Arch Orthop Trauma Surg 133(2):209–213. https://doi.org/10.1007/s00402-012-1639-8

Pierce C, O'Brien L, Griffin L, Laprade R (May 2013) Posterior cruciate ligament tears: functional and post-operative rehabilitation. Knee Surg Sports Traumatol Arthrosc 21(5):1071–1084. https://doi.org/10.1007/s00167-012-1970-1

Pourahmadi M, Delavari S, Hayden J, Keshtkar A, Ahmadi M, Aletaha A, Rubinstein S, (14. (June 2022) Does motor control training improve pain and function in adults with symptomatic lumbar disc herniation? A systematic review and meta-analysis of 861 subjects in 16 trials. Br J Sports Med. https://doi.org/10.1136/bjsports-2021-104926

Prudêncio D, Maffulli N, Migliorini F, Serafim T, Nunes L, Sanada L, Okubo R (26. January 2023). Eccentric exercise is more effective than other exercises in the treatment of mid-portion Achilles tendinopathy: systematic review and meta-analysis. BMC Sports Sci Med Rehabil 15(1):9. https://doi.org/10.1186/s13102-023-00618-2

Puntumetakul R, Saiklang P, Tapanya W, Chatprem T, Kanpittaya J, Arayawichanon P, Boucaut R. (23. July 2021) The Effects of Core Stabilization Exercise with the Abdominal Drawing-in Maneuver Technique versus General Strengthening Exercise on Lumbar Segmental Motion in Patients with Clinical Lumbar Instability: A Randomized Controlled Trial with 12-Month Follow-U. Int J Environ Res Public Health 18(15):7811. https://doi.org/10.3390/ijerph18157811

Qi X, Peng C, Fu P, Zhu A, Jiao W (19. December 2023) Correlation between physical activity and adolescent idiopathic scoliosis: a systematic review. BMC Musculoskelet Disord 24(1):978. https://doi.org/10.1186/s12891-023-07114-1

Quentin C, Bagheri R, Ugbolue U, Coudeyre E, Pélissier C, Descatha A, Dutheil F (10. August 2021) Effect of Home Exercise Training in Patients with Nonspecific Low-Back Pain: A Systematic Review and Meta-Analysis. Int J Environ Res Public Health 18(16):8430. https://doi.org/10.3390/ijerph18168430

Rafferty A, Fleming N, Kiely P, Mockler D, Dockrell S (June 2023) Does exercise therapy improve pulmonary function in patients with Adolescent Idiopathic Scoliosis? Physiother Theory Pract 39(6):1095–1105. https://doi.org/10.1080/09593985.2022.2034198

Raj 5th V, Thomas M (October 2023) Measuring transversus abdominis activity using pressure biofeedback unit-A technical report. Physiother Res Int 28(4):e2033. https://doi.org/10.1002/pri.2033

Ramos L, Callegari B, França F, Magalhães M, Nogueira Burke T, Silva A, Marques A (May2018) Comparison Between Transcutaneous Electrical Nerve Stimulation and Stabilization Exercises in Fatigue and Transversus Abdominis Activation in Patients With Lumbar Disk Herniation: A Randomized Study. J Manipulative Physiol Ther 41(4):323–331. https://doi.org/10.1016/j.jmpt.2017.10.010

Ramos L, França F, Callegari B, Burke T, Magalhães M, Marques A (May2016) Are lumbar multifidus fatigue and transversus abdominis activation similar in patients with lumbar disc herniation and healthy controls? A case control study. Eur Spine J 25(5):1435–1442. https://doi.org/10.1007/s00586-015-4375-2

Raposo F, Ramos M, Cruz A (December 2021) Effects of exercise on knee osteoarthritis: A systematic review. Musculoskeletal Care 19(4):399–435. https://doi.org/10.1002/msc.1538

Rasmussen-Barr E, Halvorsen M, Bohman T, Boström C, Dedering Å, Kuster R, Grooten W (12. October 2023) Summarizing the effects of different exercise types in chronic neck pain—a systematic review and meta-analysis of systematic reviews. BMC Musculoskelet Disord 24(1):806. https://doi.org/10.1186/s12891-023-06930-9

Renovato França F, Callegari B, Ramos L, Burke T, Magalhães M, Comachio J, Marques A (March 2019) Motor Control Training Compared With

Transcutaneous Electrical Nerve Stimulation in Patients With Disc Herniation With Associated Radiculopathy: A Randomized Controlled Trial. Am J Phys Med Rehabil 98(3):207–214. https://doi.org/10.1097/PHM.0000000000001048

Rewald S, Lenssen A, Emans P, Bie R, van Breukelen G, Mesters I (August 2020) Aquatic Cycling Improves Knee Pain and Physical Functioning in Patients With Knee Osteoarthritis: A Randomized Controlled Trial. Arch Phys Med Rehabil 101(8):1288–1295. https://doi.org/10.1016/j.apmr.2019.12.023

Rogan S, Haehni M, Luijckx E, Dealer J, Reuteler S, Taeymans J (November 2019) Effects of Hip Abductor Muscles Exercises on Pain and Function in Patients With Patellofemoral Pain: A Systematic Review and Meta-Analysis. J Strength Cond Res 33(11):3174–3187. https://doi.org/10.1519/JSC.0000000000002658

Rostron Z, Zacharias A, Semciw A, Kingsley M, Pizzari T, Woodley S, Green R (February 2023) Comparison between a targeted exercise program and a sham intervention on gluteal muscle activity in people with hip osteoarthritis: Analysis of secondary outcomes from a randomised clinical trial. Gait Posture 100:33–40. https://doi.org/10.1016/j.gaitpost.2022.11.016

Schiffke-Juhász B, Knobloch K, Vogt P, Hoy L (27. July 2021) Proprioceptive elbow training reduces pain and improves function in painful lateral epicondylitis-a prospective trial. J Orthop Surg Res 16(1):468. https://doi.org/10.1186/s13018-021-02602-3

Schneider M, Ammendolia C, Murphy D, Glick R, Hile E, Tudorascu D, Piva S. (4. January 2019) Comparative Clinical Effectiveness of Nonsurgical Treatment Methods in Patients With Lumbar Spinal Stenosis: A Randomized Clinical Trial. JAMA Netw Open 2(1):e186828. https://doi.org/10.1001/jamanetworkopen.2018.6828

Schomacher J, Falla D (October 2013) Function and structure of the deep cervical extensor muscles in patients with neck pain. Man Ther 18(5):360–366. https://doi.org/10.1016/j.math.2013.05.009

Schydlowsky P, Szkudlarek M, Madsen O (15. January 2022) Comprehensive supervised heavy training program versus home training regimen in patients with subacromial impingement syndrome: a randomized trial. BMC Musculoskelet Disord 23(1):52. https://doi.org/10.1186/s12891-021-04969-0

Sebastian D, Chovvath R, Malladi R (April 2015) Cervical extensor endurance test: a reliability study. J Bodyw Mov Ther 19(2):213–216. https://doi.org/10.1016/j.jbmt.2014.04.014

Shaarani S, O'Hare C, Quinn A, Moyna N, Moran R, O'Byrne J (September 2013) Effect of prehabilitation on the outcome of anterior cruciate ligament reconstruction. Am J Sports Med 41(9):2117–2127. https://doi.org/10.1177/0363546513493594

Shen X, Yang Z, Zhang P, Xu Y, Wang J (2023) Effects of balance training combined with Schroth therapy on adolescents with mild idiopathic scoliosis: A six-week randomized controlled trial. J Back Musculoskelet Rehabil 36(6):1365–1373. https://doi.org/10.3233/BMR-220383

Shire A, Stæhr T, Overby J, Dahl M, Jacobsen J, Christiansen D (17. April 2017). Specific or general exercise strategy for subacromial impingement syndrome-does it matter? A systematic literature review and meta analysis. *BMC Musculoskelet Disord, 18*(1), S. 158. https://doi.org/10.1186/s12891-017-1518-0

Silbernagel K, Thomeé R, Thomeé P, Karlsson J (August 2001) Eccentric overload training for patients with chronic Achilles tendon pain–a randomised controlled study with reliability testing of the evaluation methods. Scand J Med Sci Sports 11(4):197–206. https://doi.org/10.1034/j.1600-0838.2001.110402.x

Silvers-Granelli H, Bizzini M, Arundale A, Mandelbaum B, Snyder-Mackler L (October 2017) Does the FIFA 11+ Injury Prevention Program Reduce the Incidence of ACL Injury in Male Soccer Players? Clin Orthop Relat Res 475(10):2447–2455. https://doi.org/10.1007/s11999-017-5342-5

Skou S, Roos E (September-October 2019) Physical therapy for patients with knee and hip osteoarthritis: supervised, active treatment is current best practice. Clin Exp Rheumatol 120(5):112–117

Slater J, Kolber M, Schellhase K, Patel C, Rothschild C, Liu X, Hanney W, (16. February 2015) The Influence of Exercise on Perceived Pain and Disability in Patients With Lumbar Spinal Stenosis: A Systematic Review of Randomized Controlled Trials. Am J Lifestyle Med 10(2):136–147. https://doi.org/10.1177/1559827615571510

Smith T, Chester R, Cross J, Hunt N, Clark A, Donell S (September 2015) Rehabilitation following first-time patellar dislocation: a randomised controlled trial of purported vastus medialis obliquus muscle versus general quadriceps strengthening exercises. Knee 22(4):313–320. https://doi.org/10.1016/j.knee.2015.03.013

Stasinopoulos D, Stasinopoulos I (January-March 2017) Comparison of effects of eccentric training, eccentric-concentric training, and eccentric-concentric training combined with isometric contraction in the treatment of lateral elbow tendinopathy. J Hand Ther 30(1):13–19. https://doi.org/10.1016/j.jht.2016.09.001

Stensrud S, Risberg M, Roos E (June 2015) Effect of exercise therapy compared with arthroscopic surgery on knee muscle strength and functional performance in middle-aged patients with degenerative meniscus tears: a 3-mo follow-up of a randomized controlled trial. Am J Phys Med Rehabil 94(6):460–473. https://doi.org/10.1097/PHM.0000000000000209

Stensrud S, Roos E, Risberg M (November 2012) A 12-week exercise therapy program in middle-aged patients with degenerative meniscus tears: a case series with 1-year follow-up. J Orthop Sports Phys Ther 42(11):919–931. https://doi.org/10.2519/jospt.2012.4165

Straume-Næsheim T, Randsborg P-H, Mikaelsen J (October 2022) Medial patellofemoral ligament reconstruction is superior to active rehabilitation in protecting against further patella dislocations. Knee Surg Sports Traumatol Arthrosc 30(10):3428–3437. https://doi.org/10.1007/s00167-022-06934-3

Şahin M, Ayhan F, Borman P, Atasoy H (17. February 2016) The effect of hip and knee exercises on pain, function, and strength in patientswith patellofemoral pain syndrome: a randomized controlled trial. Turk J Med Sci 46(2):265–277. https://doi.org/10.3906/sag-1409-66

Taşpınar G, Angın E, Oksüz S (January 2023) The effects of Pilates on pain, functionality, quality of life, flexibility and endurance in lumbar disc herniation. J Comp Eff Res 12(1):e220144. https://doi.org/10.2217/cer-2022-0144

Tahran Ö, Yeşilyaprak S (March-April 2020) Effects of Modified Posterior Shoulder Stretching Exercises on Shoulder Mobility, Pain, and Dysfunction in Patients With Subacromial Impingement Syndrome. Sports Health 12(2):139–148. https://doi.org/10.1177/1941738119900532

Tateuchi H, Akiyama H, Goto K, So K, Kuroda Y, Ichihashi N (April 2021) Strategies for increasing gait speed in patients with hip osteoarthritis: their clinical significance and effects on hip loading. Arthritis Res Ther 23(1):129. https://doi.org/10.1186/s13075-021-02514-x

Terrell S, Lynch J (2019) Exploring Nonoperative Exercise Interventions for Individuals with Femoroacetabular Impingement. ACSM's Health & Fitness Journal 23(1):22–30. https://doi.org/10.1249/FIT.0000000000000451

Terrell S, Olson G, Lynch J (1. January 2021) Therapeutic Exercise Approaches to Nonoperative and Postoperative Management of Femoroacetabular Impingement Syndrome. J Athl Train 56(1):31–45. https://doi.org/10.4085/1062-6050-0488.19

Thorlund J, Simic M, Pihl K, Berthelsen D, Day R, Koes B, Juhl C (April 2022) Similar Effects of Exercise Therapy, Nonsteroidal Anti-inflammatory Drugs, and Opioids for Knee Osteoarthritis Pain: A Systematic Review with Network Meta-analysis. J Orthop Sports Phys Ther 52(4):207–216. https://doi.org/10.2519/jospt.2022.10490

Torstensen T, Østerås H, LoMartire R, Rugelbak G, Grooten W, Äng B (February 2023) High- Versus Low-Dose Exercise Therapy for Knee Osteoarthritis: A Randomized Controlled Multicenter Trial. Ann Intern Med 176(2):154–165. https://doi.org/10.7326/M22-2348

Tsiringakis G, Dimitriadis Z, Triantafylloy E, McLean S (December 2020) Motor control training of deep neck flexors with pressure biofeedback improves pain and disability in patients with neck pain: A systematic review and meta-analysis. Musculoskelet Sci Pract 50:102220. https://doi.org/10.1016/j.msksp.2020.102220

Turgut E, Duzgun I, Baltaci G (October 2017) Effects of Scapular Stabilization Exercise Training on Scapular Kinematics, Disability, and Pain in Subacromial Impingement: A Randomized Controlled Trial. Arch Phys Med Rehabil 98(10):1915–1923. https://doi.org/10.1016/j.apmr.2017.05.023

Turk R, Shah S, Chilton M, Thomas T, Anene C, Mousad A, Ramappa A (March 2023) Return to Sport After Anterior Cruciate Ligament Reconstruction Requires Evaluation of >2 Functional Tests, Psychological Readiness, Quadriceps/Hamstring Strength, and Time After Surgery of 8 Months. Arthroscopy 39(3):790–801. https://doi.org/10.1016/j.arthro.2022.08.038

Turner M, Hernandez D, Cade W, Emerson C, Reynolds J, Best T, (March-April 2020) The Role of Resistance Training Dosing on Pain and Physical Function in Individuals With Knee Osteoarthritis: A Systematic Review. Sports Health 12(2):200–206. https://doi.org/10.1177/1941738119887183

Tyler T, Thomas G, Nicholas S, McHugh M (September 2010) Addition of isolated wrist extensor eccentric exercise to standard treatment for chronic lateral epicondylosis: a prospective randomized trial. J Shoulder Elbow Surg 19(6):917–922. https://doi.org/10.1016/j.jse.2010.04.041

Tyler T, McHugh M, Gleim G, Nicholas S (December 1998) The effect of immediate weightbearing after anterior cruciate ligament reconstruction. Clin Orthop Relat Res 357:141–148. https://doi.org/10.1097/00003086-199812000-00019

Utsahachant N, Sakulsriprasert P, Sinsurin K, Jensen M, Sungkue S (July 2023) Effects of short foot exercise combined with lower extremity training on dynamic foot function in individuals with flexible flatfoot: A randomized controlled trial. Gait Posture 104:109–115. https://doi.org/10.1016/j.gaitpost.2023.06.013

van Doormaal M, Meerhoff G, Vlieland T, Peter W (December 2020) A clinical practice guideline for physical therapy in patients with hip or knee osteoarthritis. Musculoskeletal Care 18(4):575–595. https://doi.org/10.1002/msc.1492

van Grinsven S, van Cingel R, Holla C, van Loon C (August 2010) Knee Surg Sports Traumatol Arthrosc. Knee Surg Sports Traumatol Arthrosc 18(8):1128–1144. https://doi.org/10.1007/s00167-009-1027-2

van Melick N, van Cingel R, Brooijmans F, Neeter C, van Tienen T, Hullegie W, Nijhuis-van der Sanden M (December 2016) Evidence-based clinical practice update: practice guidelines for anterior cruciate ligament rehabilitation based on a systematic review and multidisciplinary consensus. Br J Sports Med 50(24):1506–1515. https://doi.org/10.1136/bjsports-2015-095898

Vidmar M, Baroni B, Michelin A, Mezzomo M, Lugokenski R, Pimentel G, Silva M, (September-October, (2020) Isokinetic eccentric training is more effective than constant load eccentric training for quadriceps rehabilitation following anterior cruciate ligament reconstruction: a randomized controlled trial. Braz J Phys Ther 24(5):424–432. https://doi.org/10.1016/j.bjpt.2019.07.003

Vincent K, Vincent H, (Oktober 2020) Concentric and Eccentric Resistance Training Comparison on Physical Function and Functional Pain Outcomes in Knee Osteoarthritis: A Randomized Controlled Trial. Am J Phys Med Rehabil 99(10):932–940. https://doi.org/10.1097/PHM.0000000000001450

Vincent K, Vasilopoulos T, Montero C, Vincent H (October 2019) Eccentric and Concentric Resistance Exercise Comparison for Knee Osteoarthritis. Med Sci Sports Exerc 51(10):1977–1986. https://doi.org/10.1249/MSS.0000000000002010

Viswas R, Ramachandran R, Anantkumar P (2012) Comparison of effectiveness of supervised exercise program and Cyriax physiotherapy in patients with tennis elbow (lateral epicondylitis): a randomized clinical trial. ScientificWorldJournal 2012:939645. https://doi.org/10.1100/2012/939645

Wagemans J, Bleakley C, Taeymans J, Schurz A, Kuppens K, Baur H, Vissers D (8. February 2022). Exercise-based rehabilitation reduces reinjury following acute lateral ankle sprain: A systematic review update with meta-analysis. PLoS One, 17(2):e0262023. https://doi.org/10.1371/journal.pone.0262023

Wall P, Fernandez M, Griffin D, Foster N (May2013) Nonoperative treatment for femoroacetabular impingement: a systematic review of the literature. PM R 5(5):418–426. https://doi.org/10.1016/j.pmrj.2013.02.005

Wang L, Yu G, Zhang R, Wu G, He L, Chen Y (20. January 2023) Positive effects of neuromuscular exercises on pain and active range of motion in idiopathic frozen shoulder: a randomized controlled trial. BMC Musculoskelet Disord 24(1):50. https://doi.org/10.1186/s12891-023-06173-8

Warby S, Ford J, Hahne A, Watson L, Balster S, Lenssen R, Pizzari T (January 2018) Comparison of 2 Exercise Rehabilitation Programs for Multidirectional Instability of the Glenohumeral Joint: A Randomized Controlled Trial. Am J Sports Med 46(1):87–97. https://doi.org/10.1177/0363546517734508

Warby S, Pizzari T, Ford J, Hahne A, Watson L (January 2014) The effect of exercise-based management for multidirectional instability of the glenohumeral joint: a systematic review. J Shoulder Elbow Surg 23(1):128–142. https://doi.org/10.1016/j.jse.2013.08.006

Warby S, Pizzari T, Ford J, Hahne A, Watson L (September 2016) Exercise-based management versus surgery for multidirectional instability of the glenohumeral joint: a systematic review. Br J Sports Med 50(18):1115–1123. https://doi.org/10.1136/bjsports-2015-094970

Watson L, Warby S, Balster S, Lenssen R, Pizzari T (October 2016) The treatment of multidirectional instability of the shoulder with a rehabilitation program: Part 1. Shoulder Elbow 8(4):271–278. https://doi.org/10.1177/1758573216652086

Watson L, Warby S, Balster S, Lenssen R, Pizzari T (January 2017) The treatment of multidirectional instability of the shoulder with a rehabilitation programme: Part 2. Shoulder Elbow 9(1):46–53. https://doi.org/10.1177/1758573216652087

Watson R, Sullivan B, Stone A, Jacobs C, Malone T, Heebner N, Brian Noehren B (5. May 2022) Lateral Patellar Dislocation: A Critical Review and Update of Evidence-Based Rehabilitation Practice Guidelines and Expected Outcomes. JBJS Rev 10(5). https://doi.org/10.2106/JBJS.RVW.21.00159

Weng Q, Goh S-L, Wu J, Persson M, Wei J, Sarmanova A, Zhang W (August 2023) Comparative efficacy of exercise therapy and oral non-steroidal anti-inflammatory drugs and paracetamol for knee or hip osteoarthritis: a network meta-analysis of randomised controlled trials. Br J Sports Med 57(15):990–996. https://doi.org/10.1136/bjsports-2022-105898

Wilhelm M, Donaldson M, Griswold D, Learman K, Garcia A, Learman S, Cleland J (November 2020) The Effects of Exercise Dosage on Neck-Related Pain and Disability: A Systematic Review With Meta-analysis. J Orthop Sports Phys Ther 50(11):607–621. https://doi.org/10.2519/jospt.2020.9155

Wilson F, Walshe M, O'Dwyer T, Bennett K, Mockler D, Bleakley C (December 2018) Exercise, orthoses and splinting for treating Achilles tendinopathy: a systematic review with meta-analysis. Br J Sports Med 52(24):1564–1574. https://doi.org/10.1136/bjsports-2017-098913

Winther S, Foss O, Husby O, Wik T, Klaksvik J, Husby V (June 2018) A randomized controlled trial on maximal strength training in 60 patients undergoing total hip arthroplasty. Acta Orthop 89(3):295–301. https://doi.org/10.1080/17453674.2018.1441362

Wu B, Yuan H, Geng D, Zhang L, Zhang C (July 2020) The Impact of a Stabilization Exercise on Neck Pain: A Systematic Review and Meta-analysis. J Neurol Surg A Cent Eur Neurosurg 81(4):342–347. https://doi.org/10.1055/s-0039-3400953

Xing D, Li W, Yang Z, Dong Z, Kang H, und Wang F (1. November 2022). Active exercise therapy improves the recovery of knee joint function and reduction of muscle atrophy after medial patellofemoral ligament reconstruction for recurrent patellar dislocation. Front Surg 9: 954287. https://doi.org/10.3389/fsurg.2022.954287

Yaşa M, Yıldırım N, Demir P (March 2021) The effects of a 6-Week balance training in addition to conventional physiotherapy on pain, postural control, and balance confidence in patients with cervical disc herniation: a randomized controlled trial. Somatosens Mot Res 38(1):60–67. https://doi.org/10.1080/08990220.2020.1845136

Yilmaz K, Bayramlar K, Ayhan C, Tufekci O, (January-March 2022) Investigating the effects of neuromobilization in lateral epicondylitis. J Hand Ther 35(1):97–106. https://doi.org/10.1016/j.jht.2020.11.003

Zacharias A, Pizzari T, Semciw A, English D, Kapakoulakis T, Green R (July 2020) Gluteus medius and minimus activity during stepping tasks: Comparisons between people with hip osteoarthritis and matched control participants. Gait Posture 80:339–346. https://doi.org/10.1016/j.gaitpost.2020.06.012

Zhong Y, Ding Y, Fu B, Ma G, Cui H, Li M, Guan L (2023) The effectiveness of postoperative exercise based on gait analysis compared with conventional exercise in patients with lumbar spinal stenosis: A randomized clinical trial. J Back Musculoskelet Rehabil 36(6):1399–1409. https://doi.org/10.3233/BMR-220409

Disease-Associated Test Procedures and Medical Exercise Therapy for Internal Diseases

6

Contents

Trailer

The sixth chapter navigates through the therapeutic use of physical activity in various chronic diseases and demonstrates how exercise can specifically contribute to improving health and quality of life. It provides insight into the treatment and rehabilitation of conditions affecting the cardiovascular system, respiratory system, nervous system, endocrine system, and digestive system, emphasizing the importance of individually tailored exercise programs.

S. Wolfram and R. Bauer, *Evidence-Based Medical Exercise Therapy*,
https://doi.org/10.1007/978-3-662-70774-6_6

For the cardiovascular system, it illuminates how exercise is used in the treatment and prevention of diseases such as coronary heart disease, heart failure, atrial fibrillation, myocardial infarction, angina pectoris, hypertension, atherosclerosis, and peripheral arterial occlusive disease. By promoting blood circulation and improving heart function, medical exercise therapy can help minimize the risk of future heart events and enhance overall quality of life.

In the area of the respiratory system, the positive effects of exercise on diseases such as bronchial asthma, chronic obstructive pulmonary disease (COPD), and rehabilitation after Covid-19 are highlighted. Training programs aimed at improving lung function and facilitating breathing play a crucial role in alleviating symptoms and increasing physical capacity.

For people with nervous system disorders, including Parkinson's disease, multiple sclerosis, cerebral infarction, depression, migraine, Alzheimer's disease, and dementia, the chapter offers valuable insights into how targeted exercise can bring not only physical but also psychological benefits. Exercises aimed at improving coordination, balance, and cognitive functions can help positively influence the course of these diseases.

In the endocrine system, the role of exercise therapy in metabolic syndrome and type II diabetes mellitus is discussed. By helping to regulate blood sugar levels and control weight, a tailored training regime can make a significant contribution to the treatment and prevention of these conditions.

Lastly, the importance of physical activity in combating obesity, a widespread disease of the digestive system, is emphasized. By combining endurance and strength training, affected individuals can effectively lose weight, improve their health, and reduce the risk of associated diseases.

This chapter impressively illustrates the power of medical exercise therapy as a pillar in the treatment and prevention of chronic diseases. It provides a practical guide for professionals and those affected alike to promote health and well-being through targeted exercise programs.

6.1 Cardiovascular System

6.1.1 Coronary Heart Disease/ Heart Failure

A meta-analysis from 2023 examined the influence of exercise-based rehabilitation in people with coronary heart disease. Regular physical activity can significantly reduce cardiovascular mortality and the occurrence of cardiac recurrences. In addition, the number of hospital stays can be reduced and the quality of life can be improved at the same time (see Dibben et al. 2023)

Wang et al. (2022a) advocate in their meta-analysis for the application of high-intensity interval training in the early phase of rehabilitation of people with coronary heart disease or heart failure. By practicing this, the VO2max value can be significantly increased. Furthermore, the anaerobic threshold can be shifted and the left ventricular ejection fraction can be optimized at the same time (see Wang et al. 2022a). Neto et al. (2018) also advocate for the use of high-intensity interval training in people with heart failure and accompanying reduced ejection fraction due to the targeted increase of the VO2max. This also applies to coronary heart disease (see Gomes-Neto et al. 2017). Both in heart failure and in coronary heart disease, the breaks should be actively designed at an intensity of 40–60% of the VO2max. More than two training sessions per week are recommended for coronary heart disease. More than three weekly training sessions are advised for heart failure (see García et al. 2019).

Taylor et al. (2020) confirm the application of high-intensity interval training, but also point out the positive effect of endurance training at moderate intensity (see Taylor et al. 2020). Reed et al. (2022) compared the application of high-intensity interval training, moderate endurance training, and Nordic walking in people with coronary heart disease. Training was conducted twice a week over a period of three months. The high-intensity interval training was carried out in four times four minutes at 85%-95% of the maximum heart rate. Both the moderate endurance training and the Nordic walking intervention were practiced with an increase of 20–40 beats to the resting heart rate. All three interventions were recognized as safe and successful in terms of improving the physical and mental condition (see Reed et al. January–February 2022).

Useful visualizations can be found in Fig. 6.1.

Summary for Practice
A positive effect for both diseases is provided by both regular physical activity in the form of moderate endurance training and high-intensity interval training in the early phase.

6.1.2 Atrial Fibrillation

In a randomized controlled study, high-intensity interval training was compared to a moderate to intense endurance training approach. The selected sample suffered from atrial fibrillation. The 23-minute high-intensity interval training was performed at an intensity of 80 -100 % of maximum performance. The endurance method was implemented at an intensity of 67 -95 % with a training duration of 60 minutes. The intervention period was three months. Two training sessions took place weekly. Both forms of training were able to achieve equivalent successes. The functional capacity as well as the general and disease-related quality of life could be positively influenced. In addition, the resting heart rate and the level of physical activity were positively influenced (see Reed et al. October 2022).

In their recently published meta-analysis, Yu et al. (2023) compare the effect of high-intensity interval training with moderate endurance training in people with cardiovascular diseases. After evaluating the data, it can be stated that both forms of training are similarly capable of significantly positively influencing quality of life and mental health.

Assessments include the six-minute-walk-test and the Beck-Depression-Inventory-II. The general quality of life can be assessed using the Short-Form-36. The disease-related quality of life can be assessed with the HeartQoL (see Reed et al. October 2022). More detailed information on the individual assessments can be taken from the assessment list in the appendix of this book.

Useful visualizations can be found in Fig. 6.2.

Summary for Practice
Both high-intensity interval training and moderate to intense endurance training lead to a positive influence on the functional capacity and disease-related quality of life in patients with atrial fibrillation.

Categories	Evidence-based training recommendation
Units	three or more units per week
Duration	High-intensity interval training 4x4 minutes / moderate endurance training Recommendation 20-40 minutes
Intensity	High-intensity interval training with 85-95% of maximum heart rate / moderate endurance training with 30-60 beats more than resting heart rate

Fig. 6.1 Summary of MTT in Coronary Heart Disease/Heart Failure

Categories	Evidence-based training recommendation
Units	At least 2 units per week
Duration	High-intensity interval training 23 minutes / endurance training recommendation 60 minutes
Intensity	High-intensity interval training at 80- 100% of maximum performance/ endurance training intensity at 67-95%

Fig. 6.2 Summary MTT in atrial fibrillation

6.1.3 Myocardial Infarction/Angina Pectoris

Willis et al. (2019) recognized that the combination of taking ranolazine and medical exercise therapy in patients with chronic stable angina pectoris can have a better effect than the sole use of exercise therapy. The combination of the two interventions led to an improvement in aerobic fitness, physical activity, and health-related quality of life (see Willis et al. 2019).

A meta-analysis from 2022 compared the effect of moderate endurance training and high-intensity interval training in people after a myocardial infarction. It was found that high-intensity interval training can significantly better increase the VO2max value than moderate endurance training. Regarding systolic and diastolic blood pressure, maximum and resting heart rate, left ventricular ejection fraction, left end-diastolic volume, and quality of life, no differences between the two measures could be calculated (see Qin et al. 2022).

Summary for Practice
Medical exercise therapy in the form of moderate endurance training and high-intensity interval training have a positive influence on blood pressure, resting heart rate, left ventricular ejection fraction, left end-diastolic volume, and quality of life as well as physical fitness.

6.1.4 Hypertension

In 2023, a meta-analysis was published that dealt with the influence of medical exercise therapy on resting blood pressure. A total of 270 randomized controlled studies with a total number of 15,827 subjects were integrated. It was shown that both aerobic endurance training and dynamic resistance training, as well as their combination, are capable of significantly reducing resting blood pressure. In addition, isometric and high-intensity interval training have a blood pressure-lowering effect. The best interventions include wall sitting and running (see Edwards et al. 2023).

The research results of Lopes et al. (2021) show that the application of aerobic endurance training alone and its combination with strength training, as well as the application of isometric exercises, are capable of positively influencing the stiffness of arteries and, in particular, the pulse wave velocity in patients with hypertension. Baffour-Awuah et al. (2023) also advocate the use of isometric resistance exercises in people with hypertension.

Teixeira et al. (2023) provide initial meta-analytical findings that link high-intensity interval training with a blood pressure-lowering effect. Souza Mesquita et al. (2023) also recommend high-intensity interval training to patients with stage 1 hypertension, provided they do not have any additional risk factors.

Regarding the intervention of strength training, training should be done with moderate to intense intensity, which exceeds 60% of the 1RM. Two training sessions should be completed weekly. Initial results in terms of a reduction in blood pressure can be expected after about two months (see Correia et al. 2023).

Useful visualizations can be found in Fig. 6.3.

Summary for Practice
Both aerobic endurance training and dynamic resistance training, as well as isometric and high-intensity interval training, have a blood pressure-lowering effect. These methods positively influence arterial stiffness and pulse wave velocity. Wall sitting and running are particularly recommended. Initial successes should occur after about two months.

6.1.5 Atherosclerosis

In a meta-analysis, the effect of medical exercise therapy on the disease pattern of atherosclerosis in the area of the carotid artery was examined. Both a preventive and a reversible effect were found. The method of choice is aerobic endurance training. High-intensity interval training can also make a positive contribution (see Gao et al. 2023). These findings confirm earlier research results from Wang et al. (2022b). This research group was also able to demonstrate that regular practice of aerobic endurance training can improve the atherosclerotic situation of the carotid artery. A measurable reduction in arterial wall thickness was detected after a training period of more than six months (see Wang et al. 2022).

Summary for Practice
The method of choice for patients with atherosclerosis is aerobic endurance training. High-intensity interval training can also have a positive effect on the atherosclerotic situation. A measurable decrease in wall thickness is to be expected after 6 months.

6.1.6 Peripheral Arterial Occlusive Disease

Parmenter et al. (2015) conducted a meta-analysis on the influence of medical training therapy in people suffering from peripheral arterial occlusive disease. It was found that regular endurance training is capable of extending both the pain-free walking distance and the overall walking distance. In addition, the graded performance on the treadmill improved. This leads to the recommendation of practicing endurance training in the affected area. For the upper extremity, for example, a hand ergometer could be used. In the area of the lower extremity, walking or the bicycle ergometer can be used. The intensity can vary from moderate to intense. However, during training, one should not go beyond mild pain (cf. Parmenter et al. 2015). Lyu et al. (2016) confirm the effect of intensive walking in terms of improving walking ability and establish a superiority to usual care for peripheral arterial occlusive disease (cf. Lyu et al. 2016). A superiority of Nordic walking over supervised walking could not be calculated (cf. Golledge et al. 2018).

Useful visualizations can be found in Fig. 6.4.

Categories	Evidence-based training recommendation
Units	At least 2 units per week
Intensity	Strength training with over 60% of 1RM / aerobic endurance training

Fig. 6.3 Summary of MTT in Hypertension

Categories	Evidence-based training recommendation
Units	At least 2 units per week
Intensity	moderate to intensive intensity / training should not be done beyond mild pain

Fig. 6.4 Summary of MTT in peripheral arterial occlusive disease

Summary for Practice
Regular endurance training demonstrably leads to an improvement in the pain-free walking distance as well as a general extension of the walking distance. Depending on the region of the PAOD, training can be done with a hand or bicycle ergometer, as well as by walking.

6.2 Respiratory System

6.2.1 Bronchial Asthma

A meta-analysis by Lista-Paz et al. (2023) dealt with the influence of training the inspiratory respiratory muscles on the disease pattern of bronchial asthma. If the training is carried out with an intensity of over 50% of the maximum inspiratory pressure for a period of more than six weeks, this leads to an increased performance in terms of the maximum inspiratory pressure. In addition, an improved endurance capacity of the respiratory muscles and a positive influence on emergency medication or exercise dyspnea is suggested. These results focus on adult individuals (cf. Lista-Paz et al. 2023). Regular practice of the aerobic endurance method, for example in the form of swimming or on the treadmill, improves both the lung function and the quality of life of people suffering from bronchial asthma (cf. Wu et al. 2020). Hansen et al. (2020) also mention improved lung function and optimized disease control through regular aerobic activity.

Children suffering from bronchial asthma can significantly positively influence their quality of life and physical performance by practicing interval training. The combination of respiratory muscle training and endurance training unfolds its positive effect in the sense of increased lung function (cf. Jiang et al. 2022; Liu et al. 2021).

Summary for Practice
The increase in performance of the maximum inspiratory pressure and an improvement in the general endurance function of the respiratory muscles can be achieved through targeted training of the inspiratory respiratory muscles and the regular performance of aerobic endurance training. This improves lung function as well as quality of life. Exercise dyspnea and the intake of emergency medication can also be reduced. Furthermore, interval training also has a positive influence on lung function. Initial successes can be expected after about six weeks.

6.2.2 Chronic Obstructive Pulmonary Disease

A meta-analysis examined the influence of high-intensity interval training in people with chronic obstructive pulmonary disease. In total, twelve articles with a total population of 696 people were integrated. The described form of training is capable of improving pulmonary function, performance, and quality of life in chronic obstructive pulmonary disease (see Gao et al. 2022). These results were confirmed in a more recent meta-analysis (see Wang et al. 2023). Yun et al. (2021) recommend integrating breathing exercises into the therapy of chronic obstructive pulmonary disease, with the aim of strengthening the inspiratory respiratory muscles and performance.

Strengthening the inspiratory and expiratory muscles as well as the muscles of the upper extremity contributes to a reduction in dyspnea in patients with chronic obstructive pulmonary disease (see Zhang et al. 2021; Ammous et al. 2023).

Among other things, the British-Medical-Research-Council-questionnaire, the transitional-dyspnea-index, the modified-Borg-score-during-exercise, the Chronic-Respiratory-Questionnaire-dyspnea-score, the 6-min-walking-test, and the St.-George's-Respiratory-Questionnaire serve as assessments (see Higashimoto et al. 2020). More detailed information on the individual assessments can be found in the assessment list in the appendix of this book.

Summary for Practice
High-intensity interval training improves pulmonary function, performance, and quality of life in patients with chronic obstructive pulmonary disease. During training, emphasis should be placed on the inspiratory and expiratory muscles as well as on the muscles of the upper extremity. This leads to a reduction in dyspnea.

6.2.3 Covid-19

Ahmed et al. (2022) recommend the implementation of medical exercise therapy for acutely or chronically ill Covid-19 patients. It was shown that training can improve dyspnea and at the same time increase performance. In addition to lung function, fatigue also improved.

Furthermore, regular physical activity in the form of endurance and strength training can have a preventive effect. It was shown that people who regularly perform physical training and then contract Covid-19 have a lower hospitalization rate, a lower number of intensive care stays, and a lower mortality rate (see Rahmati et al. 2022).

In the rehabilitation of Covid-19, breathing exercise programs with three training sessions per week and a minimum duration of six weeks are recommended (see Ashra et al. 2023).

Useful visualizations can be found in Fig. 6.5.

Summary for Practice
Both preventively and rehabilitatively, medical exercise therapy in the form of endurance and strength exercises as well as breathing exercise programs leads to an improvement in dyspnea, lung function, and fatigue.

6.3 Nervous System

6.3.1 Parkinson's Disease

A meta-analysis examined the effect of medical exercise therapy on people suffering from Parkinson's disease. It was found that both endurance and strength training, as well as other intensive physical exertions, evoke positive effects. In addition to improved muscle strength and performance, antidepressive and balance-improving effects can also be demonstrated (see Gamborg et al. 2022). In addition to an increase in cardiorespiratory performance, quality of life can also be improved. Assessments include the Unified-Parkinson's-Disease-Rating-Scale-III-Score

Categories	Evidence-based training recommendation
Units	At least 3 units per week, at least 6 weeks
Intensity	moderate to intensive intensity

Fig. 6.5 Summary of MTT in Covid-19

(see Uhrbrand et al. 2015). Kwok et al. (2016) meta-analytically examined the effect of mind-body training programs such as yoga, Thai-Chi, and dancing on people with Parkinson's disease. A moderate to large effect on motor symptoms, postural instability, and functional mobility in mild and moderately progressive courses of Parkinson's disease was found.

Balance training with virtual reality programs or telerehabilitation can be used after stroke, in multiple sclerosis, and in Parkinson's disease (see Truijen et al. 2022).

Assessments used included the Berg-Balance-Scale, the Timed-Up-and-Go-Test, and the Six-minute-Walk-test (see Kwok et al. 2016). For improving balance in Parkinson's disease patients, López-Liria et al. (2023) recommend practicing specific exercises to strengthen the trunk muscles. More detailed information on the individual assessments can be found in the assessment list in the appendix of this book.

Summary for Practice

Both endurance and strength training, as well as intensive physical exertion, improve quality of life, balance ability, cardiorespiratory and general performance, and muscle strength in patients with Parkinson's disease. In addition, these forms of MTT produce an antidepressive effect.

In mild to moderate courses, yoga, Thai-Chi, or dancing, as well as balance training sessions in a virtual environment, can be optimally integrated.

6.3.2 Multiple Sclerosis

In the field of multiple sclerosis, yoga, training in virtual reality, and aerobic training can be used to improve balance. Balance training with virtual reality programs or telerehabilitation can be used after stroke, in multiple sclerosis, and in Parkinson's disease (see Truijen et al. 2022).

To achieve an improvement in walking ability, water-based training programs, training in virtual reality, and aerobic endurance training can be used (see Hao et al. 2022).

Furthermore, the symptom of fatigue in multiple sclerosis can be significantly reduced by regular physical activity (see Razazian et al. 2020). With regard to the symptom of fatigue, both the execution of aerobic training and the performance of strength training lead to the goal (see Taul-Madsen et al. 2021). Training guidance in water can also be considered (see Shariat et al. 2022). Li et al. (2023b) advocate the implementation of at least three training sessions per week with a training time of 60 minutes each. The training program should include various training components. This can improve cognitive function in people with multiple sclerosis. This effect is even greater with an advanced training program or at an older age (see Li et al. 2023b). In terms of improving health-related quality of life, supervised aerobic endurance training and group training seem to be the method of choice in multiple sclerosis (see Flores et al. 2023). In addition, sensorimotor or mind-body training programs can be used (see Reina-Gutiérrez et al. 2022).

Useful visualizations can be found in Fig. 6.6.

Categories	Evidence-based training recommendation
Units	At least 3 units per week
Duration	60 minutes per training session
Intensity	Adaptable depending on your own physical condition / always vary exercises to train cognitive function

Fig. 6.6 Summary of MTT in Multiple Sclerosis

Summary for Practice
Medical exercise therapy in the form of aerobic endurance training, yoga, balance training, water-based training, and strength training has a positive influence on patients with multiple sclerosis, particularly on the symptom of fatigue. Sensorimotor exercises or mind-body training programs and group therapies also have a positive effect.

6.3.3 Brain Infarction

Training programs, which are initiated within six months after the stroke and have a weekly training time of at least 150 minutes, have a positive effect on the quality of life in stroke patients. Intervention programs, which include resistance training, proved to be the most effective (see Ali et al. 2021).

In a systematic review, Mah et al. (2022) advocate for the application of high-intensity training therapy in people in the acute and subacute rehabilitation phase after a stroke. In the first six months, high-intensity rehabilitation programs on the treadmill, stepper or bicycle ergometer, or in the sense of walking, proved helpful in improving the function of the lower extremity (see Mah et al. 2022). This confirms the findings of Luo et al. (2020).

Training of the respiratory muscles can minimize pulmonary complications after stroke and swallowing disorders (see Zhang et al. 2022b).

Aerobic training of light intensity after stroke is able to positively influence motor restrictions and at the same time increase cognitive function (see Li et al. 2023a). In addition to the general improvement of cognition, there is scientific evidence of the specific benefit of aerobic endurance training on memory, attention, and the visual spatial area (see Zheng et al. 2016). The positive effects are mainly manifested in a period of 20–40 minutes after endurance training (see Swatridge et al. 2017).

The application of training programs within virtual reality is able to improve the motor function of the upper extremity (see Chen et al. 2022). Balance training with virtual reality programs or telerehabilitation can be used after stroke, in multiple sclerosis, and in Parkinson's disease (see Truijen et al. 2022).

The Fugl-Meyer-Assessment-Upper Extremity serves as an assessment for the motor function of the upper extremity. Independence in everyday life can be assessed with the Functional-Independence-Measure and the modified-Rankin-Scale. The dexterity of the hand can be assessed with the Box-and-Block-Test. Spasticity can be classified with the Ashworth-Scale or the modified-Ashworth-Scale. The motor activity of the upper extremity is evaluated with the Wolf-Motor-Function-Test or the Manual-Function-Test or Jebsen-Hand-Function-Test. The Stroke-Impact-Scale is used to assess the quality of life (see Chen et al. 2022). More detailed information on the individual assessments can be taken from the assessment list in the appendix of this book.

Useful visualizations can be taken from Fig. 6.7.

Summary for Practice
The best effect is produced by training programs that are carried out within six months after a stroke. The focus is on resistance

Categories	Evidence-based training recommendation
Units	weekly training time of at least 50 minutes

Fig. 6.7 Summary MTT in Brain Infarction

training, high-intensity training therapy using a treadmill, stepper, and bicycle ergometer, or walking. Furthermore, training of the respiratory muscles leads to the minimization of pulmonary complications and swallowing disorders. Light aerobic training positively influences motor restrictions and balance as well as cognitive functions.

6.3.4 Depression

For both children and adults, aerobic endurance training is the most effective method of medical training therapy to combat depression. The aerobic endurance training should be applied three times a week for 40–50 minutes each training session (see Li et al. 2023c). For older depressive individuals with mild cognitive impairments, the use of mind-body exercises is additionally recommended (see Liu et al. 2023).

Physical activity is capable of improving the function of the working memory in adults with depression (see Contreras-Osorio et al. 2022).

The practice of aerobic endurance training at moderate intensity should be performed at least three times a week over a period of nine weeks to combat depression (see Stanton and Reaburn 2014). Ideally, the aerobic endurance training is supervised. Training in a group format is also considered beneficial (see Heissel et al. 2023).

Useful visualizations can be found in Fig. 6.8.

Summary for Practice
Aerobic endurance training has a positive influence on children and adults with depression. For older patients, additional mind-body training programs are recommended. Physical activity leads to improved working memory in adults with depression.

6.3.5 Migraine

A meta-analysis found that strength training is the most effective form of medical training therapy for migraines. The effectiveness of aerobic training is also mentioned (see Woldeamanuel and Oliveira 2022).

Touche et al. (2020) also recognize the benefits of aerobic endurance training in terms of intensity, frequency, and duration of pain in migraines. Additionally, the quality of life can be improved (see Touche et al. 2020). Lemmens et al. (2019) confirm the decreasing number of migraine days through the regular performance of aerobic endurance training. Training in migraine-free periods is recommended.

Summary for Practice
Both strength training and aerobic endurance training have a positive effect on patients with migraines.

6.3.6 Alzheimer's Disease

The cognitive function of people suffering from Alzheimer's disease can be improved through physical activity (see Jia et al. 2019). Endurance training can not only improve cognition but also enhance the impaired intellectual function (see Zhou et al. 2022). In addition,

Categories	Evidence-based training recommendation
Units	3 x per week
Duration	40-50 minutes per unit

Fig. 6.8 Summary of MTT in Depression

neuropsychiatric symptoms and activities of daily life can be improved with a training duration of more than 16 weeks (see Roy et al. 2023).

The duration of the endurance training should be about 30 minutes per training session. On a weekly basis, three training interventions are recommended, which should not exceed a total duration of 150 minutes (see Zhang et al. 2022a).

Strength training can also make a positive contribution in terms of improved cognition and improved memory performance (see Lv et al. 2023).

Useful visualizations can be found in Fig. 6.9.

Summary for Practice
Through physical activity in the form of endurance training and or strength training, cognitive functions, neuropsychiatric symptoms, and activities of daily life are improved.

6.3.7 Dementia

In their meta-analysis, Huang et al. (2022) report that strength training has the highest effectiveness in slowing cognitive decline. Combined forms of training also have a positive effect on cognition and executive functions (cf. Huang et al. 2022).

Furthermore, training programs that include aerobic endurance training, balance training, and flexibility exercises are capable of significantly positively influencing global cognition, executive functions, mobility, agility, muscle strength, and activities of daily living in people with dementia and mild cognitive impairment (cf. Yan et al. 2023).

Summary for Practice
Targeted strength training as well as endurance training, balance training, and flexibility exercises improve cognition, mobility, agility, and activities of daily living.

6.3.8 Amyotrophic Lateral Sclerosis

Medical training therapy is capable of slowing the deterioration of muscular status in people with amyotrophic lateral sclerosis (cf. Ortega-Hombrados et al. 2021). In addition, both functional performance and pulmonary function can be improved (cf. Meng et al. 2020). Zhu et al. (2022) advocate for a multimodal approach, which includes aerobic endurance training as well as strength training. There is a clear need for further high-quality randomized controlled studies (cf. Zhu et al. 2022; Rahmati and Malakoutinia 2021).

Summary for Practice
Medical training therapy in the form of strength and endurance training can slow deterioration as well as improve pulmonary function and overall performance.

6.4 Endocrine System

6.4.1 Metabolic Syndrome

In their meta-analysis, Liang et al. (2021) conclude that from the perspective of medical training therapy, metabolic syndrome can best be

Categories	Evidence-based training recommendation
Units	3 units per week
Duration	30-60 minutes per session, no more than 150 minutes per week

Fig. 6.9 Summary of MTT in Alzheimer's Disease

treated with a combination of regular endurance and strength training. Regarding the optimal parameters of endurance training for the therapy of metabolic syndrome, the research results of Wewege et al. (2018) provide insights. They recommend increasing the intensity of endurance training from an aerobic situation to intensive exertion. Ideally, three training sessions should be completed every week (cf. Wewege et al. 2018). In summary, the best approach against metabolic syndrome is through the sole application of aerobic endurance training or its combination with strength training (cf. Yousefabadi et al. 2021).

Useful visualizations can be found in Fig. 6.10.

Summary for Practice
Regular strength and endurance training in combination has a positive influence on metabolic syndrome.

6.4.2 Type II Diabetes Mellitus

A study by Yang et al. (2014) addressed the question of whether there is a superiority between endurance and strength training in people with type 2 diabetes mellitus. No clinically relevant difference between the two interventions was found. The recommendation is made for physical activity independent of the type of training (cf. Hou et al. 2023). Mannucci et al. (2021) advocate the use of a combination of strength and endurance training.

In overweight individuals, combined training programs have been found to improve glycemic control and insulin sensitivity. Weight loss was also recorded (cf. Zhao et al. 2021).

In their meta-analysis, Papagianni et al. (2023) point out the anti-inflammatory effect of aerobic endurance training and its relevance in type 2 diabetes mellitus.

The regular implementation of aerobic endurance training alone or in combination with strength training is capable of improving the quality of life in type 2 diabetes mellitus (cf. Sabag et al. 2023).

Summary for Practice
Medical training therapy in the form of aerobic endurance training and strength training has a positive effect on glycemic control, insulin sensitivity, and weight loss in overweight patients and has an anti-inflammatory effect. It also improves quality of life.

6.5 Digestive System

6.5.1 Obesity

It should be fundamentally noted that any form of physical activity is better than no physical activity. The best results can be achieved through a combination of high-intensity endurance training and high-intensity strength training. This can reduce abdominal belly fat, increase lean body mass, and improve cardiorespiratory fitness (cf. O'Donoghue et al. 2021).

Subcutaneous abdominal fat can be reduced by practicing the combination of endurance and strength training. Endurance training has the

Categories	Evidence-based training recommendation
Units	3 units per week
Intensity	Start aerobically and increase to intensive exertion

Fig. 6.10 Summary of MTT in Metabolic Syndrome

greater impact (cf. Yarizadeh et al. 2021). These results are transferable to both children and adults (cf. Kelley et al. 2019).

> **Summary for Practice**
> For patients with obesity, any form of physical activity in the form of high-intensity strength and/or endurance training is recommended to reduce belly fat, alleviate weight, and promote cardiorespiratory fitness.

References

Ahmed I, Mustafaoglu R, Yeldan I, Yasaci Z, Erhan B (2022, October) Effect of Pulmonary Rehabilitation Approaches on Dyspnea, Exercise Capacity, Fatigue, Lung Functions, and Quality of Life in Patients With COVID-19: A Systematic Review and Meta-analysis. Arch Phys Med Rehabil 103(10):2051–2062. https://doi.org/10.1016/j.apmr.2022.06.007

Ali A, Tabassum D, Baig S, Moyle B, Redgrave J, Nichols S, Majid A (2021, July) Effect of Exercise Interventions on Health-Related Quality of Life After Stroke and Transient Ischemic Attack: A Systematic Review and Meta-Analysis. Stroke 52(7):2445–2455. https://doi.org/10.1161/STROKEAHA.120.032979

Ammous O, Feki W, Lotfi T, Khamis A, Gosselink R, Rebai A, Kammoun S (2023, January 6) Inspiratory muscle training, with or without concomitant pulmonary rehabilitation, for chronic obstructive pulmonary disease (COPD). Cochrane Database Syst Rev 1(1):CD013778. https://doi.org/10.1002/14651858.CD013778.pub2

Ashra F, Jen H.-J, Liu D, Lee T.-Y, Pien L.-C, Chen R, Chou K.-R (2023, August) Effectiveness of respiratory rehabilitation in patients with COVID-19: A meta-analysis. J Clin Nurs 32(15–16):4972–4987. https://doi.org/10.1111/jocn.16692

Baffour-Awuah B, Pearson M, Dieberg G, Smart N (2023, April) Isometric Resistance Training to Manage Hypertension: Systematic Review and Meta-analysis. Curr Hypertens Rep 25(4):35–49. https://doi.org/10.1007/s11906-023-01232-w

Chen J, Or C, Chen T (2022, June 20) Effectiveness of Using Virtual Reality-Supported Exercise Therapy for Upper Extremity Motor Rehabilitation in Patients With Stroke: Systematic Review and Meta-analysis of Randomized Controlled Trials. J Med Internet Res 24(6): e24111. https://doi.org/10.2196/24111

Contreras-Osorio F, Ramirez-Campillo R, Cerda-Vega E, Campos-Jara R, Martínez-Salazar C, Reigal R, Campos-Jara C (2022, November 18) Effects of Physical Exercise on Executive Function in Adults with Depression: A Systematic Review and Meta-Analysis. Int J Environ Res Public Health 19(22):15270. https://doi.org/10.3390/ijerph192215270

Correia R, Veras A, Tebar W, Rufino J, Batista V, Teixeira G (2023, January 5) Strength training for arterial hypertension treatment: a systematic review and meta-analysis of randomized clinical trials. Sci Rep 13(1):201. https://doi.org/10.1038/s41598-022-26583-3

Dibben G, Faulkner J, Oldridge N, Rees K, Thompson D, Zwisler A.-D, Taylor R (2023, February 7) Exercise-based cardiac rehabilitation for coronary heart disease: a meta-analysis. Eur Heart J 44(6):452–469. https://doi.org/10.1093/eurheartj/ehac747

Edwards J, Deenmamode A, Griffiths M, Arnold O, Cooper N, Wiles J, O'Driscoll J (2023, October) Exercise training and resting blood pressure: a large-scale pairwise and network meta-analysis of randomised controlled trials. Br J Sports Med 57(20):1317–1326. https://doi.org/10.1136/bjsports-2022-106503

Flores V, Šilić P, DuBose N, Zheng P, Jeng B, Motl R (2023, July) Effects of aerobic, resistance, and combined exercise training on health-related quality of life in multiple sclerosis: Systematic review and meta-analysis. Mult Scler Relat Disord 75:104746. https://doi.org/10.1016/j.msard.2023.104746

Gamborg M, Hvid L, Dalgas U, Langeskov-Christensen M (2022, May) Parkinson's disease and intensive exercise therapy – An updated systematic review and meta-analysis. Acta Neurol Scand 145(5):504–528. https://doi.org/10.1111/ane.13579

Gao M, Huang Y, Wang Q, Liu K, Sun G (2022, January) Effects of High-Intensity Interval Training on Pulmonary Function and Exercise Capacity in Individuals with Chronic Obstructive Pulmonary Disease: A Meta-Analysis and Systematic Review. Adv Ther 39(1):94–116. https://doi.org/10.1007/s12325-021-01920-6

Gao P, Zhang X, Yin S, Tuo H, Lin Q, Tang F, Liu W (2023, January 25) Meta-Analysis of the Effect of Different Exercise Mode on Carotid Atherosclerosis. Int J Environ Res Public Health 20(3):2189. https://doi.org/10.3390/ijerph20032189

García I, Arias J, Campo D, González-Moro I, Poyatos M (2019, March) High-intensity Interval Training Dosage for Heart Failure and Coronary Artery Disease Cardiac Rehabilitation. A Systematic Review and Meta-analysis. Rev Esp Cardiol (Engl Ed) 72(3):233–243. https://doi.org/10.1016/j.rec.2018.02.015

Golledge J, Maarij K, Moxon J, Beard J, Girold S, Wrang H, Morris D (2018, October) Systematic Review and Meta-analysis of Clinical Trials Examining the Benefit of Exercise Programmes Using Nordic Walking in Patients With Peripheral Artery Disease. Eur J Vasc Endovasc Surg 56(4):534–543. https://doi.org/10.1016/j.ejvs.2018.05.026

Gomes-Neto M, Durães A, Reis H, Neves V, Martinez B, Carvalho V (2017, November) High-intensity interval training versus moderate-intensity continuous training on exercise capacity and quality of life in patients with coronary artery disease: A systematic review and meta-analysis. Eur J Prev Cardiol 24(16):1696–1707. https://doi.org/10.1177/2047487317728370

Hansen E, Pitzner-Fabricius A, Toennesen L, Rasmusen H, Hostrup M, Hellsten Y, Henriksen M (2020, July 30) Effect of aerobic exercise training on asthma in adults: a systematic review and meta-analysis. Eur Respir J, 56(1):2000146. https://doi.org/10.1183/13993003.00146-2020

Hao Z, Zhang X, Chen P (2022, June 11) Effects of Different Exercise Therapies on Balance Function and Functional Walking Ability in Multiple Sclerosis Disease Patients-A Network Meta-Analysis of Randomized Controlled Trials. Int J Environ Res Public Health 19(12):7175. https://doi.org/10.3390/ijerph19127175

Heissel A, Heinen D, Brokmeier L, Skarabis N, Kangas M, Vancampfort D, Schuch, F (2023, August) Exercise as medicine for depressive symptoms? A systematic review and meta-analysis with meta-regression. Br J Sports Med 57(16):1049–1057. https://doi.org/10.1136/bjsports-2022-106282

Higashimoto Y, Ando M, Sano A, Saeki S, Nishikawa Y, Fukuda K, Tohda Y (2020, September) Effect of pulmonary rehabilitation programs including lower limb endurance training on dyspnea in stable COPD: A systematic review and meta-analysis. Respir Investig 58(5):355–366. https://doi.org/10.1016/j.resinv.2020.05.010

Hou L, Wang Q, Pan B, Li R, Li Y, He J, Yang K (2023, January) Exercise modalities for type 2 diabetes: A systematic review and network meta-analysis of randomized trials. Diabetes Metab Res Rev 39(1):e3591. https://doi.org/10.1002/dmrr.3591

Huang X, Zhao, X, Li, B, Cai, Y, Zhang, S, Wan, Q, Yu, F (2022, March) Comparative efficacy of various exercise interventions on cognitive function in patients with mild cognitive impairment or dementia: A systematic review and network meta-analysis. J Sport Health Sci 11(2):212–223. https://doi.org/10.1016/j.jshs.2021.05.003

Jia R.-X, Liang J.-H, Xu Y, Wang Y.-Q (2019, July 2) Effects of physical activity and exercise on the cognitive function of patients with Alzheimer disease: a meta-analysis. BMC Geriatr 19(1):181. https://doi.org/10.1186/s12877-019-1175-2

Jiang J, Zhang D, Huang Y, Wu Z, Zhang W (2022, December) Exercise rehabilitation in pediatric asthma: A systematic review and network meta-analysis. Pediatr Pulmonol 57(12):2915–2927. https://doi.org/10.1002/ppul.26134

Kelley G, Kelley K, Pate R (2019, November 11) Exercise and adiposity in overweight and obese children and adolescents: a systematic review with network meta-analysis of randomised trials. BMJ Open 9(11):e031220. https://doi.org/10.1136/bmjopen-2019-031220

Kwok J, Choi K, Chan H (2016) December) Effects of mind-body exercises on the physiological and psychosocial well-being of individuals with Parkinson's disease: A systematic review and meta-analysis. Complement Ther Med 29:121–131. https://doi.org/10.1016/j.ctim.2016.09.016

Lemmens J, Pauw J, Soom T, Michiels S, Versijpt J, Breda E, Hertogh W (2019, February 14) The effect of aerobic exercise on the number of migraine days, duration and pain intensity in migraine: a systematic literature review and meta-analysis. J Headache Pain 20(1):16. https://doi.org/10.1186/s10194-019-0961-8

Li W, Luo, Z, Jiang, J, Li, K, Wu, C (2023a, June) The effects of exercise intervention on cognition and motor function in stroke survivors: a systematic review and meta-analysis. Neurol Sci 44(6):1891–1903. https://doi.org/10.1007/s10072-023-06636-9

Li G, You Q, Hou X, Zhang S, Du L, Lv Y, Yu L (2023b, June) The effect of exercise on cognitive function in people with multiple sclerosis: a systematic review and meta-analysis of randomized controlled trials. J Neurol 270(6):2908–2923. https://doi.org/10.1007/s00415-023-11649-7

Li J, Zhou X, Huang Z, Shao T (2023c, October 4) Effect of exercise intervention on depression in children and adolescents: a systematic review and network meta-analysis. BMC Public Health 23(1):1918. https://doi.org/10.1186/s12889-023-16824-z

Liang M, Pan Y, Zhong T, Zeng Y, Cheng A (2021, December 22) Effects of aerobic, resistance, and combined exercise on metabolic syndrome parameters and cardiovascular risk factors: a systematic review and network meta-analysis. Rev Cardiovasc Med 22(4):1523–1533. https://doi.org/10.31083/j.rcm2204156

Lista-Paz A, Cousillas L, Jácome C, Fregonezi G, Labata-Lezaun N, Llurda-Almuzara L, Pérez-Bellmunt A (2023, April) Effect of respiratory muscle training in asthma: A systematic review and meta-analysis. Ann Phys Rehabil Med 66(3):101691. https://doi.org/10.1016/j.rehab.2022.101691

Liu F, Liu Y.-R, Liu L (2021, October 15) Effect of exercise rehabilitation on exercise capacity and quality of life in children with bronchial asthma: a systematic review. Zhongguo Dang Dai Er Ke Za Zhi 23(10):1050–1057. https://doi.org/10.7499/j.issn.1008-8830.2104124

Liu Q, Ni W, Zhang L, Zhao M, Bai X, Zhang S, Chen L (2023, November) Comparative efficacy of various exercise interventions on depression in older adults with mild cognitive impairment: A systematic review and network meta-analysis. Ageing Res Rev 91:102071. https://doi.org/10.1016/j.arr.2023.102071

Lopes S, Afreixo V, Teixeira M, Garcia C, Leitão C, Gouveia M, Ribeiro F (2021, February 1) Exercise training reduces arterial stiffness in adults with hypertension: a systematic review and meta-analysis. J Hypertens 39(2):214–222. https://doi.org/10.1097/HJH.0000000000002619

Luo L, Meng H, Wang Z, Zhu S, Yuan S, Wang Y, Wang Q (2020, January) Effect of high-intensity exercise on cardiorespiratory fitness in stroke survivors: A systematic review and meta-analysis. Ann Phys Rehabil Med 63(1):59–68. https://doi.org/10.1016/j.rehab.2019.07.006

López-Liria R, Vega-Tirado S, Valverde-Martínez M, Calvache-Mateo A, Martínez-Martínez A, Rocamora-Pérez P (2023 February 6) Efficacy of Specific Trunk Exercises in the Balance Dysfunction of Patients with Parkinson's Disease: A Systematic Review and Meta-Analysis. Sensors (Basel) 23(4):1817. https://doi.org/10.3390/s23041817

Lv S, Wang Q, Liu W, Zhang X, Cui M, Li X, Xu Y (2023, December) Comparison of various exercise interventions on cognitive function in Alzheimer's patients: A network meta-analysis. Arch Gerontol Geriatr 115:105113. https://doi.org/10.1016/j.archger.2023.105113

Lyu X, Li S, Peng S, Cai H, Liu G, Ran X (2016, May) Intensive walking exercise for lower extremity peripheral arterial disease: A systematic review and meta-analysis. J Diabetes 8(3):363–77. https://doi.org/10.1111/1753-0407.12304

Mah S, Goodwill A, Seow H, Teo W.-P (2022, December 22) Evidence of High-Intensity Exercise on Lower Limb Functional Outcomes and Safety in Acute and Subacute Stroke Population: A Systematic Review. Int J Environ Res Public Health 20(1):153. https://doi.org/10.3390/ijerph20010153

Mannucci E, Bonifazi A, Monami M (2021, June 30) Comparison between different types of exercise training in patients with type 2 diabetes mellitus: A systematic review and network metanalysis of randomized controlled trials. Nutr Metab Cardiovasc Dis 31(7):1985–1992. https://doi.org/10.1016/j.numecd.2021.02.030

Meng L, Li X, Li C, Tsang R, Chen Y, Ge Y, Gao Q (2020, September) Effects of Exercise in Patients With Amyotrophic Lateral Sclerosis: A Systematic Review and Meta-Analysis. Am J Phys Med Rehabil 99(9):801–810. https://doi.org/10.1097/PHM.0000000000001419

Neto M, Durães A, Conceição L, Saquetto M, Ellingsen Ø, Carvalho V (2018 June 15) High intensity interval training versus moderate intensity continuous training on exercise capacity and quality of life in patients with heart failure with reduced ejection fraction: A systematic review and meta-analysis. Int J Cardiol 261:134–141. https://doi.org/10.1016/j.ijcard.2018.02.076

O'Donoghue G, Blake C, Cunningham C, Lennon O, Perrotta C (2021, February) What exercise prescription is optimal to improve body composition and cardiorespiratory fitness in adults living with obesity? A network meta-analysis. Obes Rev 22(2):e13137. https://doi.org/10.1111/obr.13137

Ortega-Hombrados L, Molina-Torres G, Galán-Mercant A, Sánchez-Guerrero E, González-Sánchez M, Ruiz-Muñoz M (2021, January 26) Systematic Review of Therapeutic Physical Exercise in Patients with Amyotrophic Lateral Sclerosis over Time. Int J Environ Res Public Health 18(3):1074. https://doi.org/10.3390/ijerph18031074

Papagianni G, Panayiotou C, Vardas M, Balaskas N, Antonopoulos C, Tachmatzidis D, Kadoglou N (2023, April) The anti-inflammatory effects of aerobic exercise training in patients with type 2 diabetes: A systematic review and meta-analysis. Cytokine 164:156157. https://doi.org/10.1016/j.cyto.2023.156157

Parmenter B, Dieberg G, Smart N (2015, February) Exercise training for management of peripheral arterial disease: a systematic review and meta-analysis. Sports Med 45(2):231–44. https://doi.org/10.1007/s40279-014-0261-z

Qin Y, Bundhun P, Yuan Z.-L, Chen M.-H (2022, March 25) The effect of high-intensity interval training on exercise capacity in post-myocardial infarction patients: a systematic review and meta-analysis. Eur J Prev Cardiol 29(3):475–484. https://doi.org/10.1093/eurjpc/zwab060

Rahmati M, Malakoutinia F (2021) December) Aerobic, resistance and combined exercise training for patients with amyotrophic lateral sclerosis: a systematic review and meta-analysis. Physiotherapy 113:12–28. https://doi.org/10.1016/j.physio.2021.04.005

Rahmati M, Shamsi M, Khoramipour K, Malakoutinia F, Woo W, Park S, Smith L (2022, September) Baseline physical activity is associated with reduced mortality and disease outcomes in COVID-19: A systematic review and meta-analysis. Rev Med Virol 32(5):e2349. https://doi.org/10.1002/rmv.2349

Razazian N, Kazeminia M, Moayedi H, Daneshkhah A, Shohaimi S, Mohammadi M, Salari N (2020, March 13) The impact of physical exercise on the fatigue symptoms in patients with multiple sclerosis: a systematic review and meta-analysis. BMC Neurol 20(1):93. https://doi.org/10.1186/s12883-020-01654-y

Reed J, Terada T, Vidal-Almela S, Tulloch H, Mistura M, Birnie D, Pipe A (2022, October 3) Effect of High-Intensity Interval Training in Patients With Atrial Fibrillation: A Randomized Clinical Trial. JAMA Netw Open 5(10):e2239380. https://doi.org/10.1001/jamanetworkopen.2022.39380

Reed J, Terada T, Cotie L, Tulloch H, Leenen F, Mistura M, Pipe A (2022b January-February) The effects of high-intensity interval training, Nordic walking and moderate-to-vigorous intensity continuous training on functional capacity, depression and quality of life in patients with coronary artery disease enrolled in cardiac rehabilitation: A ra. Prog Cardiovasc Dis 70:73–83. https://doi.org/10.1016/j.pcad.2021.07.002

Reina-Gutiérrez S, Cavero-Redondo I, Martínez-Vizcaíno V, Arenas-Arroyo S, López-Muñoz P, Álvarez-Bueno C, Torres-Costoso, A (2022, May) The type of exercise most beneficial for quality of life in people with multiple sclerosis: A network meta-analysis. Ann Phys Rehabil Med 65(3):101578. https://doi.org/10.1016/j.rehab.2021.101578

Roy S, Wang J.-J, Xu Y.-M (2023, July) Effects of exercise interventions in Alzheimer's disease: A meta-analysis. Brain Behav, 13(7):e3051. https://doi.org/10.1002/brb3.3051

Sabag A, Chang C, Francois M, Keating S, Coombes J, Johnson N, Lopez J (2023, August 1) The Effect of Exercise on Quality of Life in Type 2 Diabetes: A Systematic Review and Meta-analysis. Med Sci Sports Exerc 55(8):1353–1365. https://doi.org/10.1249/MSS.0000000000003172

Shariat A, Najafabadi M, Fard Z, Nakhostin-Ansari A, Shaw B (2022, December) A systematic review with meta-analysis on balance, fatigue, and motor function following aquatic therapy in patients with multiple sclerosis. Mult Scler Relat Disord 68:104107. https://doi.org/10.1016/j.msard.2022.104107

Souza Mesquita F, Gambassi B, Silva M, Moreira S, Neves V, Gomes-Neto M, Schwingel P (2023, July-August) Effect of High-Intensity Interval Training on Exercise Capacity, Blood Pressure, and Autonomic Responses in Patients With Hypertension: A Systematic Review and Meta-analysis. Sports Health 15(4):571–578. https://doi.org/10.1177/19417381221139343

Stanton R, Reaburn P (2014, March) Exercise and the treatment of depression: a review of the exercise program variables. J Sci Med Sport 17(2):177–82. https://doi.org/10.1016/j.jsams.2013.03.010

Swatridge K, Regan K, Staines W, Roy E, Middleton L (2017, December) The Acute Effects of Aerobic Exercise on Cognitive Control among People with Chronic Stroke. J Stroke Cerebrovasc Dis 26(12):2742–2748. https://doi.org/10.1016/j.jstrokecerebrovasdis.2017.06.050

Taul-Madsen L, Connolly L, Dennett R, Freeman J, Dalgas U, Hvid L (2021, October) Is Aerobic or Resistance Training the Most Effective Exercise Modality for Improving Lower Extremity Physical Function and Perceived Fatigue in People With Multiple Sclerosis? A Systematic Review and Meta-analysis. Arch Phys Med Rehabil 102(10):2032–2048. https://doi.org/10.1016/j.apmr.2021.03.026

Taylor J, Holland D, Keating S, Leveritt M, Gomersall S, Rowlands A, Coombes J (2020, December 1) Short-term and Long-term Feasibility, Safety, and Efficacy of High-Intensity Interval Training in Cardiac Rehabilitation: The FITR Heart Study Randomized Clinical Trial. JAMA Cardiol 5(12):1382–1389. https://doi.org/10.1001/jamacardio.2020.3511

Teixeira J, Motta-Santos D, Milanovic Z, Pereira R, Krustrup P, Póvoas S (2023, April) Intermittent high-intensity exercise for pre- to established hypertension: A systematic review and meta-analysis. Scand J Med Sci Sports 33(4):364–381. https://doi.org/10.1111/sms.14299

Touche R, Pérez J, Acosta A, Campodónico L, García S, Juárez D, Paris-Alemany A (2020, June) Is aerobic exercise helpful in patients with migraine? A systematic review and meta-analysis. Scand J Med Sci Sports 30(6):965–982. https://doi.org/10.1111/sms.13625

Truijen S, Abdullahi A, Bijsterbosch D, Zoest E, Conijn M, Wang Y, Saeys W (2022, May) Effect of home-based virtual reality training and telerehabilitation on balance in individuals with Parkinson disease, multiple sclerosis, and stroke: a systematic review and meta-analysis. Neurol Sci 43(5):2995–3006. https://doi.org/10.1007/s10072-021-05855-2

Uhrbrand A, Stenager E, Pedersen M, Dalgas U (2015) Parkinson's disease and intensive exercise therapy–a systematic review and meta-analysis of randomized controlled trials. J Neurol Sci 353(1–2):9–19. https://doi.org/10.1016/j.jns.2015.04.004

Wang C, Xing J, Zhao B, Wang Y, Zhang L, Wang Y, Liu G (2022a, June) The Effects of High-Intensity Interval Training on Exercise Capacity and Prognosis in Heart Failure and Coronary Artery Disease: A Systematic Review and Meta-Analysis. Cardiovasc Ther 2022:4273809. https://doi.org/10.1155/2022/4273809

Wang Y, Wu H, Sun J, Wei M, Wang J, Li H, Wu J (2022b, October 18) Effect of Exercise on Carotid Artery Intima-Media Thickness in Adults: A Systematic Review and Meta-Analysis. J Phys Act Health 19(12):855–867. https://doi.org/10.1123/jpah.2022-0372

Wang H, Liu Q, Liu L, Cao J, Liang Q, Zhang X (2023, March) High-intensity interval training improves the outcomes of patients with chronic obstructive pulmonary disease: A meta-analysis of randomized controlled trials. Respir Med 208:107128. https://doi.org/10.1016/j.rmed.2023.107128

Wewege M, Thom J, Rye K-A, Parmenter B (2018) July) Aerobic, resistance or combined training: A systematic review and meta-analysis of exercise to reduce cardiovascular risk in adults with metabolic syndrome. Atherosclerosis 274:162–171. https://doi.org/10.1016/j.atherosclerosis.2018.05.002

Willis L, Slentz C, Johnson J, Kelly L, Craig K, Hoselton, A, Kraus W (2019, September 1) Effects of Exercise Training With and Without Ranolazine on Peak Oxygen Consumption, Daily Physical Activity, and Quality of Life in Patients With Chronic Stable Angina Pectoris. Am J Cardiol 124(5):655–660. https://doi.org/10.1016/j.amjcard.2019.05.063

Woldeamanuel, Y, Oliveira, A (2022, October 13) What is the efficacy of aerobic exercise versus strength training in the treatment of migraine? A systematic review and network meta-analysis of clinical trials. J Headache Pain 23(1):134. https://doi.org/10.1186/s10194-022-01503-y

Wu X, Gao S, Lian Y (2020, September) Effects of continuous aerobic exercise on lung function and quality of life with asthma: a systematic review and meta-analysis. J Thorac Dis 12(9):4781–4795. https://doi.org/10.21037/jtd-19-2813

Yan J, Li X, Guo X, Lin Y, Wang S, Cao Y, Liu W (2023, December) Effect of Multicomponent Exercise on Cognition, Physical Function and Activities of Daily Life in Older Adults With Dementia or Mild Cognitive Impairment: A Systematic Review and Meta-analysis. Arch Phys Med Rehabil 104(12):2092–2108. https://doi.org/10.1016/j.apmr.2023.04.011

Yang Z, Scott C, Mao C, Tang J, Farmer A (2014, April) Resistance exercise versus aerobic exercise for type 2 diabetes: a systematic review and meta-analysis. Sports Med 44(4):487–99. https://doi.org/10.1007/s40279-013-0128-8

Yarizadeh H, Eftekhar R, Anjom-Shoae J, Speakman J, Djafarian K (2021, February 1) The Effect of Aerobic and Resistance Training and Combined Exercise Modalities on Subcutaneous Abdominal Fat: A Systematic Review and Meta-analysis of Randomized Clinical Trials. Adv Nutr 12(1):179–196. https://doi.org/10.1093/advances/nmaa090

Yousefabadi H, Niyazi A, Alaee S, Fathi M, Rahimi G (2021, April) Anti-Inflammatory Effects of Exercise on Metabolic Syndrome Patients: A Systematic Review and Meta-Analysis. Biol Res Nurs 23(2):280–292. https://doi.org/10.1177/1099800420958068

Yu H, Zhao X, Wu X, Yang J, Wang J, Hou L (2023, August 25) High-intensity interval training versus moderate-intensity continuous training on patient quality of life in cardiovascular disease: a systematic review and meta-analysis. Sci Rep 13(1):13915. https://doi.org/10.1038/s41598-023-40589-5

Yun R, Bai Y, Lu Y, Wu X, Lee S.-D (2021, January 29) How Breathing Exercises Influence on Respiratory Muscles and Quality of Life among Patients with COPD? A Systematic Review and Meta-Analysis. Can Respir J 2021:1904231. https://doi.org/10.1155/2021/1904231

Zhang F, Zhong Y, Qin Z, Li X, Wang W (2021, March 5) Effect of muscle training on dyspnea in patients with chronic obstructive pulmonary disease: A meta-analysis of randomized controlled trials. Medicine (Baltimore) 100(9):e24930. https://doi.org/10.1097/MD.0000000000024930

Zhang S, Zhen K, Su Q, Chen Y, Lv Y, Yu L (2022a, November 25) The Effect of Aerobic Exercise on Cognitive Function in People with Alzheimer's Disease: A Systematic Review and Meta-Analysis of Randomized Controlled Trials. Int J Environ Res Public Health 19(23):15700. https://doi.org/10.3390/ijerph192315700

Zhang W, Pan H, Zong Y, Wang J, Xie Q (2022b, June) Respiratory Muscle Training Reduces Respiratory Complications and Improves Swallowing Function After Stroke: A Systematic Review and Meta-Analysis. Arch Phys Med Rehabil 103(6):1179–1191. https://doi.org/10.1016/j.apmr.2021.10.020

Zhao X, He Q, Zeng Y, Cheng L (2021, October 6) Effectiveness of combined exercise in people with type 2 diabetes and concurrent overweight/obesity: a systematic review and meta-analysis. BMJ Open 11(10):e046252. https://doi.org/10.1136/bmjopen-2020-046252

Zheng G, Zhou W, Xia R, Tao J, Chen L (2016, November) Aerobic Exercises for Cognition Rehabilitation following Stroke: A Systematic Review. J Stroke Cerebrovasc Dis 25(11):2780–2789. https://doi.org/10.1016/j.jstrokecerebrovasdis.2016.07.035

Zhou X.-P, Zhang L.-M, Chen G.-Q, Wang S.-W, He J.-F, Li Z, Zhang B.-S (2022, October 21) Meta analysis of aerobic exercise improving intelligence and cognitive function in patients with Alzheimer's disease. Medicine (Baltimore) 101(42):e31177. https://doi.org/10.1097/MD.0000000000031177

Zhu Y, Xu Y, Xuan, R, Huang J, István B, Fekete G, Gu Y (2022, July 11) Mixed Comparison of Different Exercise Interventions for Function, Respiratory, Fatigue, and Quality of Life in Adults With Amyotrophic Lateral Sclerosis: Systematic Review and Network Meta-Analysis. Front Aging Neurosci 14:919059. https://doi.org/10.3389/fnagi.2022.919059

7 Influencing Factors of Medical Exercise Therapy

Contents

Trailer

In the seventh chapter of the book, the focus is on the diverse factors that can influence the effectiveness and success of medical training therapy. It emphasizes that in addition to physical training, other lifestyle aspects such as fluid intake, nutrition, mental state, sleep, and even the interaction between the halves of the body play a significant role.

Fluid intake is presented as a fundamental element for optimal performance and recovery. Adequate hydration not only supports physical performance but also cognitive function and overall health.

Nutrition takes a central place, with a detailed look at the importance of macro and micronutrients. The discussion includes various nutritional strategies such as carbohydrate restriction, the use of high-fat diets, BCAA supplementation, as well as the benefits of protein, leucine, vitamin D, and omega-3 fatty acids. Special attention is given to the role of a weight-reducing diet in promoting health and supporting therapy goals.

The influence of mental training is recognized as a critical factor for motivation and perseverance. Techniques and strategies that promote a positive attitude and increase mental strength can improve adherence to the training program and the overall effectiveness of the therapy.

S. Wolfram and R. Bauer, *Evidence-Based Medical Exercise Therapy*,
https://doi.org/10.1007/978-3-662-70774-6_7

The interaction of the halves of the body and the reciprocal training effect are highlighted as fascinating aspects of neurological adaptation to training. This concept underscores how exercises on one side of the body can also influence performance and recovery on the opposite side.

The muscle memory effect is presented as a key component for long-term training benefits and the body's ability to "remember" previous training states. This effect supports the rapid restoration of muscle mass and function after breaks or injuries.

Sleep, often underestimated, is highlighted as a fundamental part of recovery and physical progress. Sufficient and high-quality sleep promotes healing, regeneration, and can directly influence performance in training.

Overall, the chapter provides a comprehensive understanding of how a holistic approach, encompassing nutrition, hydration, psychological factors, sleep, and physiological interactions, is crucial for the success of medical training therapy. It clarifies that the path to optimal health and performance goes far beyond training and requires an integrative consideration of all areas of life.

7.1 Fluid Intake

A 2015 meta-analysis recognizes the training-associated relevance of adequate hydration status. Hypohydration manifests itself in terms of deteriorated endurance and strength performance. Anaerobic performance and anaerobic capacity are also limited by it (see Savoie et al. 2015). Deshayes et al. (2020) meta-analytically confirm the negative consequences of hypohydration on endurance performance.

Fluid intake between 0.15 and 0.34 ml/kg body weight/min during cycling for an hour at high intensity is associated with a reduction in endurance performance. However, if cycling is practiced at moderate intensity within a timeframe between one and two hours, a fluid intake of 0.15–0.20 ml/kg body weight/min can increase endurance performance by at least 2%. If the duration of cycling exceeds two hours and is performed at the same time at moderate intensity, fluid intake at will or at a rate of 0.14–0.27 ml/kg body weight/min can increase endurance performance by at least three percent (see Holland et al. 2017).

Regarding beverage selection, Rowlands et al. (2022) recommend the use of carbohydrate- and electrolyte-rich hypotonic drinks.

Endurance performance at temperatures above 27°C can be improved by the intake of 6 mg/kg body weight of caffeine one hour before the start of training (see Naulleau et al. 2022). Consumption recommendations vary depending on the literature source between 3–6 mg/kg body weight. The effect of caffeine manifests itself through improved aerobic and anaerobic endurance performance in heat or altitude (see Guest et al. 2021).

7.2 Nutrition

7.2.1 Carbohydrate Restriction/Low-Carbohydrate and High-Fat Diet/BCAA Supplementation

Margolis and Pasiakos (2023) discuss the effects of carbohydrate restriction on metabolism. It has been shown that a reduced intake of carbohydrates leads to increased fat oxidation. This reduces fat mass. In addition to fat oxidation, protein oxidation is also stimulated. As a result, a reduced intake of carbohydrates restricts the available amino acids. This is the case for branched-chain amino acids (BCAA) after 24 hours of carbohydrate restriction. As a result, muscle protein synthesis cannot proceed optimally during the recovery period. If the reduced intake of carbohydrates is practiced over a period of eight to twelve weeks, this has negative effects on anabolic signaling, protein synthesis, and myogenesis. In summary, it can be stated that a restriction of carbohydrates has a negative effect on anaerobic performance and muscle hypertrophy (cf. Margolis and Pasiakos 2023).

Based on the results of a randomized controlled study, Dudgeon et al. (2016) recommend BCAA supplementation in trained strength athletes during a hypocaloric diet. This aims to maintain existing muscle mass while simultaneously losing fat. (cf. Dudgeon et al. 2016).

Gillen et al. (2019) confirm the increased protein requirement for endurance activities, which are associated with a previous restrictive intake of carbohydrates. Even with a low-carbohydrate and high-fat diet, sufficient protein intake should be ensured (cf. Howard and Margolis, 2020).

A low-carbohydrate and high-fat diet impairs performance in professional race walkers (cf. Burke et al. 2017).

Low-carbohydrate and high-fat diets are unable to increase aerobic capacity or training performance (cf. Cao et al. 2021). The combination of a low-carbohydrate and high-fat diet offers no advantages over other dietary strategies in terms of lean mass, body fat percentage, body mass, VO2max, and aerobic performance (cf. Wang et al. 2022).

7.2.2 Supplementation of Protein, Leucin, and Vitamin D

As soon as strength training is practiced, sufficient protein intake should be ensured. With a daily protein intake of 1.6–2.0 g of protein per kilogram of body weight, it does not matter for muscular metabolism whether the protein comes from an animal or non-animal source (cf. Hevia-Larraín et al. 2021; Monteyne et al. 2023). Morton et al. (2018) recognize the positive influence of protein supplementation on muscle strength and muscle size in people who perform regular recurring strength training. The effectiveness increases with the fitness level of the trainees and decreases with increasing age. A daily protein intake of more than 1.6 g per kilogram of body weight does not seem to bring any additional effect in terms of increasing lean body mass (cf. Morton et al. 2018).

In a randomized controlled study, the effect of supplementation with protein, leucine, and vitamin D in overweight people in their seventh decade of life was tested. The supplementation was given to the intervention group in parallel with a daily calorie deficit of 600 kcal and was compared to the control group, which worked exclusively with a calorie deficit. Supplementation with protein, leucine, and vitamin D significantly better maintained muscle mass during the diet. Therefore, supplementation during a hypocaloric diet in older people is recommended for the prevention of sarcopenia (cf. Verreijen et al. 2015). In another study, supplementation with protein, leucine, and vitamin D was found to increase lower extremity muscle mass over a 13-week period in sarcopenic patients (cf. Bauer et al. 2015). Furthermore, the combination of sufficient protein, leucine, and vitamin D intake can increase walking speed in older people (cf. Lin et al. 2021). In summary, it can be stated that the supplementation of protein, leucine, and vitamin D in combination with a training program is capable of increasing muscle mass in people with sarcopenia (cf. Chang and Choo 2023).

7.2.3 Supplementation of Omega-3 Fatty Acids

In a meta-analysis by Cornish et al. (2022), the supplementation of omega-3 fatty acids is attributed a strength and function enhancing effect on the lower extremity of older people. Omega-3 fatty acids are capable of positively affecting muscle mass when supplemented with over 2 g daily. With long-term intake, an improvement in walking speed can also be achieved (cf. Huang et al. 2020).

The supplementation of long-chain, polyunsaturated omega-3 fatty acids has a positive effect on muscle mass and muscle strength in people with sarcopenia (cf. Bird et al. 2021). Ma et al. (2021) indicate that further future research work on this topic is necessary.

7.2.4 Supplementation of Creatine

In a meta-analysis by Delpino et al. (2022), it was recognized that the supplementation of creatine in combination with strength training can contribute to an increase in lean body mass. In this case, male subjects respond more clearly than female study participants. Burke et al. (2023) recognized that the combination of creatine supplementation and resistance training can positively influence the hypertrophy of the skeletal musculature of the upper and lower extremity. Forbes et al. (2021) mention the optional use of a preparation phase in which more than 20 g per day is consumed over a period of 5-7 days. Subsequently, the dosages diverge at more or less than 5 g daily.

7.2.5 Supplementation of Magnesium

A meta-analysis by Wang et al. (2017) concludes that the supplementation of magnesium in athletes and physically active people does not increase muscular performance. Only people who have a proven deficit of magnesium, such as frequently alcohol-dependent people, can benefit from supplementation (cf. Wang et al. 2017). This is supported by earlier research findings by Newhouse and Finstad (2000).

7.2.6 Supplementation of Vitamin K2

In a randomized controlled study, the effect of a supplementation of Vitamin K2 on endurance-trained male and female athletes was investigated. In week 1 to 4, 300 mg per day were consumed and in week 5 to 8, 150 mg per day were consumed. The training behavior was individually maintained during this period. The intervention group showed a significant improvement of the maximum cardiac heart performance by 13% after the intervention period (cf. McFarlin et al. 2017).

7.2.7 Weight-Reducing Diet

A ketogenic diet is capable of causing a highly significant weight reduction in people with overweight and the diagnosis of type 2 diabetes mellitus. The ketogenic diet is characterized by a reduced carbohydrate intake of less than 50 g per day. In addition, high amounts of fat and moderate amounts of protein are consumed. This approach leads, based on a meta-analytical evaluation, to an improvement of the fat metabolism in addition to a reduction of body weight (cf. Zhou et al. 2022; Luo et al. 2022; Choi et al. 2020).

Roth et al. (2022) describe the high relevance of sufficient protein intake during a training-associated diet and underline with their research work statements, which were already made in Sect. 7.2.1. If sufficient protein intake is present, the loss of lean mass in overweight adults can be best contained (cf. Roth et al. 2022).

Johnston et al. (2014) meta-analytically compared a low-carbohydrate diet to a low-fat diet. Both strategies led to a significant weight loss in overweight adults. No superiority of one approach was recognized.

For a better stimulation of the fat metabolism during aerobic endurance training, Vieira et al. (2016) recommend performing it in a fasting state.

Flore et al. (2022) point out that weight loss is only the first step of a long-term process. The recurrence rate of weight gain after a diet is about 50%. Therefore, a long-term change in diet and an increase in nutrition and health-specific education is inevitable.

7.3 Influence of Mental Training

In a comparative study, Ranganathan et al. (2004) examined the effect of purely mental training. The training unit was thus carried out without physical activity, using only the power of imagination. Over a period of 12 weeks, mental training was conducted five times a week for 15 minutes each time. Depending on the group assignment, purely mental training of the Musculus abductor digiti minini or the elbow flexors was practiced. In addition, a physical training of the Musculus abductor digiti minimi was carried out by another group. Another control group did not perform either mental or physical training. After the three-month intervention period, a significant increase in strength could be measured in both training groups. The mental training group of the Musculus abductor digiti minimi was able to achieve a strength increase of 35%. The mental training group of the elbow flexors achieved a strength increase of 13.5%. The group which physically trained the Musculus abductor digiti minimi achieved a strength increase of 53% (cf. Ranganathan et al. 2004). These results show the great influence of the output performance of the central nervous system and its optimization through mental training.

Parsowith et al. (2023) also found that the mental motor imagination of strength training leads to increased corticospinal excitability.

In another study, the effect of a mental exercise program for strengthening the hip abductors was examined. The mental training was carried out over a period of two weeks, five times a week, with a respective training time of 30 minutes. After the intervention period, both the bilateral strength ability of the hip abductors could be significantly improved and an increase in the power of imagination could be achieved (cf. Alenezi et al. 2023).

Mental training can be most effectively used when the trainee imagines the movements of their own body or their own overcoming of resistances in the course of movement. Thus, the "inner" perspective should be adopted. This is important because the effectiveness of assuming a mental observer position in the sense of a third person observing the training "from the outside" achieves less good results (cf. Yao et al. 2023).

▶ **Practical Tip**

The mental focus should be on the training or one's own body perception during the training time. Any mental distractions should be prevented as much as possible.

7.4 Interaction of Body Halves and Mutual Training Effect

In their research work, Lee et al. (2009) provide insight into the effects of training the upper extremity of one half of the body on the other untrained upper extremity of the opposite side. It was shown that unilateral strength training of the wrist extensors increases the strength ability of the extensors on the opposite side. While the strength on the trained side increased on average by 31.5%, the untrained side also recorded a strength increase of 8.2%. This effect is attributed to an increased cortical excitability after unilateral training, which transfers to the opposite side (cf. Lee et al. 2009).

In a meta-analysis, further research of this kind was summarized to assess the strength of this cross-body effect. It was calculated that the strength of the untrained extremity increased by about 7.8% during the study periods. This is 35.1% of the strength gain on the trained side (cf. Munn et al. 2004).

For the maximum exploitation of this effect, Munn et al. (2005) recommend a fast exercise execution and at least three sets.

▶ **Practical Tip**

If training of extremities is temporarily not possible due to diseases or injuries, training the opposite extremity is a suitable means to slow down the loss of strength due to inactivity.

7.5 The Muscle Memory Effect

When the skeletal muscles are trained, this leads to structural, genetic, and neuronal adaptations of the body (see Snijders et al. 2020). If a phase occurs after a training period in which no training is carried out, there is a gradual loss of strength or mass of the muscles (see Blocquiaux et al. 2020). However, this does not mean that all training-induced adaptations disappear with the loss of strength or mass. If there is a training break of several weeks after a training phase, the skeletal muscle does not start at the starting point, but can draw on adaptations generated in the past and thus increase its performance in a new training phase more quickly to its old training level. This phenomenon is referred to in the literature as the muscle memory effect.

The sample of Seaborne et al. (2018) practiced intensive strength training over a period of seven weeks. As a result, strength could be increased by 9.3% and muscle growth by 6.5% significantly compared to the initial value. The training was then discontinued for a period of seven weeks. After the seven-week break, both the strength and muscle growth reduced to the initial value. After the seven-week break, another seven weeks of intensive strength training was practiced. After the second training phase, the strength increased by 18% and the muscle growth by 12.4% significantly compared to the initial value (see Seaborne et al. 2018).

In a randomized controlled study, Ogasawara et al. (2013) were able to show that there is no significant difference between a continuous 24-week strength training and a recurring change between six weeks of training and three weeks of break over a period of 24 weeks in terms of muscular hypertrophy.

From a physiological point of view, the muscle memory effect seems to be due to different processes. In addition to neural and genetic adaptations, the hypothesis of persisting myonuclei during training-free periods is often discussed (see Sharples and Adam 2023). Further research work is necessary for a more precise clarification of these mechanisms, although these findings only have a minor influence on the clinical relevance of medical training therapy. More interesting for improving training control are information about the duration, intensity, influencing factors, and optimal evocability of the muscle memory effect.

> **Practical Tip**
> The better the skeletal muscles were trained before disease-, injury- or surgery-related training breaks, the faster the previous performance level can be reached when re-entering medical training therapy. Past efforts prove their worth in the present and future.

7.6 Sleep

The performance within the training therapy and the quality of sleep interact with each other (see Fullagar et al. 2015; Yang et al. 2012). While Yang et al. (2012) were able to demonstrate that the practice of medical training therapy has a positive effect on sleep quality in people from the age of 40, Fullagar et al. (2015) established the negative consequences of complete sleep deprivation in athletes in terms of performance within the training therapy. Based on a study of ten women aged between 18 and 35 years, the performance-reducing effect of sleep reduction in strength training was determined (see Knowles et al. 2022). For optimal endurance performance, Roberts et al. (2019) recommend a sleep duration of more than eight hours.

With a sleep duration of three hours each for two consecutive nights, Brotherton et al. (2019) were able to demonstrate the effectiveness of a one-hour power nap, which ended three hours before training, in terms of performance improvement in submaximal strength training.

For a maximum training-induced improvement in sleep quality, Hasan et al. (2022) recommend the practice of endurance training in combination with walking. Strength training can also have a positive effect on sleep quality (see Kovacevic et al. 2018).

Frimpong et al. (2021) were able to show that high-intensity training in the evening in a period of two to four hours before sleep has no negative effects on the sleep quality of healthy young and middle-aged people. These results were confirmed by Yue et al. (2022).

In addition to sleep quality, physical training can also positively influence the autonomous function of the heart in people over the age of 40 (see Tseng et al. 2020).

References

Alenezi M, Hayes A, Lawrence G, Kubis H-P (7 September 2023) Influence of motor imagery training on hip abductor muscle strength and bilateral transfer effect. Front Physiol 14:1188658. https://doi.org/10.3389/fphys.2023.1188658

Bauer J, Verlaan S, Bautmans I, Brandt K, Donini L, Maggio M, Cederholm T (1 September 2015) Effects of a vitamin D and leucine-enriched whey protein nutritional supplement on measures of sarcopenia in older adults, the PROVIDE study: a randomized, double-blind, placebo-controlled trial. J Am Med Dir Assoc 16(9):740–747. https://doi.org/10.1016/j.jamda.2015.05.021

Bird J, Troesch B, Warnke I, Calder P (December 2021) The effect of long chain omega-3 polyunsaturated fatty acids on muscle mass and function in sarcopenia: A scoping systematic review and meta-analysis. Clin Nutr ESPEN 46:73–86. https://doi.org/10.1016/j.clnesp.2021.10.011

Blocquiaux S, Gorski T, Roie E, Ramaekers M, Thienen R, Nielens H, Thomis M (May 2020) The effect of resistance training, detraining and retraining on muscle strength and power, myofibre size, satellite cells and myonuclei in older men. Exp Gerontol 133:110860. https://doi.org/10.1016/j.exger.2020.110860

Brotherton E, Moseley S, Langan-Evans C, Pullinger S, Robertson C, Burniston J, Edwards B (March 2019) Effects of two nights partial sleep deprivation on an evening submaximal weightlifting performance; are 1 h powernaps useful on the day of competition? Chronobiol Int 36(3):407–426. https://doi.org/10.1080/07420528.2018.1552702

Burke L, Ross M, Garvican-Lewis L, Welvaert M, Heikura I, Forbes S, Hawley J (1 May 2017) Low carbohydrate, high fat diet impairs exercise economy and negates the performance benefit from intensified training in elite race walkers. J Physiol 595(9):2785–2807. https://doi.org/10.1113/JP273230

Burke R, Piñero A, Coleman M, Mohan A, Sapuppo M, Augustin F, Schoenfeld B (28 April 2023) The Effects of Creatine Supplementation Combined with Resistance Training on Regional Measures of Muscle Hypertrophy: A Systematic Review with Meta-Analysis. Nutrients 15(9):2116. https://doi.org/10.3390/nu15092116

Cao J, Lei S, Wang X, Cheng S (23 August 2021) The Effect of a Ketogenic Low-Carbohydrate, High-Fat Diet on Aerobic Capacity and Exercise Performance in Endurance Athletes: A Systematic Review and Meta-Analysis. Nutrients 13(8):2896. https://doi.org/10.3390/nu13082896

Chang M, Choo Y (19 January 2023) Effects of Whey Protein, Leucine, and Vitamin D Supplementation in Patients with Sarcopenia: A Systematic Review and Meta-Analysis. Nutrients 15(13):521. https://doi.org/10.3390/nu15030521

Choi Y, Jeon S-M, Shin S (6 July 2020) Impact of a Ketogenic Diet on Metabolic Parameters in Patients with Obesity or Overweight and with or without Type 2 Diabetes: A Meta-Analysis of Randomized Controlled Trials. Nutrients 12(7):2005. https://doi.org/10.3390/nu12072005

Cornish S, Cordingley D, Shaw K, Forbes S, Leonhardt T, Bristol A, Chilibeck P (26 May 2022) Effects of Omega-3 Supplementation Alone and Combined with Resistance Exercise on Skeletal Muscle in Older Adults: A Systematic Review and Meta-Analysis. Nutrients 14(11):2221. https://doi.org/10.3390/nu14112221

Delpino F, Figueiredo L, Forbes S, Candow D, Santos H (November-December 2022) Influence of age, sex, and type of exercise on the efficacy of creatine supplementation on lean body mass: A systematic review and meta-analysis of randomized clinical trials. Nutrition 111791:103–104. https://doi.org/10.1016/j.nut.2022.111791

Deshayes T, Jeker D, Goulet E (March 2020) Impact of Pre-exercise Hypohydration on Aerobic Exercise Performance, Peak Oxygen Consumption and Oxygen Consumption at Lactate Threshold: A Systematic Review with Meta-analysis. Sports Med 50(3):581–596. https://doi.org/10.1007/s40279-019-01223-5

Dudgeon W, Kelley E, Scheett T (5 January 2016) In a single-blind, matched group design: branched-chain amino acid supplementation and resistance training maintains lean body mass during a caloric restricted diet. J Int Soc Sports Nutr 13:1. https://doi.org/10.1186/s12970-015-0112-9

Flore G, Preti A, Carta M, Deledda A, Fosci M, Nardi A, Velluzzi F (16 March 2022) Weight Maintenance after Dietary Weight Loss: Systematic Review and Meta-Analysis on the Effectiveness of Behavioural Intensive Intervention. Nutrients 14(6):1259. https://doi.org/10.3390/nu14061259

Forbes S, Candow D, Ostojic S, Roberts M, Chilibeck P (2 June 2021) Meta-Analysis Examining the Importance of Creatine Ingestion Strategies on Lean Tissue Mass and Strength in Older Adults. Nutrients 13(6):1912. https://doi.org/10.3390/nu13061912

Frimpong E, Mograss M, Zvionow T, Dang-Vu T (December 2021) The effects of evening high-intensity exercise on sleep in healthy adults: A systematic review and meta-analysis. Sleep Med Rev 60:101535. https://doi.org/10.1016/j.smrv.2021.101535

Fullagar H, Skorski S, Duffield R, Hammes D, Coutts A, Meyer T (February 2015) Sleep and athletic performance: the effects of sleep loss on exercise performance, and physiological and cognitive responses to exercise. Sports Med 45(2):161–186. https://doi.org/10.1007/s40279-014-0260-0

Gillen J, West D, Williamson E, Fung H, Moore D (November 2019) Low-Carbohydrate Training Increases Protein Requirements of Endurance Athletes. Med Sci Sports Exerc 51(11):2294–2301. https://doi.org/10.1249/MSS.0000000000002036

Guest N, VanDusseldorp T, Nelson M, Grgic J, Schoenfeld B, Jenkins N, Campbell B (2 January 2021) International society of sports nutrition position stand: caffeine and exercise performance. J Int Soc Sports Nutr 18(1):1. https://doi.org/10.1186/s12970-020-00383-4

Hasan F, Tu Y-K, Lin C-M, Chuang L-P, Jeng C, Yuliana L, Chiu H-Y (October 2022) Comparative efficacy of exercise regimens on sleep quality in older adults: A systematic review and network meta-analysis. Sleep Med Rev 65:101673. https://doi.org/10.1016/j.smrv.2022.101673

Hevia-Larraín V, Gualano B, Longobardi I, Gil S, Fernandes A, Costa L, Roschel H (June 2021) High-Protein Plant-Based Diet Versus a Protein-Matched Omnivorous Diet to Support Resistance Training Adaptations: A Comparison Between Habitual Vegans and Omnivores. Sports Med 51(6):1317–1330. https://doi.org/10.1007/s40279-021-01434-9

Holland J, Skinner T, Irwin C, Leveritt M, Goulet E (November 2017) The Influence of Drinking Fluid on Endurance Cycling Performance: A Meta-Analysis. Sports Med 47(11):2269–2284. https://doi.org/10.1007/s40279-017-0739-6

Howard E, Margolis L (19 August 2020) Intramuscular Mechanisms Mediating Adaptation to Low-Carbohydrate. High-Fat Diets during Exercise Training. Nutrients 12(9):2496. https://doi.org/10.3390/nu12092496

Huang Y-H, Chiu W-C, Hsu Y-P, Lo Y-L, Wang Y-H (4 December 2020) Effects of Omega-3 Fatty Acids on Muscle Mass, Muscle Strength and Muscle Performance among the Elderly: A Meta-Analysis. Nutrients 12(12):3739. https://doi.org/10.3390/nu12123739

Johnston B, Kanters S, Bandayrel K, Wu P, Naji F, Siemieniuk R, Mills E (3 September 2014) Comparison of weight loss among named diet programs in overweight and obese adults: a meta-analysis. JAMA 312(9):923–933. https://doi.org/10.1001/jama.2014.10397

Knowles O, Drinkwater E, Roberts S, Alexander S, Abbott G, Garnham A, Aisbett B (1 December 2022) Sustained Sleep Restriction Reduces Resistance Exercise Quality and Quantity in Females. Med Sci Sports Exerc 54(12):2167–2177. https://doi.org/10.1249/MSS.0000000000003000

Kovacevic A, Mavros Y, Heisz J, Singh M (June 2018) The effect of resistance exercise on sleep: A systematic review of randomized controlled trials. Sleep Med Rev 39:52–68. https://doi.org/10.1016/j.smrv.2017.07.002

Lee M, Gandevia S, Carroll T (April 2009) Unilateral strength training increases voluntary activation of the opposite untrained limb. Clin Neurophysiol 120(4):802–808. https://doi.org/10.1016/j.clinph.2009.01.002

Lin C-C, Shih M-H, Chen C-D, Yeh S-L (March 2021) Effects of adequate dietary protein with whey protein, leucine, and vitamin D supplementation on sarcopenia in older adults: An open-label, parallel-group study. Clin Nutr 40(3):1323–1329. https://doi.org/10.1016/j.clnu.2020.08.017

Luo W, Zhang J, Xu D, Zhou Y, Qu Z, Yang Q, Lv Q (13 December 2022) Low carbohydrate ketogenic diets reduce cardiovascular risk factor levels in obese or overweight patients with T2DM: A meta-analysis of randomized controlled trials. Front Nutr 9:1092031. https://doi.org/10.3389/fnut.2022.1092031

Ma W-J, Li H, Zhang W, Zhai J, Li J, Liu H, Li D (February 2021) Effect of n-3 polyunsaturated fatty acid supplementation on muscle mass and function with aging: A meta-analysis of randomized controlled trials. Prostaglandins Leukot Essent Fatty Acids 165:102249. https://doi.org/10.1016/j.plefa.2021.102249

Margolis L, Pasiakos S (1 July 2023) Low carbohydrate availability impairs hypertrophy and anaerobic performance. Curr Opin Clin Nutr Metab Care 26(4):347–352. https://doi.org/10.1097/MCO.0000000000000934

McFarlin B, Henning A, Venable A (July 2017) Oral Consumption of Vitamin K2 for 8 Weeks Associated With Increased Maximal Cardiac Output During Exercise. Altern Ther Health Med 23(4):26–32

Monteyne A, Coelho M, Murton A, Abdelrahman D, Blackwell J, Koscien C, Wall B (June 2023) Vegan and Omnivorous High Protein Diets Support Comparable Daily Myofibrillar Protein Synthesis Rates and Skeletal Muscle Hypertrophy in Young Adults. J Nutr 153(6):1680–1695. https://doi.org/10.1016/j.tjnut.2023.02.023

Morton R, Murphy K, McKellar S, Schoenfeld B, Henselmans M, Helms E, Phillips S (March 2018) A systematic review, meta-analysis and meta-regression of the effect of protein supplementation on resistance training-induced gains in muscle mass and strength in healthy adults. Br J Sports Med 52(6):376–384. https://doi.org/10.1136/bjsports-2017-097608

Munn J, Herbert R, Gandevia S (May 2004) Contralateral effects of unilateral resistance training: a meta-analysis. J Appl Physiol 96(5):1861–1866. https://doi.org/10.1152/japplphysiol.00541.2003

Munn J, Herbert R, Hancock M, Gandevia S (November 2005) Training with unilateral resistance exercise increases contralateral strength. J Appl Physiol 99(5):1880–1884. https://doi.org/10.1152/japplphysiol.00559.2005

Naulleau C, Jeker D, Pancrate T, Claveau P, Deshayes T, Burke L, Goulet E (October 2022) Effect of Pre-Exercise Caffeine Intake on Endurance Performance and Core Temperature Regulation During Exercise in the Heat: A Systematic Review with Meta-Analysis. Sports Med 52(10):2431–2445. https://doi.org/10.1007/s40279-022-01692-1

Newhouse I, Finstad E (July 2000) The effects of magnesium supplementation on exercise performance. Clin J Sport Med 10(3):195–200. https://doi.org/10.1097/00042752-200007000-00008

Ogasawara R, Yasuda T, Ishii N, Abe T (April 2013) Comparison of muscle hypertrophy following 6-month of continuous and periodic strength training. Eur J Appl Physiol 113(4):975–985. https://doi.org/10.1007/s00421-012-2511-9

Parsowith E, Stock M, Girts R, Beausejour J, Alberto A, Carr J, Harmon K (25 November 2023) The Influence of Resistance Training Experience on the Efficacy of Motor Imagery for Acutely Increasing Corticospinal Excitability. Brain Sci 13(12):1635. https://doi.org/10.3390/brainsci13121635

Ranganathan V, Siemionow V, Liu J, Sahgal V, Yue G (2004) From mental power to muscle power–gaining strength by using the mind. Neuropsychologia 42(7):944–956. https://doi.org/10.1016/j.neuropsychologia.2003.11.018

Roberts S, Teo W-P, Aisbett B, Warmington SA (December 2019) Extended Sleep Maintains Endurance Performance Better than Normal or Restricted Sleep. Med Sci Sports Exerc 51(12):2516–2523. https://doi.org/10.1249/MSS.0000000000002071

Roth A, Sattelmayer M, Schorderet C, Gafner S, Allet L (5 January 2022) Effects of exercise training and dietary supplement on fat free mass and bone mass density during weight loss – a systematic review and meta-analysis. F1000Res 11:8 https://doi.org/10.12688/f1000research.75539.3

Rowlands D, Kopetschny B, Badenhorst C (February 2022) The Hydrating Effects of Hypertonic, Isotonic and Hypotonic Sports Drinks and Waters on Central Hydration During Continuous Exercise: A Systematic Meta-Analysis and Perspective. Sports Med 52(2):349–375. https://doi.org/10.1007/s40279-021-01558-y

Savoie F-A, Kenefick R, Ely B, Cheuvront S, Goulet E (August 2015) Effect of Hypohydration on Muscle Endurance, Strength, Anaerobic Power and Capacity and Vertical Jumping Ability: A Meta-Analysis. Sports Med 45(8):1207–1227. https://doi.org/10.1007/s40279-015-0349-0

Seaborne R, Strauss J, Cocks M, Shepherd S, O'Brien T, Someren K, Sharples A (30 January 2018) Human Skeletal Muscle Possesses an Epigenetic Memory of Hypertrophy. Sci Rep 8(1):1898. https://doi.org/10.1038/s41598-018-20287-3

Sharples A, Turner D (1 June 2023) Skeletal muscle memory. Am J Physiol Cell Physiol 324(6):C1274–C1294. https://doi.org/10.1152/ajpcell.00099.2023

Snijders T, Aussieker T, Holwerda A, Parise G, Loon L (July 2020) The concept of skeletal muscle memory: Evidence from animal and human studies. Acta Physiol (Oxf) 229(3):e13465. https://doi.org/10.1111/apha.13465

Tseng T-H, Chen H-C, Wang L-Y, Chien M-Y (September 2020) Effects of exercise training on sleep quality and heart rate variability in middle-aged and older adults with poor sleep quality: a randomized controlled trial. J Clin Sleep Med 16(9):1483–1492. https://doi.org/10.5664/jcsm.8560

Verreijen A, Verlaan S, Engberink M, Swinkels S, Bosch J-V, Weijs P (February 2015) A high whey protein-, leucine-, and vitamin D-enriched supplement preserves muscle mass during intentional weight loss in obese older adults: a double-blind randomized controlled trial. Am J Clin Nutr 101(2):279–286. https://doi.org/10.3945/ajcn.114.090290

Vieira A, Costa R, Macedo R, Coconcelli L, Kruel L (October 2016) Effects of aerobic exercise performed in fasted v. fed state on fat and carbohydrate metabolism in adults: a systematic review and meta-analysis. Br J Nutr 116(7):1153–1164 https://doi.org/10.1017/S0007114516003160

Wang R, Chen C, Liu W, Zhou T, Xun P, He K, Chen P (1 November 2017) The effect of magnesium supplementation on muscle fitness: a meta-analysis and systematic review. Magnes Res 30(4):120–132. https://doi.org/10.1684/mrh.2018.0430

Wang Y, Zhou K, Wang V, Bao D, Zhou J (14 September 2022) The Effects of Concurrent Training Combined with Low-Carbohydrate High-Fat Ketogenic Diet on Body Composition and Aerobic Performance: A Systematic Review and Meta-Analysis. Int J Environ Res Public Health 19(18):11542. https://doi.org/10.3390/ijerph191811542

Yang P-Y, Ho K-H, Chen H-C, Chien M-Y (2012) Exercise training improves sleep quality in middle-aged and older adults with sleep problems: a systematic review. J Physiother 58(3):157–163. https://doi.org/10.1016/S1836-9553(12)70106-6

Yao W, Ge S, Zhang J, Hemmat P, Jiang B, Liu X, Yue G (2 June 2023) Bilateral transfer of motor performance as a function of motor imagery training: a systematic review and meta-analysis. Front Psychol 14:1187175. https://doi.org/10.3389/fpsyg.2023.1187175

Yue T, Liu X, Gao Q, Wang Y (14 December 2022) Different Intensities of Evening Exercise on Sleep in Healthy Adults: A Systematic Review and Network Meta-Analysis. Nat Sci Sleep 14:2157–2177. https://doi.org/10.2147/NSS.S388863

Zhou C, Wang M, Liang J, He G, Chen N (22 August 2022) Ketogenic Diet Benefits to Weight Loss, Glycemic Control, and Lipid Profiles in Overweight Patients with Type 2 Diabetes Mellitus: A Meta-Analysis of Randomized Controlled Trails. Int J Environ Res Public Health 19(16):10429. https://doi.org/10.3390/ijerph191610429

Glossary List

Apoptosis	Apoptosis refers to programmed cell death, a controlled process through which cells die in an orderly manner. This process is crucial for the development and maintenance of the health of organisms by removing damaged or unnecessary cells.
Autophagy	Autophagy is a cellular cleaning process in which cells break down and recycle their own damaged or unnecessary components. This mechanism helps to maintain cell health and plays an important role in the response to cell stress and in disease prevention.
auxoton	Auxoton describes the mechanism that during a muscle contraction, both the length and the tension of the muscle change simultaneously.
Risk of Bias	The risk of bias refers to the danger that systematic errors in data collection, analysis, or interpretation lead to a distortion of the results. Such distortions can affect the validity and reliability of study results and lead to erroneous conclusions.
epicritic	Epicritic refers to a type of sensory perception that allows particularly fine detail recognition, such as the distinction of touches or temperatures on the skin.
evoked	cause, provoke
Giving Way	"Giving Way" describes a phenomenon where a joint, particularly the knee, suddenly gives way or becomes unstable, often leading to a feeling of sinking or uncertainty when standing or walking.
helical	Helical refers to a shape or structure that has a spiral or screw-like configuration.
Hip moment	Hip moment refers to the torque that acts around the hip axis of a person, typically during movements such as walking or running.
Inclinometer	An inclinometer is an instrument used to measure angles or inclinations relative to gravity.
isometric	Muscle contraction in which the tension changes and the length of the muscle remains the same.
isotonic	Muscle contraction in which the tension of the muscle remains constant and the muscle length changes.

S. Wolfram and R. Bauer, *Evidence-Based Medical Exercise Therapy*,
https://doi.org/10.1007/978-3-662-70774-6

Knee moment	Knee moment refers to the torque that acts on the knee joint axis during movements such as walking, running, or jumping.
Comorbidities	Comorbidities refer to the simultaneous presence of two or more diseases or medical conditions in a person. These can influence each other and complicate the diagnosis, treatment, and course of the individual diseases.
Mind-Body Program	A mind-body program is a therapeutic approach that combines techniques for mental and physical health promotion to improve overall well-being. Such programs may include practices like meditation, yoga, breathing exercises, and relaxation techniques, and aim to strengthen the connection between mind and body and promote health benefits.
Motility	Motility refers to the ability of cells, organisms, or their specific parts to move or actively relocate themselves. This ability to move is essential for many biological processes, such as the locomotion of microorganisms, the function of muscle cells, or the transport of nutrients and cells in the body.
Plyometrics	Plyometrics refers to a form of training aimed at increasing power through explosive movements such as jumps and sprints. This training utilizes muscle elongation immediately followed by a muscle contraction to improve neuromuscular efficiency and enhance athletic performance.
protopathic	Protopathic refers to a type of sensory perception that is primarily specialized in recognizing coarse, diffuse sensations such as pain or temperature. This form of sensitivity is less precise than epicritic perception, but plays an important role in warning the body of potential damage or dangers.
Reliability	Reliability refers to the dependability and consistency with which a measuring instrument or test procedure delivers the same results under the same conditions. It is a central quality indicator in empirical research and serves to assess the stability and accuracy of measurements.
Syncytium	A syncytium is a multinucleated cell that is formed by the fusion of several individual cells, with the cell membranes between them disappearing. This structure is often found in certain tissues, such as muscle tissue or during placenta development, and allows efficient communication and metabolic activity across large cell associations.
Validity	Validity refers to the extent to which a test or measurement instrument actually measures what it purports to measure. It is a crucial criterion for the quality and significance of research results, as it confirms the accuracy and relevance of the measurement in relation to the construct being investigated.
Valsalva Maneuver	The Valsalva maneuver is a breathing technique where one inhales deeply and then forcefully exhales against a closed airway, leading to increased pressure in the chest and abdominal cavity.
VO2max	VO2max stands for maximum oxygen uptake and is a measure of how much oxygen the body can process at maximum during intense physical exertion. It is an important indicator of a person's aerobic endurance and cardiovascular fitness and is often used to assess performance in sports and medicine.

MIX
Papier aus verantwortungsvollen Quellen
Paper from responsible sources
FSC® C105338

If you have any concerns about our products,
you can contact us on
ProductSafety@springernature.com

In case Publisher is established outside the EU,
the EU authorized representative is:
Springer Nature Customer Service Center GmbH
Europaplatz 3, 69115 Heidelberg, Germany

Printed by Libri Plureos GmbH
in Hamburg, Germany